T0135377

Trauma and Migration

Meryam Schouler-Ocak

Editor

Trauma and Migration

Cultural Factors in the Diagnosis and Treatment of Traumatised Immigrants

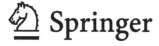 Springer

Editor
Meryam Schouler-Ocak
Department of Psychiatry and
Psychotherapy of the Charité
St. Hedwig Hospital
Berlin
Germany

ISBN 978-3-319-35010-3   ISBN 978-3-319-17335-1   (eBook)
DOI 10.1007/978-3-319-17335-1

Springer Cham Heidelberg New York Dordrecht London
© Springer International Publishing Switzerland 2015
Softcover reprint of the hardcover 1st edition 2015

Printed on acid-free paper

Springer International Publishing AG Switzerland is part of Springer Science+Business Media
(www.springer.com)

Foreword

Many migrants experience traumatisation when leaving their countries and moving to a new location. This is particularly true for refugees. However, different factors including discrimination and social exclusion can traumatise all migrants, including those who have a secure legal status. This book focuses on these various ways in which refugees and migrants can be traumatised, describes the epidemiology of post-traumatic stress disorders among refugees and migrants, discusses challenges in cross-cultural diagnosis and communication and elucidates the role of stigmatisation on the one hand and resilience on the other, which impact on the ability of refugees to cope with the challenges of migration and social exclusion. A special focus is given to gender issues and challenges of specific settings and experiences such as torture and incarceration. Finally, specific treatment issues are discussed and include a description of the relevance of cultural competence, the need to orient towards resilience and coping capacities of migrants and to integrate such approaches in best practice models for traumatised refugees.

Altogether, this book gives an excellent overview over the epidemiology and relevance of the topic, shows ways how to diagnose trauma in different cultural and social settings and discusses best practice approaches for treating traumatised migrants. This topic is highly relevant given the increasing number of racist attacks on refugees, but also in view of the changing landscape of legal requirements and border policies in Europe and other parts of the world. Meryam Schouler-Ocak, the head of the outpatient unit of the Department of Psychiatry and Psychotherapy of the Charité, St. Hedwig Hospital, Berlin, managed to bring together an excellent group of experts in epidemiology, diagnosis and treatment of trauma among refugees and other migrants. The book includes views and voices from Turkey and Israel, Canada, Sweden, Denmark, the Netherlands, Germany and Spain and thus spans northern and southern, eastern and western regions of Europe and its neighbouring regions and links them with a global perspective. European societies dedicated to humanitarian ideals have to respond to the question how to adequately deal with the weakest members of society. Traumatised refugees and other migrants are among these subjects, which deserve special attention and care. May this book help to provide them with the best available support!

Berlin, Germany   Andreas Heinz

Contents

Part III   Trauma and Migration: Treatment Issues

Part I

Trauma and Migration: Epidemiological and Conceptual Issues

Introduction: The Relevance of Trauma Among Immigrants

1

Meryam Schouler-Ocak

According to the United Nations High Commissioner for Refugees (UNHCR), a global total of 15.4 million refugees sought asylum in 2012 (UNHCR 2013). From a global perspective, 48.9 % of all asylum applications were made within the European Union (Eurostat 2014), the majority of these in Germany, France, Sweden, the UK and Italy (UNHCR 2014). Whether in crisis areas in their native countries, during the journey of migration itself or on arrival in their host countries, most of these people have had experiences which may result not only in adjustment disorders, but also in chronic psychiatric disorders such as anxiety, depression and somatoform disorders (Lindert et al. 2009; Hansson et al. 2012).

Wirtgen (2009) reports that the majority of refugees and asylum seekers are in a very poor physical and mental condition when they arrive in the host country (Wirtgen 2009). Various studies point out that the rate of post-traumatic stress disorder (PTSD) is around ten times higher among refugees and asylum seekers than among the general population of the host country (Fazel et al. 2005; Crumlish and O'Rourke 2010). Statistics on PTSD are very high, with studies reporting an incidence of anything between 3 and 86 %. Commonly mentioned causes are escape from crisis areas, physical and sexual violence, torture, loss of family members and persecution. One meta-analysis described the rate of mental illness as being twice as high among refugees and asylum seekers compared to those who migrated for economic reasons (40 % vs. 21 %) (Lindert et al. 2009).

Moreover, various authors (Laban et al. 2004; Porter and Haslam 2005; Hallas et al. 2007) report that the prevalence of mental disorders and physical health problems increases in proportion to the length of the asylum procedure, while their quality of life and satisfaction decrease accordingly (Laban et al. 2004, 2005, 2007,

M. Schouler-Ocak
Department of Psychiatry and Psychotherapy of the Charité, St. Hedwig Hospital,
Berlin, Germany
e-mail: meryam.schouler-ocak@charite.de

© Springer International Publishing Switzerland 2015
M. Schouler-Ocak (ed.), *Trauma and Migration:*
Cultural Factors in the Diagnosis and Treatment of Traumatised Immigrants,
DOI 10.1007/978-3-319-17335-1_1

2008). It would appear that their resources are not activated; this process is characterised by a lack of access to healthcare, the low quality of life in the institutions which receive them, perceived discrimination and stigmatisation, and the absence of permission to work, hindering both the acquisition of financial resources and the basic structuring of everyday life. The related financial worries have a heavy impact on the overall situation (Laban et al. 2004; Noh et al. 1999).

Studies report on the multiple and highly complex stressors with which refugees are often faced and which are at risk of having a lasting impact on their mental health (Bhugra et al. 2014). These might be experiences of traumatisation before, during and after the actual journey of migration. If they succeed in leaving the crisis area, this journey is often a long and tortuous one on which they may be exposed to other traumatic events. When they finally arrive in the host country that they may have long been yearning for, they usually have to deal with sharing cramped accommodation, often with very poor sanitary facilities, next door to strangers from other cultures and unable to make themselves understand (Wirtgen 2009). A lack of future perspectives exacerbates the situation.

Access to the healthcare system varies greatly between countries. In Germany, the current Law on Benefits for Asylum Seekers only enables medical treatment for acute symptoms or life-threatening cases (Wirtgen 2009). The pressure and stress that refugees and asylum seekers are exposed to in the host country have the effect of complicating or delaying recovery (Porter and Haslam 2005; Silove et al. 1997; Momartin et al. 2006). Although numerous studies have shown that precisely this difficulty in gaining access to healthcare contributes to further deterioration in general health and especially in mental disorders among refugees and asylum seekers (Laban et al. 2004, 2005, 2007, 2008; Bhui et al. 2006; Gerritsen et al. 2006), no uniform solution has been found so far.

In addition, in most countries, especially in psychiatric care for refugees and asylum seekers, linguistic and culture-related factors that have a significant influence on diagnosis and treatment also form significant barriers to entry (Tribe 2002; Priebe et al. 2013; Penka 2013; Heinz and Kluge 2011). Other barriers to access constitute discrimination motivated by racism, with adverse effects on physical health (Pascoe and Smart Richman 2009; Williams and Neighbors 2001) and especially mental health (van Dijk et al. 2010; Igel et al. 2010; Pascoe and Smart Richman 2009).

Indeed, in a study conducted in Germany, Igel et al. (2010) demonstrated that 43.4 % of immigrants were frequently exposed to experiences of discrimination, regardless of their specific country of origin. At the same time, in the group of migrants originating from the former states of the Soviet Union, the researchers found a relationship between these experiences of discrimination and mental health (Igel et al. 2010).

Lederbogen et al. (2011) report that stigma and social exclusion also affect the recovery process and social participation itself, including in the healthcare system (Lederbogen et al. 2011). Other major barriers to access include cultural misunderstandings (Heinz and Kluge 2011; Penka 2013; Penka et al. 2012), different expectations and explanatory models (Heinz and Kluge 2011; Penka et al. 2008; Kleinman

1980) and diagnostic blurriness arising in the course of using psychiatric instruments and during verbal communication (Heinz and Kluge 2011; Penka 2013; Penka et al. 2012; Haasen et al. 1999).

As a consequence of these barriers, refugees and asylum seekers are likely only to be offered an appointment with a general medical practitioner, even if they have mental health problems (Fenta et al. 2007), meaning that they often only reach crucial professional treatment after much delay (Laban et al. 2004, 2005, 2007, 2008). Laban et al. report that this is also commonly caused by a lack of knowledge within the medical institutions, not only about culture-specific variations in the presentation of symptoms, but also about the basic symptoms of common mental disorders ('health literacy') such as depression or post-traumatic stress disorder (Laban et al. 2004, 2005, 2007, 2008). The authors also report that refugees and asylum seekers are very unlikely to have access to social networks and therefore to the kind of social support that could help them to overcome the barriers to accessing mental health services.

Bhugra et al. (2014) emphasise that refugees and asylum seekers constitute one of the highest-risk groups in terms of developing mental disorders and are one of the most vulnerable groups in society. Although the worldwide numbers of refugees and asylum seekers show an upward trend and, as already mentioned, the proportion of traumatised people with a serious mental disorder is very high, the available healthcare systems are not prepared for this specialised group of traumatised migrants.

There are still significant access barriers and those working in the healthcare systems are on the whole inadequately trained and are unqualified to diagnose and treat traumatised refugees and asylum seekers. Both the WPA (Bhugra et al. 2011) and the EPA (Bhugra et al. 2014) have published guidelines for the treatment of mentally ill migrants, including refugees and asylum seekers.

The precarious situation which many of the afflicted find themselves in means that it is even more important to bring refugees and asylum seekers under the spotlight of diagnostic and therapeutic attention (Schouler-Ocak et al. 2015). This is exactly what this book is for. The title *Trauma and Migration* refers here primarily to people who were exposed to a traumatic event before, during or after migration, and refugees and asylum seekers are focussed on in particular.

The book gives an overview on how traumatised migrants are dealt with in various different contexts. Authors from various countries, namely, Germany, the Netherlands, Denmark, Spain, Sweden, Turkey, Israel and Canada have contributed to the book. In addition to epidemiological data and conceptual considerations, the focus is on diagnostic and therapeutic approaches to the treatment of refugees and asylum seekers.

The first group of topics presents an introduction to the subject, illustrating its relevance in today's psychiatry and psychotherapy; an emphasis is laid on the necessity to rethink healthcare for traumatised migrants and ensure the provision of additional resources for the care and treatment of refugees and asylum seekers. In his chapter *Rethinking Trauma as a Global Challenge*, Duncan Pedersen focusses on our current concept of trauma and raises questions pertaining to this.

Marion C. Aichberger offers an overview in her article *The Epidemiology of Post-Traumatic Stress Disorder – a focus on refugee and immigrant populations*. Sofie Baarnhielm and Mike Mosko report on *Cross-cultural Communication with Traumatised Immigrants*, while Levent Küey's chapter, *Trauma and Migration: the Role of Stigma*, elaborates on the importance of stigma in this context. Antonio Ventriglio and Dinesh Bhugra emphasise the relevance of *Trauma, Migration and Resilience*.

In the section on diagnostic features, Ibrahim Özkan and Maria Belz's contribution on *Clinical Diagnosis of Traumatised Immigrants* and Ferdinand Haenel's *Special problems in the assessment of psychological sequelae of torture and incarceration*. Inci User's chapter illuminates the relationship between *Gender and Trauma*. In their contribution *Forced Migration to Israel: Exposure to Trauma, Mental Health and Acculturation*, Ido Lurie and Ora Nakash offer an insight into the treatment of migrants who emigrated involuntarily to Israel. In the section on *Therapeutic Aspects*, Adil Qureshi, Irene Falgas, Khalid Ghali and Francisco Collazos focus on the subject of *Cultural Competence in Trauma*, while Meryam Schouler-Ocak introduces a special method of therapy for traumatised migrants in her chapter on *Intercultural Trauma-Centered Psychotherapy and the Application of the EMDR Method*. Cornelis J. Laban presents features of *Resilience-oriented Treatment of Traumatized Asylum seekers and Refugees*, followed by Johanna Winkler with her report on *Traumatised Immigrants in an Outpatient Clinic* and Ljiljana Joksimovic, Monika Schröder and Eva van Keuk with their contribution on *Psychotherapy with Immigrants and Refugees from Crisis Zones*. Finally, Marianne C. Kastrup and Klement Dymi finish the book with their manuscript on a *Therapy Model for Traumatised Refugees in Denmark*.

The authors bear responsibility for their own chapters.

It is my hope that this book will help bring the subjects of trauma and migration, traumatised migrants and in particular refugees and asylum seekers increasingly to our attention and that this very vulnerable group will be treated with due sensitivity. The book contains not only scientific contributions, but also contributions from practice, particularly examples of 'good clinical practice'. It also recounts specific features in the diagnosis and treatment of traumatised migrants in the hope that it can be of assistance in therapeutic work with this group of the population.

References

Bhugra D, Gupta S, Bhui K, Craig T, Dogra N, Ingleby JD et al (2011) WPA guidance on mental health and mental health care in migrants. World Psychiatry 10(1):2–10

Bhugra D, Gupta S, Schouler-Ocak M, Graeff-Calliess I, Deakin NA, Qureshi A, Dales J, Moussaoui D, Kastrup M, Tarricone I, Till A, Bassi M, Carta M (2014) EPA guidance mental health care of migrants. Eur Psychiatry 29(2):107–115

Bhui K, Audini B, Singh S, Duffett R, Bhugra D (2006) Representation of asylum seekers and refugees among psychiatric inpatients in London. Psychiatr Serv 57(2):270–272

Crumlish N, O'Rourke K (2010) A systematic review of treatments for post-traumatic stress disorder among refugees and asylum-seekers. J Nerv Ment Dis 198(4):237–251

EUROSTAT (2014) Asylum applicants and first instance decisions on asylum applications: 2013. Population and social conditions. Eurostat. http://ec.europa.eu/eurostat/documents/4168041/5948845/KS-QA-13-016-EN.PDF/0d5aedee-fb25-4c9b-9818-407372bb0870

Fazel M, Wheeler J, Danesh J (2005) Prevalence of serious mental disorder in 7000 refugees resettled in western countries: a systematic review. Lancet 365(9467):1309–1314

Fenta H, Hyman I, Noh S (2007) Health service utilization by Ethiopian immigrants and refugees in Toronto. J Immigr Minor Health 9(4):349–357

Gerritsen AAM, Bramsen I, Devillé W, Van Willigen LHM, Hovens JE, Van der Ploeg HM (2006) Use of health care services by Afghan, Iranian, and Somali refugees and asylum seekers living in The Netherlands. Eur J Public Health 16(4):394–399

Haasen C, Kraft M, Yagdiran O (1999) Auswirkungen von Sprachproblemen in der stationären Behandlung von Migranten. Krankenhauspsychiatrie 10:91–95

Hallas P, Hansen AR, Staehr MA, Munk-Andersen E, Jorgensen HL (2007) Length of stay in asylum centres and mental health in asylum seekers: a retrospective study from Denmark. BMC Public Health 7:288

Hansson EK, Tuck A, Lurie S, McKenzie K (2012) Rates of mental illness and suicidality in immigrant, refugee, ethnocultural, and racialized groups in Canada: a review of the literature. Can J Psychiatry 57(2):111–121

Heinz A, Kluge U (2011) Ethnologische Ansätze in der transkulturellen Psychiatrie. In: Machleidt W, Heinz A (eds) Praxis der Interkulturellen Psychiatrie und Psychotherapie. Migration und psychische Gesundheit. Elsevier, Urban &Fischer, München

Igel U, Brähler E, Grande G (2010) Der Einfluss von Diskriminierungserfahrungen auf die Gesundheit von Migranten. Psychiatr Prax 37:183–190

Kleinman A (1980) Major conceptual and research issues for cultural (anthropological) psychiatry. Cult Med Psychiatry 4(1):3–23

Laban CJ, Gernaat HBPE, Komproe IH, Schreuders GA, De Jong JTVM (2004) Impact of a long asylum procedure on the prevalence of psychiatric disorders in Iraqi asylum seekers in the Netherlands. J Nerv Ment Dis 192:843–852

Laban CJ, Gernaat HBPE, Komproe IH, Van Tweel I, De Jong JTVM (2005) Post migration living problems and common psychiatric disorders in Iraqi asylum seekers in the Netherlands. J Nerv Ment Dis 193:825–832

Laban CJ, Komproe IH, Gernaat HB, de Jong JT (2007) The impact of a long asylum procedure on quality of life, disability and physical health in Iraqi asylum seekers in the Netherlands. Soc Psychiatry Psychiatr Epidemiol 43(7):507–515

Laban CJ, Komproe IH, Gernaat HBPE, De Jong JTVM (2008) Impact of a long asylum procedure on quality of life, disability and physical health in Iraqi asylum seekers in the Netherlands. Soc Psychiatry Psychiatr Epidemiol 43:507–515

Lederbogen F et al (2011) City living and urban upbringing affect neural social stress processing in humans. Nature 474:498–501

Lindert J, Ehrenstein OS, Priebe S, Mielck A, Brähler E (2009) Depression and anxiety in labor migrants and refugees – a systematic review and meta-analysis. Soc Sci Med 69(2):246–257

Momartin S, Steel Z, Coello M, Aroche J, Silove DM, Brooks R (2006) A comparison of the mental health of refugees with temporary versus permanent protection visas. Med J Aust 185(7):357–361

Noh S, Beiser M, Kaspar V, Hou F, Rummens J (1999) Perceived racial discrimination, depression, and coping: a study of Southeast Asian refugees in Canada. J Health Soc Behav 40(3):193–207

Pascoe EA, Smart Richman L (2009) Perceived discrimination and health: a meta-analytic review. Psychol Bull 135(4):531–554

Penka S (2013) Zugangsbarrieren von Personen mit Migrationshintergrund zum Suchthilfesystem-Konsequenzen für die Praxis. In: Koch E, Müller MJ, Schouler-Ocak M (eds) Sucht und Migration. Lambertus-Verlag, Freiburg i. Br

Penka S, Heimann H, Heinz A, Schouler-Ocak M (2008) Explanatory models of addictive behaviour among native German, Russian-German, and Turkish Youth. Eur Psychiatry 23(1):S36–S42

Penka S, Schouler-Ocak M, Heinz A, Kluge U (2012) Interkulturelle Aspekte der Interaktion und Kommunikation im psychiatrisch/psychotherapeutischen Behandlungssetting. Bundesgesundheitsblatt 55:1168–1175

Porter M, Haslam N (2005) Predisplacement and postdisplacement factors associated with mental health of refugees and internally displaced persons: a meta-analysis. JAMA 294(5):602–612

Priebe S, Matanov A, Barros H, Canavan R, Gabor E, Greacen T, Holcnerová P, Kluge U, Nicaise P, Moskalewicz J, Díaz-Olalla JM, Strassmayr C, Schene AH, Soares JJ, Tulloch S, Gaddini A (2013) Mental health-care provision for marginalized groups across Europe: findings from the PROMO study. Eur J Public Health 23(1):97–103

Schouler-Ocak M, Graef-Calliess IT, Tarricone I, Qureshi A, Kastrup M, Bhugra D (2015) EPA Guidance on Cultural Competence Training. Eur Psychiatry 30(3):431–40

Silove D, Sinnerbrink I, Field A, Manicavasagar V, Steel Z (1997) Anxiety, depression and PTSD in asylum-seekers: associations with pre-migration trauma and post-migration stressors. Br J Psychiatry 170:351–357

Tribe R (2002) Mental health of refugees and asylum-seekers. Advances in Psychiatric Treatment, vol. 8, pp. 240–248

UNHCR (2013) UNHCR asylum trends 2012. United Nations High Commissioner of Refugees, Geneva

UNHCR (2014) UNHCR global reports 2013. United Nations High Commissioner for Refugees, Geneva

van Dijk TK, Agyemang C, de Wit M, Hosper K (2010) The relationship between perceived discrimination and depressive symptoms among young Turkish-Dutch and Moroccan-Dutch. Eur J Public Health 21(4):477–483

Williams DR, Neighbors H (2001) Racism, discrimination and hypertension: evidence and needed research. Ethn Dis 11(4):800–816

Wirtgen W (2009) Traumatisierte Flüchtlinge: Psychische Probleme bleiben meist unerkannt. Dtsch Arztebl 106(49):A-2463/B-2115/C-2055

Rethinking Trauma as a Global Challenge

2

Duncan Pedersen

Introduction

Trauma is a term originally applied to physical injuries and some of its immediate effects. The first mention of the term 'traumatic' was recorded in the Oxford English Dictionary edition of 1656, in which trauma is defined as '… pertaining to wounds or the cure of wounds'. It is since the late 1800s that 'trauma' has come to refer to a range of psychological impacts of the experience or threat of violence, injury and loss.

Events that are considered potentially traumatic include a wide range of intentional and non-intentional acts of violence such as violent personal assault, rape, physical or sexual abuse, severe automobile accidents, natural or biotechnological disasters, being kidnapped or taken hostage, being diagnosed with a life-threatening illness, exposed to military combat or terrorist attacks, torture, incarceration as prisoner of war or seclusion in a concentration camp, among others. The term 'trauma' (referred to as psychological or 'mental') is highlighted as a common denominator for all these dissimilar events, with much overlapping in between events, although it is clear that each one has its own languages of affliction, so-called idioms of distress, in addition to different attributions of causality, and specific features and meanings associated with certain effects and outcomes.

Traumatic events vary widely in terms of the nature of the threat or injury, its frequency and duration, its personal significance (which may change over time), the relationship of the victim to the perpetrator (in the case of interpersonal violence or abuse) and the broader collective meaning and social response. What constitutes a

D. Pedersen
Division of Social and Transcultural Psychiatry,
Douglas Hospital Research Centre, McGill University,
6875 LaSalle Blvd., Montreal, QC H4H 1R3, Canada
e-mail: duncan.pedersen@mcgill.ca
URL: http://www.mcgill.ca/tcpsych/research/global-mental-health-research

© Springer International Publishing Switzerland 2015
M. Schouler-Ocak (ed.), *Trauma and Migration:*
Cultural Factors in the Diagnosis and Treatment of Traumatised Immigrants,
DOI 10.1007/978-3-319-17335-1_2

'trauma' then is not entirely dependent on the nature of the event but also on the personal meaning assigned and the social interpretation of the event, including responses of the affected person, their family and community, as well as the society at large.

Over the last two decades, the language of violence, terror and dislocation has often been conflated with the discourse of trauma. In Western popular and professional discourses, 'trauma' has undergone a true metamorphosis and has become a dominant category to explain not only the origins or cause of other health-related problems but also the consequence of exposure to violence. It is especially after the 9/11 events in the USA that trauma has become an emblematic category that is invasive in everyday life and has reached epidemic proportions: the media, the lay public and the medical professions, the sports and the arts are all claiming the universality of trauma as a unique and unavoidable outcome of exposure to violence. In this context, trauma has almost become synonymous with post-traumatic stress disorder in both popular and scientific thought.

The Genealogy of Trauma as a Mental Injury

The first allusion to a 'mental wound' makes its appearance in the late eighteenth century, when John Erichsen, a British surgeon, first referred to the notion of 'trauma' as a mental injury in his book *On Railway and Other Injuries of the Nervous System*, published in 1866 (Young 1995).[1] It was then that Erichsen, who was in charge of assessing cases of train accidents requesting compensation, described that powerful blows or 'shocks', or simple shaking and jarring of railroad shocks and derailments, would result either as visible lesions (in the post-mortem) or, in some damage, invisible to the naked eye, produced by the nervous shock or bruising of the spinal cord, which he called the *railway spine* syndrome. The main symptoms were pallor, faint, tremor and palpitations, unmotivated crying and insomnia, among others, which – according to Erichsen – occurred as a state of 'natural perturbation of the mind' after an accident or derailment. The nervous system injury was explained by an analogy comparing the spinal lesions with the scattering effects of a magnetic charge of a magnet when hit by a mallet or hammer blow.

It is attributed to J-M. Charcot the earliest psychological account of the 'railway spine', when he classified these cases under the category of 'hysteria'. By the early twentieth century and the years after World War I, Sigmund Freud turned his attention to trauma as the origin of hysterical attacks, which later were described as 'traumatic neurosis'. Moving away from the neurological explanations of his predecessors, Freud attributed hysterical symptoms as the result of memories of childhood traumatic experiences, the so-called traumatic memory. These were the forerunners of what was later described during World War I as 'war neurosis' or

---

[1] The initial part of this section is largely based on the works of Allan Young, in his book *The Harmony of Illusions: Inventing Post-traumatic Stress Disorder*. Princeton: Princeton University Press, 1995.

'shell shock' among the soldiers of the British army, characterised by symptoms such as numbness, anaesthesia, pain hypersensitivity, palpitations, muscle twitching and paralysis and gastrointestinal symptoms, among others. This set of polymorphic signs and symptoms was most often attributed to the dreadful conditions of warfare in the trenches and exposure to explosives in the front lines. It is interesting to note that the explanation of *shell shock* was in many ways similar to the *railway spine* syndrome, in that exposure to shock waves produced by the proximity to an explosion would cause concussions and vascular disorders in the nervous system, causing damage to the histological structures of the brain and microscopic spinal cord injuries.

Over the years, researchers were influenced by historical events representing massive trauma (i.e. the trenches of World War I, the genocide perpetrated by the Nazi doctors in World War II, the survivors of Hiroshima, the Korean War and returning Vietnam veterans), where different approaches were used in an attempt to build a conceptual framework for trauma studies.

During World War II, the Allied troops, including a large number of American soldiers who were exposed to combat, developed a variety of symptoms that were classified under the general rubric of *shell shock*. Many of these cases were described as clinical syndromes and labelled as 'conversion states', 'somatic regressions' or 'psychosomatic disorders' and therefore treated with a wide range of therapies (e.g. abreactive therapy, induced sleep drugs, electroshocks, psychotherapy and occupational therapy were some of the most used). To this list, it was among the veterans of the wars in Korea and then Vietnam, between 1965 and 1969, where the first cases of 'post-traumatic syndromes' were described. In 1980, post-traumatic stress disorder (PTSD) appeared in the Diagnostic and Statistical Manual of Mental Disorders (DSM), the official publication of the American Psychiatry Association. A few years after, the so-called Gulf syndrome would be the label transiently applied to the PTSD symptom cluster experienced among veterans of the Gulf War.

The medical model of trauma that prevailed at that time was largely generated and enacted by military doctors and psychiatrists, holding a particular vision of the phenomenon, limiting their attention to the veterans or 'victims' among the military population and interpreting their symptoms and reactions as abnormal or psychopathological problems in response to exposure to traumatic events, which were then subject to the appropriate diagnosis and treatment in order to reassign them promptly to the battlefront and/or reintegrate them into the civil society and the workforce.

In the early 1990s, an important shift occurred by which trauma was no longer a category restrained to the military, but it was extended to civilian populations. Therapeutic interventions followed the same path, changing their focus from the military into civilians, targeting entire 'war-traumatised communities', a shift that was later followed by the rise of the 'therapeutic state' in the post-war period (Moon 2009), as discussed below. War atrocities, lethal violence and its consequences were from now on framed through the 'morally neutral' sciences of memory and psychology (Hacking 1996; Summerfield 2004).

In short, the explanatory model to explain the outcomes of exposure to traumatic events was gradually medicalised, as part of secularisation of life, while psychology displaced religion as a source of explanation to life adversities. The 'psychological man' emerged and replaced the nineteenth-century 'economic man' and its predecessors: the 'religious man' as a pre-Enlightenment figure of Judeo-Christian heritage and the 'political man' at the centre of public life in classical antiquity (Rieff 1966; Moon 2009).

It is now generally accepted that victims react to the experience of trauma according to the meaning that this represents for them, and therefore not all reactions should be regarded as necessarily pathological or abnormal. In fact, it can be argued that many of the reactions to trauma are 'normal' and represent a rather healthy response, from which defence mechanisms evolve and healing processes are constructed. This new frame has implications for the research agenda of trauma and stress, where the focus of analysis has shifted from the 'victims' to 'survivors' and the occurrence of trauma has been transferred from the battleground to the public space.

In summary, the social, political and cultural realities structure the context in which trauma is experienced and influence individual and collective reactions at various levels: the perception, interpretation and subjective meaning of traumatic events, the modes of expressing distress and explaining adversities, the coping responses and adaptation and, finally, the help-seeking patterns and treatment responses. The important concept to retain here is that society and culture assign significance and attach meanings to the traumatic event, which can give to and make sense of the traumatic experience, so that in turn it could somehow mitigate, reduce or even amplify its impact.

Trauma and PTSD

From an evolutionary perspective, human beings have long lived under the threat of violence, injury and death throughout their existence as a group, to the extent that we might expect reactions, responses and mechanisms have evolved to help us adapt to threats that fail to destroy us. The most common response to mild or moderate levels of trauma is an acute distress reaction rapidly followed by recovery. We are biologically primed to learn to be fearful and avoidant of potentially life-threatening situations. When threats are more severe, sustained and inescapable, other mechanisms come into play such as dissociation or cognitive process of blocking out or compartmentalising memory and experience (Konner 2007).

Although trauma can aggravate any psychiatric condition, certain disorders are presumed to have a direct causal link to trauma exposure. When confronting a traumatic event, some individuals will have more severe or incapacitating acute symptoms of short duration, while some will go on to have chronic distress and long-term disability. Others may do well initially but manifest significant symptoms at a later time. These pathological outcomes reflect both individual and social vulnerabilities. Among the problems specifically linked to trauma are grief and other normal forms of reactive distress, depressive and anxiety disorders and post-traumatic stress disorder (PTSD).

Trauma exposure may result in a variety of short- and long-term adaptive and pathological responses. Common responses during or immediately after the traumatic event include intense autonomic arousal associated with fear, agitated behaviour or 'freezing' and dissociative symptoms, with an altered sense of time speeding up or slowing down, and feelings of derealisation and depersonalisation, until extinction (Bouton and Waddell 2007).

PTSD is one of the few psychiatric constructs having an explicit causal mechanism built into its diagnostic criteria: exposure to an unexpected or unpredictable event that involves possible serious injury or death to oneself or others leads to appraisal of the event as threatening and so leads to intense fear, helplessness, horror and other negative emotions (i.e. shame, guilt, anger). These effects in turn influence memory and other cognitive-emotional-sensory processing of the event such that it leaves lasting traces in brain and behaviour. A major component of the PTSD syndrome is subserved by a conditioned emotional response of 'fear'. Reminders of the context where threat originally occurred evoke anxiety, and this is managed by cognitive and behavioural efforts to avoid such contextual cues, resulting in emotional numbing and withdrawal (Kirmayer et al. 2007).

Fear conditioning can be long-lasting, but in the ordinary course of events, repeated exposure to the same cues without any fearsome outcome eventually results in a decrease in conditioned fear, hyperarousal and avoidance behaviour – a process called 'extinction'. It is now known that extinction involves a type of learning distinct from fear conditioning, involving different neural pathways. In fact, the original conditioned fear is not erased or replaced but simply suppressed by extinction learning.

The two types of learning have different characteristics; fear conditioning is quicker and generalises more easily than extinction learning. As a result, a small change in environmental cues can reinstate the originally learned fear. This helps to account for the phenomenon of triggering or reactivation of symptoms in patients with PTSD (Barad and Cain 2007).

These biological mechanisms are important for understanding the causes, course and chronicity of PTSD, the dynamics of triggering and re-experiencing and the effectiveness of exposure therapy as a treatment, but PTSD involves additional cognitive and behavioural responses mediated by forms of learning and memory, as well as processes of recall and narrative elaboration that are regulated by the personal meaning of the traumatic events. Both recollection and narration also involve social process so that traumatic outcomes reflect the culturally sanctioned occasions for remembering, accumulating and forgetting.

The Diagnostic and Statistics Manual of Mental Disorders, in its 4th edition (DSM-IV), introduced the diagnosis criteria for acute stress disorder (ASD), limiting its occurrence within the first 4 weeks of trauma exposure. ASD is similar to PTSD but with prominent dissociative symptoms. A severe ASD response is a predictor of longer-term distress, including PTSD (APA 1994).

DSM-IV-TR classifies PTSD as an anxiety disorder that is characterised by the '… reexperiencing of an extremely traumatic event accompanied by symptoms of increased arousal and by avoidance of stimuli associated with the trauma'

(APA 2000). According to the DSM 4th edition, the essential features of PTSD are the development of specific symptoms following exposure to an event that involved actual or threatened death, or serious injury, to which the person responded with 'intense fear, helplessness or horror'.

In addition to the stressor criterion A, PTSD includes three additional criteria classified in main symptom clusters: (criterion B) intrusive recollection (intrusive thoughts, distressing dreams, reliving or dissociative 'flashbacks', psychological distress and physiological reactivity when exposed to reminders), (criterion C) avoidance/numbing (efforts to avoid thoughts, feelings, conversations or activities associated with the stressor, difficulty remembering the traumatic event, social withdrawal and emotional numbing) and (criterion D) hyperarousal (sleep problems, irritability or angry outbursts, concentration problems, hypervigilance and an exaggerated startle response). The diagnostic criteria for PTSD in the International Classification of Diseases (ICD-10) are similar, but the latter does not include numbing and does not require functional impairment; these differences are likely to result in higher prevalence rates for PTSD when using ICD-10 criteria.

The wording of PTSD used in the DSM-IV (APA 1994) implies a causal relationship between the traumatic triggering event (criterion A) and the symptom clusters that follow. In other words, the symptoms that comprise the syndrome are connected by a simple logic: criterion A causes B, and criterion B causes C, and probably D (arousal). In other words, a traumatic event can lead to painful memories, and the individual adapts to recurrent memories and excitement through behavioural avoidance and numbing (Young and Breslau in print). This causation path (A-B-C) is most frequently cited in the stories of survivors, as well as in descriptions made by outside observers or clinicians (Shalev 2007).

The DSM, 5th edition (DSM-5) (APA 2013), has undergone a few modifications over the previous version. The changes in the diagnostic criteria for PTSD are relatively minor but may have an impact in the calculation of prevalence rates and current diagnostic procedures. The cumulative effects of the changes introduced remain to date unclear, and the new DSM-5 has been criticised for both reliability and validity, as well as potential legal implications (Zoellner et al. 2013). Changes can be summarised as follows: (1) PTSD has been shifted from 'anxiety disorder' to a new category of 'trauma and stressor-related disorders'; (2) the traumatic event (criterion A) has been redefined and as such may create ambiguities and additional problems of interpretation; and (3) the symptom clusters have been changed, with the addition of more symptoms – negative beliefs/expectations, distorted blame, persistent negative emotions, reckless or self-destructive behaviour and the creation of a dissociative subtype.

These changes have resulted in a lower inter-rater agreement yet, according to the DSM-5 field trials, it has retained very good reliability (Kappa = 0.67) (Regier et al. 2013).

DSM-5 revised the parameters of criterion A1, whereby indirect exposure is defined more specifically as 'learning that the traumatic event occurred to a close family member or close friend' in which the 'actual or threatened death must have been violent or accidental' (APA 2013). The definition of traumatic event has been expanded to include 'experience or extreme exposure to aversive details of the traumatic event' such as first responders involved in the collection of human remains and police officers exposed repeatedly to details of child abuse. It has further excluded the category of 'virtual trauma' in previous DSM versions, such as witnessing traumatic events through electronic media (TV, video games, movies, pictures, etc.).

However, these changes in the definition of traumatic stressor leave gaps and do not remove the ambiguities of previous versions. The so-called bracket creep of criterion A remains open to misinterpretation and malingering with expanding the definition of what constitutes a traumatic stressor beyond its intended boundaries (McNally 2009). The addition of 'new' symptoms (from 17 to 20) may introduce new sources of heterogeneity of PTSD and increase the risk of PTSD over diagnosis, as the number of possible combinations of symptoms rises significantly and differential diagnosis becomes more difficult.

According to Allen Frances, former Chair of the DSM-IV, all the DSM-5 changes loosen diagnosis and threaten to turn our current diagnostic inflation into a diagnostic hyperinflation (except for autism). Psychiatric diagnosis has become too important in selecting treatments, determining eligibility for benefits and services, allocating resources, guiding legal judgments and influencing personal expectations to be left in the hands of a few experts endorsing a system of classification of dubious validity. New diagnoses in psychiatry, whether based on the DSM, the ICD or any classificatory system, are possibly more dangerous than new drugs because ultimately they influence whether or not millions of people are diagnosed and placed on psychotropic drugs, often prescribed by primary health-care workers after brief and simplified clinical assessment. Before their introduction, new diagnoses deserve the same level of attention to safety that is devoted to new drugs (Frances 2012).

Although the trauma construct appears to be homogeneous, in fact it has been described in many different ways over the past three decades. The ever-growing and inclusive definition of trauma has made problematic the objective evaluation of their existence, and caution should be exercised when attempting to measure the construct 'trauma' in different contexts, especially those that can be called non-Western societies.

Today, some authors challenge the presumption that PTSD is actually homogeneous with respect to the A-B-C pathway discussed above. In fact, PTSD is an heterogeneous disorder that is often incorrectly perceived as being homogeneous in its manifestations and universal in its distribution, resulting in symptoms described as the same, regardless of culture or historical period of observation (Bracken and Thomas 2001; Young 1995).

It is now well established that symptom clusters constituting PTSD have grown and vanished in importance across time. As shown above, the DSM-5 changed criterion A, eliminating criterion A2, while qualifying symptoms were increased from 17 to 20. These variations in symptom clusters and their frequency distribution reflect advances of medical theories as much as new knowledge and changes in the clinical assessment, medical diagnosis and treatment practices. Interestingly, criterion A, the traumatic event creating the distressful memory, has been questioned with regard to its utility and demarcation but remained so far untouched in the recent versions of the DSM.

To explain the heterogeneity of the phenomenon, an argument often invoked is the encoding and recovery of memory. The first refers to multiple types of logical memory associated with post-traumatic stress. Distressing memories, generating unease and anxiety, are inherently considered malleable representations. The retrieval of memory (also called reconsolidation) is a process in which the memory traces of a traumatic experience again rebuild and recalibrate and possibly become reclassified or outlined.

Recent research in neurosciences suggests that the malleability of memory and the process of reconsolidation are products of evolutionary biology. The process of retrieval or memory reconsolidation seems to be a means to improve the body's ability to respond to new or unforeseen emergencies, rather than a means of providing faithful copies of the past. This is a complex but promising field of research in PTSD, which may lead to more effective and culturally appropriate therapeutic interventions aimed to interfere or block the reconsolidation process (Brunet et al. 2011).

Turning to the epidemiology of PTSD, about 15–20 % of people exposed to traumatic events have symptoms and impairment lasting for several days or weeks (Breslau 1998). Epidemiological studies in the general population show that the psychological trauma does not occur in all those who have experienced traumatic events but appears in a fraction of the exposed, and the traumatic event itself does not sufficiently explain why post-traumatic stress disorder develops or persists (or dies) with the passage of time (Yehuda 1998).

It is recognised that combat exposure usually explains less than 25 % of the variance in PTSD symptoms and often even much less (Miller and Rasmussen 2010). Moreover, the prevalence of PTSD in the general population has been estimated as low, which may be explained by differences in the sensitivity of the instruments used to measure the presence of PTSD but may also reflect the presence of other 'hidden' factors involved in its pathogenesis (Shalev and Yehuda 1998). In short, it may be concluded that the traumatic event itself is a necessary but not sufficient cause to explain the occurrence of PTSD.

Risk factors for PTSD may be divided into two main categories: (1) those relevant to the traumatic event (i.e. severity and duration of the type of trauma) and (2) those relating to the person who experiences the event (i.e. gender, income, educational level, previous traumatic experiences, child sexual abuse, etc.). Studies have found that higher rates of PTSD symptoms are associated with the degree of direct violence of the war and exposure to a larger number of traumatic experiences (Scholte et al. 2004). This feature is called dose-response, and it is argued that people could develop PTSD regardless of other risk factors once the trauma load reaches a certain threshold (Neuner et al. 2004).

Empirical studies among war-affected populations have shown that repeated exposure to trauma is cumulative and makes a person more vulnerable to developing PTSD (Kolassa et al. 2010). Similarly, researchers have found the cumulative effect of traumatic events on PTSD symptoms and frequency in different populations (Marshall et al. 2005; Cardozo et al. 2000; Eytan et al. 2004). That is, they found a linear decrease in the mental health and social functioning proportional to the increase in traumatic events.

Moreover, post-traumatic reactions persisted beyond such as the presence of the stressor and the passage of time. While the intensity of the initial traumatic reaction tends to decrease in the days, weeks or months after exposure, reduction of symptoms takes a different rate depending on the nature of the traumatic event.

Re-examining the Impact of Organised Violence, Armed Conflict and War on Population Health

There is a growing body of evidence suggesting that the short- and long-term consequences of organised violence, endemic conflict and war on civilian populations are more complex than initially thought. In the strict sense, the impact of a war cannot be solely examined by the sheer number of casualties, the numbers of refugees and forcibly displaced populations or the material losses and breakdown of social services resulting from it. There are significant effects expressed in the lingering, additional burden of disease, disability and death, as well as other less evident but more pervasive ecological, social and economic consequences, such as family disintegration and attrition of social support networks, environmental degradation, dislocation of food production systems, disruption of the local economies and exodus of the workforce, all of which have profound implications in the health and well-being of survivors (Pedersen and Kienzler 2008).

Evidences from studies conducted in the aftermath of World War II and, more recently, in central Asia (i.e. Iraq, Afghanistan) and some countries of the African and Latin American and Caribbean regions have consistently shown that exposure to multiple physiological stressors – including famine-induced malnutrition – occurring in utero or early infancy, may lead to chronic diseases later in life, ranging from osteoporosis to cardiovascular disease and diabetes (Markowitz 1955; Toole and Waldman 1997; Gluckman and Hanson 2005).

Sharp declines of childhood growth and stunting have been shown in many European countries during World War II. For example, a study by Bruntland et al. (1980) conducted in Oslo, Norway, revealed a significant but transient decline in height of school children in the mid-1940s, as a direct consequence of food shortages and adversities experienced during the German occupation. In Guatemala, high stunting rates were reported among Mayan and Ladino children during a period where extreme violence and massacres were inflicted in the civilian population along with increased levels of poverty, ethnic conflict, nutritional deprivation and rising social inequalities (Bogin and Keep 1999).

In short, as exposure to environmental stressors is stratified along socioeconomic levels and birth weight is proven to predict developmental outcomes, prenatal exposure to acute environmental stressors such as protracted conflict and war may also have not only short- but also long-term effects, thus contributing to the intergenerational reproduction of inequality with poor health outcomes for both mothers and children.

Another spill-over effect of armed conflict and war is the apparent increase of interpersonal violence, armed assaults, homicides and other drug-related crimes in the post-war. The 'dirty wars' (see below the section on contemporary wars) often result in a breakdown of the state, creating territories controlled by local warlords who provide safe haven for the illegal production and trade of drugs. It is estimated that some 95 % of the hard drug primary production, mainly *opium* and *coca*, is concentrated in countries undergoing conflict and civil war (i.e. Afghanistan) or in post-conflict scenarios (i.e. Colombia, Peru) (Collier et al. 2009). The drug trade, in turn, has worldwide rippling effects and creates multiple niches of endemic lethal violence with significant negative repercussions in population health.

More recently, researchers have begun to explore how trauma is both a marker and product of social inequality and exclusion. Studies on narratives of distress have emphasised the taxonomies of stress, pain and suffering but have not sufficiently contributed to our understanding of the many interrelations between poverty and exposure to violence as health determinants. This is so, despite the recognition that the effects of war cannot be separated from those of other forces such as structural violence and social injustice, unemployment, falling commodity prices, unbridled environmental exploitation and landlessness. Moreover, a wealth of data is available showing that imposed structural adjustment packages most often result in slashed budgets for health, education and social welfare on which the poorest are most dependent on. The neoliberal economic model may undermine the social fabric no less effectively than armed conflicts and wars (Stuckler and Basu 2013; Labonte et al. 2011).

Structural violence is embedded in 'ubiquitous social structures, normalized by stable institutions and regular experience' (Gilligan 1997) and as such may be unintentional yet closely related to intentional forms of violence (i.e. interpersonal) (Blau and Blau 1982). The effects of income inequality on violence and criminality have been given some empirical support. A multi-country study by Wolf et al. (2014) concluded that income inequality, as measured by the Gini coefficient, is associated with certain violent outcomes and found a correlation between alcohol consumption with self-reported assault rates in all 169 countries of their study. Wilkinson and Pickett (2006, 2009) have also shown evidence in 23 high-income countries where homicide rates are associated with income inequality as measured by the Gini index (Pickett et al. 2005; Wilkinson and Pickett 2009).

In short, when trying to explain poor health outcomes (i.e. disease occurrence, distress, trauma-related disorders and social suffering) in relation to collective violence and contemporary wars, the issues of poverty and social inequalities cannot be ignored, as they are the most important co-determinants.

It is within this context a few questions may be raised regarding the impact of exposure to massive traumatic events in population health. How is organised violence linked to poor health outcomes at the individual and at the community levels? Are post-traumatic stress disorder (PTSD) and other trauma-related disorders a unique, universal and unavoidable outcome of exposure to violence? What about the role of other forces at play such as resilience, coping skills and social cohesion and the density and quality of social support networks? What is the role of other social ills, such as racism and extreme nationalism, alongside poverty and inequalities, in determining the health and disease equation? What is the social production of collective and individual suffering? These are some of the crucial questions shaping the global mental health research agenda in the current times.

As we have seen above, the implications of contemporary wars in the collective health status and well-being of affected populations, at home or in exile, go well beyond the loss of life and destruction of physical infrastructure: the devastation of the social and cultural fabric, the people's history and life trajectories, their identity and value systems (which are in many ways vital for their survival) are under threat to fade away or disappear. The instilled terror, social polarisation and forced militarisation of daily life (Martin-Baró 1994) lead to significant changes both in the lifestyle and quality of life of civilian populations that are difficult to measure and attribute significance in terms of well-being, life expectancy or resulting morbidity and burden of illness. On the other hand, the collective responses in confronting extreme violence and death represent a range of critical mechanisms for restoration and survival, which should not be underestimated.

The literature focussing on long-term effects of war and atrocities has attempted to establish direct linkages between the original experience of trauma and persistence of certain symptoms in some individuals, at times for as long as 50 years, interpreted as anxiety, depression, alcohol and drug abuse and chronic PTSD. However, we should be more cautious in making false attributions and drawing erroneous conclusions while ignoring the presence of confounding variables in the chain of events leading to poor mental health outcomes or emotional states accompanied by vivid and painful memories of the past (Summerfield 1999). In phenomenological terms, these emotional states are not necessarily psychopathological but rather illustrate aspects of normal cognitive functioning and fall within the range of normal responses to adversity (Bracken and Petty 1998).

The Global Impact of War and Violence

There is growing consensus that crime and lethal violence in their various manifestations are emerging public health problems, closely related to certain social characteristics, including poverty and social inequalities. Across time, the societies with higher levels of intentional violence are also those mostly poor, with high inequalities in the distribution of wealth, less educated, more intolerant to racial differences, living under autocratic regimes and less likely to engage in commerce and trade. Conversely, the more peaceful societies also tend to be richer and more equalitarian, living under more democratic governments, healthier and better educated, more respectful of their women and more likely to engage in trade and nonviolent exchanges (Pinker 2011).

Lethal and intentional violence in particular has become one of the leading causes of death worldwide for men aged 15–44 years (Krug et al. 2002). Of the total number of global injury-related deaths, about two thirds are of non-intentional origin (e.g. traffic accidents), while one third are due to intentional violence, including

Table 2.1 Estimated global (intentional) violent-related deaths (WHO 2000)

World distribution and type of lethal event	Number	Rate per 100,000	Percentage %
Low- and middle-income countries	1,510,000	32.1	91.1
High-income countries	149,000	14.4	8.9
Homicide	520,000	8.8	31.3
Suicide	815,000	14.5	49.1
War related	310,000	5.2	18.6
Total	1,659,000	28.8	100.0

Source: WHO Burden of Disease project for 2000, Version 1

suicides, homicides and organised violence (i.e. terrorism, wars and armed conflict, genocide and ethnic cleansing) (WHO 2000; Murray et al. 2002) (see Table 2.1).

Both the frequency and the numbers of people killed by intentional violence (homicides and organised violence) have shown a tendency to decline over the last half-century, especially after the 1990s, while the proportion of survivors has risen significantly (Pedersen and Kienzler 2008; Center for Research on the Epidemiology of Disasters 2009). This means that compared to the previous years, today there are many more survivors who may have been exposed to and affected psychologically by traumatic events resulting in poor mental health outcomes (Desjarlais et al. 1995).

Today, the overall homicide rate estimated by the WHO for the entire world hovers around $8.8 \times 100,000$ per year (Krug et al. 2002), a figure that compares favourably with the triple-digit values for pre-state societies and the double-digit values for medieval Europe (Pinker 2011). Of the estimated global (intentional) violent-related deaths, homicides represent almost one third (31.3 %), while suicides reach almost half (49.1 %) of all deaths (see Table 2.2).

According to Pinker (2011), as one becomes aware of the global and historical decline in lethal and intentional violence, the world begins to look much different: the past seems less innocent and innocuous and the present less sinister and ominous. Thus, instead of asking what are the causes and why is there so much violence and wars in the world today, we might start asking what are the foundations for a durable peace as well as why is there much peace and goodwill around us (Pinker 2011).

People day-to-day perceptions of the global levels of violence are usually disconnected from the actual proportions and real prevalence. But this does not mean to say that we should be at ease with the steady violence decline per se, but we should remain engaged in trying to explain why the decline has occurred and commit ourselves to reduce even further the still unacceptably high current levels of lethal violence among certain population segments, low-income countries and regions, to the lowest possible levels, if not to their total eradication (Pinker 2011).

This approach would hopefully lead us into a different and more fruitful direction. Our most serious contemporary problems – including mental health – should be seen as an intricate part of globalisation and the global crisis: global warming, resource depletion, ecosystem degradation, poverty and social inequalities,

Table 2.2 Estimated global homicide and suicide rates (per 100,000) by age group and sex (WHO 2000)

Age group (years)	Homicide rates		Suicide rates	
	Males	Females	Males	Females
0–4	5.8	4.8	0	0
5–14	2.1	2.0	1.7	2.0
15–29	19.4	4.4	15.6	12.2
30–44	18.7	4.3	21.5	12.4
45–59	14.8	4.5	28.4	12.6
60+	13.0	4.5	44.9	22.1
Total (age standardised)	13.6	4.0	18.9	10.6

Source: WHO Burden of Disease project for 2000, Version 1

violence, conflict and war are the fundamental problems inherent in the basic cultural patterns of our now global-scale civilisation.

If we limit this review of violence, conflict and wars to the last two centuries only, wars with a long-lasting – so-called transformational – effect on the course of world history, leading to important changes in the global order, represent an estimated total of 42 years of conflicts, with a conservative estimate of about 95 million deaths, including both combatants and civilians (Smil 2008). Another estimate shows that since the end of World War II, a total of 240 armed conflicts have been active in 151 locations throughout the world (Harbom and Wallensteen 2009). While the number of interstate wars has been declining since the early 1990s, the number of intrastate wars, most often fought between ethnic groups or loosely connected networks, most often challenging poor and underdeveloped states or even powerful nation-states, has increased both in frequency and in levels of organised violence, inflicted atrocities and psychological warfare. According to Holsti (1996), the classical and persistent Clausewitzian conception of war 'as the continuation of politics by other means' which was predominant in Europe for almost three centuries (1648–1945) bears little relevance to the analysis of today's contemporary wars.

The emergence of the so-called low-intensity wars,[2] which are at once 'a war of resistance and a campaign to politicize the masses whose loyalty and enthusiasm must sustain a post-war regime' (Holsti 1996), represents the prevailing forms of armed conflict today. In these contemporary wars, the target is not the territory but the local population, mostly the poor, often including those who have an added symbolic value (e.g. local leaders, priests, health workers, local civil authorities and teachers) (Pedersen 2002). Social conflicts are however persistent and in some cases escalating, where the lives of ethnic groups and indigenous peoples are increasingly under threat as they attempt to defend their land and possessions from incursions by insurgent groups and the military, mining and timber companies, drug traffickers

---

[2] Low-intensity warfare has been defined as a 'total war at the grass roots level', where the local population and not the territory is the target for psychological warfare, terrorisation and other traumatic experiences.

and drug enforcement operations, corrupted government officials and disruptive development projects (Pedersen 1999).

Contemporary Wars and the Emergence of New Forms of Warfare

Contemporary wars and changes in war strategic targets and warfare styles and technologies, such as aerial bombing and unmanned aerial vehicles (UAV), known as 'drones', have led to a significant increase in the number of civilian casualties, now making up approximately 90 % of all war-related deaths (Pedersen and Kienzler 2008).[3] The global impact in numbers of accumulated civilian deaths is thus considerable. Psychological warfare is a devastatingly effective central feature in these contemporary wars, where terror is infused and atrocities are committed, including massacres and mass executions, desecration of corpses, disappearances, torture and gang rape are the norm (Summerfield 1995, 1998; Pedersen 2002).

These new forms of warfare and their devastating consequences can be observed across all regions of the world. In Africa, the style of warfare has shifted dramatically in recent years. Emerging rebel movements are mushrooming, and the continent is now plagued by countless small-scale 'dirty wars' with no front lines, no battlefields and no distinctions between combatants and civilians. Many of the recruits are children and young adolescents who are engaged in a vicious circle of gang rape, pillage and crime, leaving behind a trail of mutilation and murder, trauma, deaths, despair and suffering (Reno 2012).

The Arab league countries also have a distinct experience of revolt and rebellion against authoritarian regimes and a recent history of violent military repression, with a high death toll among civilians engaged in massive demonstrations and exposed to different forms of organised violence. The siege and bombardment of cities and the use of heavy artillery and aerial bombing, chemical weapons and other abusive and repressive measures, including harassment, jail, torture, suicide bombings and summary executions, are common occurrence in countries such as Syria, Libya, Yemen, Egypt and the occupied Palestinian territories, among others, resulting in large numbers of civilians killed and wounded, yet the total number of fatalities remains unknown. According to recent UNHCR estimates, the number of refugees from the Syrian long-standing civil war is now over 2.5 million peoples, which is one of the highest numbers of refugees in the region's recorded history.

In South and Central Asia, apart from the two major wars being fought in Iraq and Afghanistan which are responsible for thousands of lives lost and millions of displaced populations and refugees, numerous protracted ethnic conflicts have erupted and continue to engulf the region in organised violence, resulting in high death tolls, particularly among civilians and enrolled militias, resulting in massive population internal displacements and increasing numbers of refugees. Prime examples of these are the ongoing ethnic conflicts in the Kashmir region between India

---

[3] In recent war scenarios, such as in the former Yugoslavia and Somalia, about nine out of every ten people injured or killed were civilians.

and Pakistan, Tibet in southern China, Bhutan, Nepal and Sri Lanka. In the case of Nepal, there were more than 10,000 people killed and an estimated 100,000 suffered torture (CVICT 2008), rape and other form of physical and psychological abuse. Sri Lanka has been shaken by a long-standing ethnic conflict between the Sri Lankan Sinhalese majority government forces and the Liberation Tigers of Tamil Eelam (LTTE) which divided the country in a brutal conflict and war that lasted well over two decades (1983–2009). The conflict ended with more than 300,000 Tamils held hostage in the northeastern part of the island, in what became for a few months one of the largest concentration camps in recorded history, where systematic violations of human rights were enforced by government forces.

In the Latin American region, there are many recent examples of ethnic conflicts and internal wars resulting in high death tolls, particularly among indigenous peoples: the almost four decades of violent conflict and massive killing of more than 200,000 civilians, mostly of Mayan origins in Guatemala; the extrajudicial executions of Miskito Indians in Nicaragua; the murder of Tzotzils in Chiapas, Mexico, and Yanomami Indians along the border between Venezuela and Brazil; and the annihilation and disappearance of 70,000 civilians, mostly Quechua-speaking peasants in the Peruvian highlands, undertaken by Shining Path guerrillas and the military repression (Pedersen et al. 2003), are some of the exemplary cases in point.

Refugees and Internally Displaced Populations (IDPs)

Despite a decreasing trend of armed conflict and wars and the mounting number of civilian war casualties, the post-cold era is characterised for growing and significant global flows of refugees and internally displaced persons (IDPs). For example, the UNHCR Global Trends Report (2011) shows that globally there were 43.7 million forcibly displaced people at the end of 2010. The global number of people affected by conflict-induced international displacement increased from 24.4 to 26 million, and available information suggests that a total of 67 million people had been forcibly displaced at the end of 2007. The number of IDPs keeps growing – mostly because the ongoing Syrian civil war now responsible for over 2.5 million refugees – and has been more recently estimated at 54 million worldwide, where about 30 million were displaced as a result of armed conflict and war and another 24 million by natural disasters. In addition, while often not considered as being displaced per se, it is estimated that there are some 12 million stateless people worldwide (UNHCR 2011). Although demographic information on displaced populations is not always available for all countries, the available data by sex indicates that women represent about half (47 %) of most populations falling under UNHCR's responsibility.

Furthermore, around one third of all refugees are residing in countries in the Asia and Pacific region, with 80 % of them being Afghans. The Middle East and North Africa regions are host to more than a quarter of all refugees, primarily from Iraq and Syria, while Africa and Europe hosted, respectively, 20 and 14 % of the world's refugees. The Americas region had the smallest share of refugees (9 %), with Colombians constituting the largest number for this region (UNHCR 2009).

Whether internally or cross-nationally, the majority of refugees are clearly made up of women, children and the elderly. They are often subject to various forms of social exclusion, exploitation, rape and sexual abuse and are exposed to political violence and torture. The conditions found in sheltered zones, in larger cities or across the border in neighbouring countries are not necessarily better than the ones left behind. The lack of sanitation, food and water shortages, loss of family and social support networks, crowding and overall deprivation experienced in refugee camps impose additional health risks and increased mortality and morbidity and inflict further distress and suffering among survivors. Outbreaks of cholera, dysentery, tuberculosis, acute respiratory infections and other viral diseases, such as measles, are common occurrence in most refugee camps. Pregnancy, sexually transmitted diseases and AIDS are also on the increase among refugee women and young adolescents who have experienced sexual abuse. According to UNICEF (1996), in Rwanda virtually every adolescent girl who had survived the genocide of 1994 was subsequently raped. Rape and commercial sex is also widespread in refugee camps, often resulting in unsafe abortions and the spread of sexually transmitted diseases, including AIDS. The displaced are usually deprived from social, material and emotional support systems, which may make them more fragile and vulnerable to environmental adversities and social distress.

Humanitarian Interventions Aimed at Civilian Populations in War-Torn Countries and Conflict Zones

To close this chapter, we would like to discuss briefly the nature and content of humanitarian interventions being used in civilian populations in the aftermath of organised violence, armed conflict and war-related adversities.

The aftermath of contemporary wars is partly characterised by the overall reordering of post-conflict post-war politics and the emergence of what has been called a 'therapeutic moral order', which is largely driven by the false premise that not only combatants but entire civilian populations exposed to the adversities of endemic violence and armed conflict are traumatised and would require therapeutic management of one kind or the other (Moon 2009). That is, in the post-conflict and post-disaster operations, psychiatric teams or trauma counsellors are often mobilised under the assumption that trauma-related disorders will necessarily affect most if not all of the exposed.

At the same time, it is acknowledged that states recently emerging from armed conflict or under endemic and protracted organised violence have inadequate mental health resources due to a lack of funding, reduced health budgets and a shortage and inequitable distribution of mental health professionals (Allden et al. 2009; Al-Obaidi et al. 2010). In order to ameliorate this situation, the funding and delivery of humanitarian assistance is increasingly organised by bilateral aid, as well as international and local NGOs, and most current therapeutic interventions are exported from Western countries and adopted by the recipients from to war-torn societies worldwide with little adaptation if any.

While various forms of mental health intervention may have a role to play in post-conflict or post-disaster recovery, the medicalisation of psychosocial intervention programmes in terms of PTSD and related constructs often leads to the uncritical application of symptom check lists and provision of 'trauma counselling' (Dwyer and Santikarma 2007). This approach reflects our limited understanding of the relationships among the range of possible health outcomes after exposure to catastrophic and traumatic events (Young 1995, 2000). Moreover, at a clinical level, we know little of who should (or should not) receive individual intervention and still less about how and why it may work in some cases and not in others. Most ongoing efforts and humanitarian interventions carried out by government agencies and NGOs have not been assessed in terms of health outcomes and overall impact in the quality of life and well-being of local communities and potential beneficiaries.

There is now a wide repertoire of therapies to deal with trauma-related disorders ranging from cognitive-behavioural therapy (prolonged exposure therapy) to meditative techniques derived from Eastern traditions aimed at relieving suffering through spiritual development to the use of psychopharmacological agents, such as antidepressants or medications that interfere with fear conditioning or beta-blockers interfering with consolidation of traumatic memory. At present, the effectiveness of these therapies, both psychosocial and pharmacological, in diverse populations, remains uncertain. For many patients exposed to massive trauma, the complete remission of symptoms may be an unattainable treatment goal (Marshall et al. 1998). While it is possible that aspects of PTSD might be prevented or treated by medication and exposure therapy, in the case of long-standing violence and enduring social disruption, such focussed interventions are bound to have limited impact.

Practitioners and scholars in the field of humanitarian assistance largely agree that despite the plethora of available treatment options, there remains an absence of a solid evidence base for most mental health and psychosocial support interventions (Allden et al. 2009). A similar claim was raised by the Institute of Medicine (IOM), who in 2008 published a report with a systematic review of the scientific evidence on treatment modalities for PTSD. The report states that for all drug classes and specific drugs reviewed in each of the classes, the evidence is inadequate to determine efficacy in the treatment of PTSD among war veterans. With regard to psychotherapies, the committee states that only for exposure therapies is there sufficient evidence to conclude its efficacy in the treatment of PTSD (IOM 2008).

There is a long-standing controversy among researchers, health professionals and health planners involved in post-conflict/post-disaster interventions about the relevance and cross-cultural applicability of conventional psychiatric constructs of trauma, particularly PTSD. While international experts and organisations have argued that there is growing consensus regarding traumatic events and stressors resulting in universally recognisable patterns, including diagnosable medical conditions of acute stress disorder and chronic PTSD, that are amenable to Western standard treatments (Mollica et al. 2004; van Ommeren et al. 2005), the critique from health and social scientists working within affected communities suggests that traumatic events have far broader, more varied and complex meanings and effects than are recognised by conventional psychiatric nosology or practice (Kirmayer 1996;

Bracken and Petty 1998). These effects, in turn, evoke a wide range of culturally specific adaptive strategies that are still poorly understood.

Among the most important implications of the emergence of a therapeutic moral order is that for collective interventions to be meaningful, they should reflect a macro perspective that recognises not only the direct consequences of war and natural disasters but also the transnational impacts of globalisation and growing social inequalities on the mental health of survivors. We remain convinced that it is equally important to address both local and national health-care issues within the global context and, at the same time, pay attention to how these multiple macro-level forces play out locally, in the lives of individuals, families and communities.

Thus, we would argue that in order to provide meaningful psychosocial assistance to individuals and communities in need, including IDPs and refugees, interventionists have to learn more about mental health problems and psychosocial stressors that community members identify as most important, as well as about the impact of other forms of violence such as structural violence, institutionalised racism, gender-based discrimination and so on may have on mental health. To live up to the complexities involved, community interventions should combine both *emic* and *etic* approaches by taking existing healing strategies, initiatives and programmes into consideration 'in a participatory, empowering and ownership manner' (Aro et al. 2008).

Concluding Remarks

In this chapter, it has been argued that in order to rethink and re-examine the notion of trauma as a global challenge and its related intervention strategies, three key issues have to be taken into consideration: First, it is crucial to examine the effects of intentional violence and wars not only in terms of the immediate stressful events and economic and political hardships that are their inevitable precursors but also for making the link between these and the broad social structures in which they originate (Gibson 1989; Pedersen 2010). Second, there is a need to document non-Western patterns of trauma-related conditions such as local idioms of distress and other adaptive and strategic responses to trauma on the individual and the collective level. And finally, it is crucial to assess the circumstances in which medical or humanitarian interventions help or hinder long-term recovery from traumatic experiences such as torture and war atrocities and related adversities (Pedersen 2010).

Moreover, it has to be kept in mind that mental disorders such as PTSD are not monolithic biomedical categories, but heterogeneous entities that are subject to interpretation in that they are differently understood across diverse cultural and social settings. Mental disorders may be seen as only one facet of suffering and do not account for other forms of distress that are related to a combination of traumatic events and stressful life experiences. Local idioms of distress attest to that and the ways individuals, families and entire communities explain adversity and develop coping strategies and ways of healing (Pedersen et al. 2010).

Based on this understanding, multiple pathways can be seen through which social inequalities, discrimination and violence may translate into poor mental health outcomes. While psychosocial pathways seem to be most important, there is growing evidence of the physiological channels though which stressful negative environmental changes can affect endocrine and immunological processes (Dressler et al. 2005; Wilkinson 1996). This makes apparent that it is important to integrate both psychosocial and biological approaches in order to better understand the causality of the pathways (Bolton 2010; Dohrenwend 2000), that is, the complex relations and interdependencies, and the various ways in which these interactions influence the distress and disease occurrence, illness experience and well-being of individuals, families and communities (Buitrago and Cuellar 2004; Martin-Baro 1994).

We may conclude that it is through the development of critical frames of analysis and transdisciplinary approaches, that we will eventually gain better understanding of how distress, mental illness and social suffering are transformed into nosographic categories and eventually absorbed in the realm of the psychiatric domain of practices. We also acknowledged how the medico-psychiatric science and medical technologies have been used both in the medicalisation of the 'problem' and as a form of social control often in detriment of local, endogenous resources.

Finally, it remains essential to move beyond critical thinking and promote innovation and a greater heterogeneity of models, theories and concepts as a counterweight to the increasing homogenisation of medical and psychiatric scientific knowledge and practice. The critical perspectives presented here in examining distress and social suffering, trauma and PTSD may also be of relevance to a broad range of disease conditions, thus cutting across all areas pertaining to the global mental health and well-being of populations (Pedersen and Kienzler 2015).

References

Allden K, Jones L, Weissbecker I et al (2009) Mental health and psychosocial support in crisis and conflict: report of the mental health working group. Prehosp Disaster Med 24(Suppl 2):s217–s227

Al-Obaidi A, Budosan B, Jeffrey L (2010) Child and adolescent mental health in Iraq: current situation and scope of promotion of child and adolescent mental health policy. Intervention 8(1):40–51

American Psychiatry Association (2000) Diagnostic and statistical manual of mental disorders, 4th edn, Text Revision. APA, Washington, DC

American Psychiatry Association (1994) Diagnostic and statistical manual of mental disorders, 4th edn. APA, Washington, DC

American Psychiatry Association (2013) Diagnostic and statistical manual of mental disorders, 5th edn. APA, Arlington

Aro AR, Smith J, Dekker J (2008) Contextual evidence in clinical medicine and health promotion. Eur J Public Health 18(6):548–549

Barad M, Cain CK (2007) Mechanisms of fear extinction: toward improved treatment for anxiety. In: Kirmayer LK, Lemenson R, Barad M (eds) Understanding trauma: integrating biological, clinical and cultural perspectives. Cambridge University Press, New York, pp 78–97

Blau JR, Blau PM (1982) The cost of inequality: metropolitan structure and violent crime. Am Sociol Rev 47:114–129

Bogin B, Keep R (1999) Eight thousand years of economic and political history in Latin America, revealed by anthropometry. Ann Hum Biol 19(5):631–642

Bolton D (2010) Social, biological and personal constructions of mental illness. In: Morgan C, Bhugra D (eds) Principles of social psychiatry. Wiley, Hoboken, pp 39–50

Bouton ME, Wadell J (2007) Some biobehavioural insights into persistent effects of emotional trauma. In: (2008) Contextual evidence in clinical medicine and health promotion. Eur J Public Health 18(6):548–549

Bracken P, Petty C (eds) (1998) Rethinking the trauma of war. Free Association Books, London

Bracken P, Thomas P (2001) Post-psychiatry: a new direction for mental health. Br Med J 322:724–727

Breslau N (1998) Epidemiology of trauma and posttraumatic stress disorder. In: Yehuda R (ed) Psychological trauma. American Psychiatric Press, Washington, DC, pp 1–26

Brunet A, Poundja J, Tremblay J, Bui E, Thomas E, Orr S, Azzoug…Pitman RK (2011) Trauma reactivation under the influence of propranolol decreases posttraumatic stress symptoms and disorder: 3 open-label trials. J Clin Psychopharmacol 31(4):547–550

Bruntland GH, Liestol K, Walloe L (1980) Height, weight and menarcheal age of Oslo schoolchildren during the last 60 years. Ann Hum Biol 7(4):307–322

Buitrago C (2004) Internationally displaced Colombians: the recovery of victims of violence within a psychosocial framework. In: Miller K, Rasco L (eds) The mental health of refugees: ecological approaches to healing and adaptation. Lawrence Erlbaum Associates, Mahwah, N J, pp 229–262

Cardozo B, Vergara A, Agani F et al (2000) Mental health, social functioning, and attitudes of Kosovar Albanians following the war in Kosovo. JAMA 284(5):569–577

Center for Research on the Epidemiology of Disasters (2009) EM-DAT: emergency events database. Université Catholique de Louvain – Ecole de Santé Publique, Louvain. Retrieved from: http://www.emdat.be/Database/terms.html

Centre for Victims of Torture – Nepal (CVICT) (2008) (unpublished manuscript). A report on torture victims in Nepal

Collier P, Chauvet L, Hegre H (2009) The security challenge in conflict-prone countries. In: Lomborg B (ed) Global crises, global solutions. Cambridge University Press, Cambridge, pp 58–103

Desjarlais R, Eisenberg L, Good B, Kleinman A (1995) World mental health: problems and priorities in low-income countries. Oxford University Press, New York

Dohrenwend B (2000) The role of adversity and stress in psychopathology, some evidence and its implications for theory and research. J Health Soc Behav 41:1–19

Dressler W, Oths K, Gravlee C (2005) Race and ethnicity in public health research models to explain health disparities. Annu Rev Anthropol 34:231–252

Dwyer L, Santikarma D (2007) Posttraumatic politics: violence, memory, and biomedical discourse in Bali. In: Kirmayer LJ, Lemelson R, Barad M (eds) Understanding trauma: biological, psychological and cultural perspectives. Cambridge University Press, New York, pp 403–432

Eytan A, Gex-Fabry M, Toscani L, Deroo L, Loutan L, Bovier P (2004) Determinants of postconflict symptoms in Albanian Kosovars. J Nerv Ment Dis 192:664–671

Frances AJ (2012) DSM5 in distress: the DSM's impact on mental health practice and research. Psychol Today. http://www.psychologytoday.com/blog/dsm-5-in-distress/201212. Accessed 16 May 2014

Gibson K (1989) Children in political violence. Soc Sci Med 28(7):659–668

Gilligan J (1997) Violence: reflections on a national epidemic. Vintage Books, New York

Gluckman PD, Hanson MA (2005) The fetal matrix: evolution, development and disease. Cambridge University Press, Cambridge

Hacking I (1996) Rewriting the soul: multiple personality and the sciences of memory. Princeton University Press, Princeton

Harbom L, Wallensteen P (2009) Armed conflicts, 1946–2008. J Peace Res 46(4):577–587

Holsti KJ (1996) The state, war, and the state of war. Cambridge University Press, Cambridge

IOM (2008) Treatment of posttraumatic stress disorder. An assessment of the evidence. The National Academies Press, Washington, DC

Kirmayer LJ (1996) Landscapes of memory: Trauma, narrative and dissociation. In: P Antze and M Lambek (eds), Tense past: cultural essays of memory and trauma. Routledge, London, pp 173–198

Kirmayer LK, Lemenson R, Barad M (eds) (2007) Understanding trauma: integrating biological, clinical and cultural perspectives. Cambridge University Press, New York, pp 41–59

Kolassa I-T, Ertl V, Eckart C, Kolassa S, Onyut LP, Elbert T (2010) Spontaneous remission from PTSD depends on the number of traumatic event types experienced. Psychol Trauma Theory Res Pract Policy 2(3):169–174

Konner M (2007) Trauma, adaptation and resilience: a cross-cultural and evolutionary perspective. In: Kirmayer LK, Lemenson R, Barad M (eds) Understanding trauma: integrating biological, clinical and cultural perspectives. Cambridge University Press, New York, pp 300–338

Krug EG, Dahlberg LL, Mercy JA, Zwi AB, Lozano R (2002) World report on violence and health. World Health Organization, Geneva. Retrieved from: http://www.who.int/violence_injury_prevention/violence/world_report/en/

Labonté R, Mohindra K, Schrecker T (2011) The growing impact of globalization for health and public health practice. Annu Rev Public Health 32:263–283

Markowitz SD (1955) Retardation in growth of children in Europe and Asia during World War II. Hum Biol 27(4):258–273

Marshall RD, Davidson JRT, Yehuda R (1998) Pharmacotherapy in the treatment of PTSD and other trauma-related syndromes. In: Yehuda R (ed) Psychological trauma. American Psychiatric Press, Washington, DC, pp 133–178

Marshall GN, Schell TL, Elliott MN et al (2005) Mental health of Cambodian refugees two decades after resettlement in the United States. JAMA 294(5):571–579

Martin-Baro I (1994) War and mental health. Translated by Anne Wallace. In: Mishler EG (ed) Writings for a liberation psychology. Harvard University Press, Cambridge, pp 108–121

McNally RJ (2009) Can we fix PTSD in DSM-5? Depress Anxiety 26:597–600

Miller KE, Rasmussen A (2010) War exposure, daily stressors, and mental health in conflict and post-conflict settings: bridging the divide between trauma-focused and psychosocial frameworks. Soc Sci Med 70(1):7–16

Mollica RF, Lopez Cardozo B, Osofsky HJ, Raphael B, Ager A, Salama P (2004) Mental health in complex emergencies. Lancet 364(9450):2058–2067

Moon C (2009) Healing past violence: traumatic assumptions and therapeutic interventions in war and reconciliation. J Human Rights 8:71–91

Murray CJL, King G, Lopez AD, Tomijima N, Krug EG (2002) Armed conflict as a public health problem. Br Med J 324(9):346–349

Neuner F, Schauer M, Karunakara U, Klaschik C, Robert C, Elbert T (2004) Psychological trauma and evidence for enhanced vulnerability for posttraumatic stress disorder through previous trauma among West Nile refugees. BMC Psychiatry 4(1):34

Pedersen D (1999) Surviving Amerindian nations: the impact of political violence and wars. (Unpublished manuscript). 10th summer course of social and transcultural psychiatry. McGill University. Montreal

Pedersen D (2002) Political violence, ethnic conflict and contemporary wars: broad implications for health and social well-being. Soc Sci Med 55:175–190

Pedersen D (2010) Secuelas de la pobreza, el racismo y la violencia organizada entre los pueblos indo-americanos. Academia Nacional de Medicina, Lima

Pedersen D, Kienzler H (2008) Ethnic conflict and public health. In: Heggenhougen HK, Quah SR (eds) International encyclopedia of public health, vol 2. Academic, San Diego, pp 508–518

Pedersen D, Kienzler H (2015) Exploring Pathways of Distress and Mental Disorders: the Case of the Highland Quechua Populations in the Peruvian Andes. In D E Hinton and B J Good (eds) Culture and PTSD. University of Pennsylvania Press, Philadelphia, pp 240–274

Pedersen D, Gamarra J, Planas ME, Errazuriz C (2003) Violencia Política y Salud Mental en las Comunidades Altoandinas de Ayacucho, Perú. In: Cáceres C, Cueto M, Ramos M, Vallenas S (eds) La salud como derecho ciudadano. Perspectivas y propuestas desde América Latina. Universidad Peruana Cayetano Heredia, Lima, pp 289–307

Pedersen D, Kienzler H, Gamarra J (2010) Llaki and Ñakary: idioms of distress and suffering among the highland Quechua in the Peruvian Andes. Cult Med Psychiatry 34(2):279–300

Pickett K, Mookherjee J, Wilkinson R (2005) Adolescent birth rates, total homicides, and income inequality in rich countries. Am J Public Health 95:1181

Pinker S (2011) The better angels of our nature. Penguin Books Ltd., New York

Regier DA, Narrow WE, Clarke DE, Kraemer HC, Kuramoto SJ, Kuhl EA, Kupfer DJ (2013) DSM-5 field trials in the United States and Canada, part II: test–retest reliability of selected categorical diagnoses. Am J Psychiatry 170:59–70

Reno W (2012) Warfare in independent Africa. Cambridge University Press, Cambridge

Rieff P (1966) The triumph of the therapeutic: uses of faith after Freud. Chatto and Windus, London

Scholte WF, Olff M, Ventevogel P, de Vries GJ, Jansveld E, Cardozo BL et al (2004) Mental health symptoms following war and repression in eastern Afghanistan. JAMA 292(5):585–593

Shalev AY (2007) PTSD: a disorder of recovery? In: Kirmayer LK, Lemenson R, Barad M (eds) Understanding trauma: integrating biological, clinical and cultural perspectives. Cambridge University Press, New York, pp 207–223

Shalev AY, Yehuda R (1998) Longitudinal development of traumatic stress disorders. In: Yehuda R (ed) Psychological trauma. American Psychiatric Press, Washington, DC, pp 31–66

Smil V (2008) Global catastrophes and trends: the next 50 years. The MIT Press, Cambridge

Stuckler D, Basu S (2013) Preface. In: The body economic: why austerity kills. HarperCollins Publishers Ltd, Toronto, pp ix–xv

Summerfield D (1995) Addressing human response to war and atrocity. In: Kleber RJ, Figley CR, Gersons BPR (eds) Beyond trauma: cultural and societal dynamics. Plenum Press, New York, pp 17–29

Summerfield D (1998) The social experience of war and some issues for the humanitarian field. In: Bracken P, Petty C (eds) Rethinking the trauma of war. Free Association Books, New York, pp 9–37

Summerfield D (1999) Critique of seven assumptions behind psychological trauma programmes in war affected areas. Soc Sci Med 48:1449–1462

Summerfield D (2004) Cross-cultural perspectives on the medicalization of human suffering. In: Rosen G (ed) Posttraumatic stress disorder. Issues and controversies. Wiley, West Sussex, pp 233–245

Toole MJ, Waldman RJ (1997) The public health aspects of complex emergencies and refugee situations. Annu Rev Public Health 18:283–312

UNHCR (2009) 2008 Global trends: refugees, asylum-seekers, returnees, internally displaced and stateless persons. UNHCR, Geneva

UNHCR (2011) A year in crisis and reports. In: UNHCR global trends 2010. UNHCR, Geneva

UNICEF (1996) Impact of armed conflict on children. Retrieved from: http://www.unicef.org/graca/a51-306_en.pdf

van Ommeren M, Saxena S, Saraceno B (2005) Mental and social health during and after acute emergencies emerging consensus? Bull World Health Organ 83(1):71–77

WHO (2000) Global burden of disease. WHO, Geneva

Wilkinson R (1996) Unhealthy societies. The afflictions of inequality. Routledge, London

Wilkinson R, Pickett K (2006) Income inequality and population health: a review and explanation of the evidence. Soc Sci Med 62:1768–1784

Wilkinson R, Pickett K (2009) The spirit level: why more equal societies almost always do better. Allen Lane, London

Wolf A, Gray R, Fazel S (2014) Violence as a public health problem: an ecological study of 169 countries. Soc Sci Med 104:220–227

Yehuda R (ed) (1998) Psychological trauma. American Psychiatric Press, Washington, DC

Young A (1995) Harmony of illusions: inventing post-traumatic stress disorder. Princeton University Press, New Jersey

Young A (2000) An alternative history of traumatic stress. In: Yehuda R et al (eds) International handbook of human response to trauma. Kluwer Academic, New York, pp 51–66

Young A, Breslau N (2015) What is PTSD? The heterogeneity thesis. In: Hinton DE, Good BJ (eds) Culture and PTSD. University of Pennsylvania Press, Philadelphia, Penn, pp 135–154

Zoellner LA, Bedard-Gilligan MA, Jun JJ, Marks LH, Garcia NM (2013) The evolving construct of posttraumatic stress disorder (PTSD): DSM-5 criteria changes and legal implications. Psychol Inj Law 6(4):277–289

The Epidemiology of Post-traumatic Stress Disorder: A Focus on Refugee and Immigrant Populations

Marion C. Aichberger

Background

Post-traumatic stress disorder (PTSD) has been added to the official psychiatric classification systems only in the early 1980s. The diagnosis was first introduced under its current name in the Diagnostic and Statistical Manual of the American Psychiatric Association DSM-III and under the same name only in the International Classification of Diseases ICD-10 (Turnbull 1998). Before the introduction of PTSD in DSM-III, ICD-9 only included the diagnoses 'acute reaction to stress' and 'adjustment reaction', which were viewed as being associated with exceptional physical or mental stress, e.g. battle and natural disaster (Turnbull 1998). Some aspects of its definition and the associated traumatic events have changed since the diagnosis was incorporated into DSM and ICD (Breslau 2009; Keane et al. 2006; Turnbull 1998), thus affecting prevalence and incidence estimates over the decades (Keane et al. 2006).

The syndrome's first revised definition in DSM-III-R regarded the traumatic events to be extraordinary stressors that were beyond normal human experience (American Psychiatric Association 1980). Later DSM-IV only required the traumatic event to be '...a confrontation/threat of death, serious injury or a threat to the physical integrity of self and others...' which creates '...intense fear, helplessness, or horrors...' (Breslau 2009). DSM-V now defines the traumatic event to be a '...exposure to real or threatened death, injury, or sexual violence...' (American Psychiatric Association 2013). In ICD-10 the traumatic situation has to be '...of exceptionally threatening or catastrophic nature "..." likely to cause pervasive distress in almost anyone...' (World Health Organization 1992). ICD does include a

M.C. Aichberger, MSc
Department of Psychiatry and Psychotherapy, Campus Mitte,
Charité University Medicine Berlin, Berlin, Germany
e-mail: marion.aichberger@charite.de

© Springer International Publishing Switzerland 2015
M. Schouler-Ocak (ed.), *Trauma and Migration:*
Cultural Factors in the Diagnosis and Treatment of Traumatised Immigrants,
DOI 10.1007/978-3-319-17335-1_3

time criterion relating to the maximum time that may have passed since the traumatic event and the onset of symptoms (6 months).

Prevalence of PTSD and Traumatic Events

These changes in definition over time and between the classification systems have to be kept in mind when comparing prevalence rates of PTSD. The exposure to potentially traumatizing events and situations in the general population has been shown to exceed the number of persons who then develop a PTSD by far (Breslau 2009; Brewin et al. 2000; Keane et al. 2006). Kessler et al. (1995) examined 5,877 persons aged 15–54 years in the United States for the National Comorbidity Survey, a survey in the US general population which aimed to depict the overall prevalence of mental disorders in the community (Kessler et al. 1995). The lifetime prevalence rate for PTSD was 7.8 % for both genders, with 10.4 % higher in women than in men, where the rate was 5.0 %. In the follow-up survey, the National Comorbidity Survey Replication, Kessler et al. (2005) found a lifetime prevalence for PTSD of 6.8 % (Kessler et al. 2005). The highest lifetime prevalence Kessler et al. (2005) reported in the age-group 45–59 years with 9.2 % and the age-group 30–44 years with 8.2 %. In the Detroit area survey, a representative survey of 2,181 persons in the metropolitan area of Detroit, the risk of PTSD was highest when related to assaultive violence, with a rate of 35.7 % in women and 6.0 % in men, while the rate associated with any trauma was 13.0 % in women and 6.2 % in men (Breslau 2009). Criminal victimization, such as assault or rape, in women has been found to be associated with higher lifetime prevalence of PTSD with 26 % versus 12 % among those who did not experience these kinds of traumatic events (Keane et al. 2006).

Prevalence of PTSD in Refugee Populations

The experiences prior and during migration may put refugees and asylum seekers under particular risk for the deterioration of mental health. So have studies suggested that refugees show elevated rates of anxiety and depressive disorders (Lindert et al. 2009). Fazel et al. (2005) performed a comprehensive review of psychiatric surveys which examined psychiatric disorders prevalence in refugee populations between 1966 and 2002 (Fazel et al. 2005). The authors included a total of 20 surveys with 6,743 persons from seven countries, including refugees from Southeast Asia, former Yugoslavia, the Middle East and Central America. The overall PTSD prevalence was 9 % (99 % Confidence Interval: 8–10 %). Fazel et al. found a great heterogeneity in the reported PTSD prevalences which could partly be explained by ethnicity, age, host country, duration of displacement, sample size, method of diagnosis and sampling and interview language. The authors further identified five studies on PTSD in children and adolescents, including data from 260 children from Bosnia, Central America, Iran, Rwanda and Kurdistan resettled in Canada, the United States and Sweden. The pooled prevalence rate of PTSD for refugee children in these studies was 11.0 % (99 % CI 7.0–17.0 %). Another systematic review focused on mental health in refugees, conducted by Steel et al. (2009), identified 145 surveys reporting estimates of PTSD prevalence in refugees and further examined the influence of torture on the these rates (Steel et al. 2009). The review included surveys published between 1980 and May 2009 of studies including populations aged 18 years and older, which had a minimum sample size of $n = 50$. Thus, a total of $n = 64{,}332$ persons were included in the meta-analysis on PTSD conducted by Steel et al. The PTSD prevalence rates ranged from 0 % to 99 %; the overall weighted PTSD prevalence across all surveys was 30.6 % (95 % CI 26.3–35.2 %). The prevalence of torture, which was reported by a subset of 84 surveys, was estimated to be 21.0 % (95 % CI 17.0–26.0 %). A meta-regression of factors associated with PTSD prevalence showed that experiences of torture explained the greatest intersurvey variance with 23.6 %. Surveys with a high rate of reported history of torture were associated with an odds ratio of 4.03 (95 % CI 2.31–7.04) for PTSD compared to surveys with a low rate (>40.0 % vs. <20.0 %). Surveys conducted within an ongoing conflict found a higher PTSD prevalence than those conducted in subsequent years (39.9 % vs. 2.3 years, 22.1 %; 3–5 years, 27.0 %; >5 years, 22.3 %). The countries/regions of origin with the highest PTSD prevalence were Africa (including 16 African nations; 33.5 %, 95%CI 14.2–60.7 %), Kosovo (31.6 %, 95 % CI 11.9–61.3 %) and Cambodia (30.3 %, 95 % CI 10.6–61.3 %). The lowest prevalence was found in one study of $n = 2{,}422$ persons in Vietnam with 10.0 %. High rates of PTSD have also been found in refugee populations exposed to political violence, such as, e.g. Armenian refugees from Azerbaijan who were exposed to the pogrom in Sumgait, Azerbaijan, in 1988 (Goenjian et al. 1994).

Refugees who had to flee from countries and regions in war or civil unrest, conditions which increase the likelihood of being exposed to potentially traumatizing situations, may show increased mental distress and some may also have a history of PTSD. Lopes Cardozo et al. (2000) found in a study on the psychiatric morbidity of the Albanian population related to the Kosovo war in 1999 that the rate of PTSD was 17.1 % (95 % CI 13.2–21.0 %) while the overall psychiatric morbidity was much higher with an estimated prevalence of 43.0 % (Lopes Cardozo et al. 2000). Some studies also suggest that overall asylum seekers (and refugees) display higher levels of PTSD than immigrants (Lindert et al. 2009; Silove et al. 1997). Yet, in particular studies focusing on the PTSD prevalence in immigrant populations without a history of displacement have been conducted to a lesser extent.

Risk Factors Associated with PTSD

As has been mentioned above, the findings on prevalence rates of PTSD are quite heterogeneous and may also vary within the same population over time. Risk factors for PTSD may be more consistent over time and population group studied. Among the factors most frequently found to be associated with increased risk for PTSD is having a psychiatric history prior to the trauma (Breslau 2009; Brewin et al. 2000; Lopes Cardozo et al. 2000). A meta-analysis by Brewin et al. (2000) also found childhood abuse and a family history of psychiatric disorders to be consistently associated with PTSD risk (Brewin et al. 2000). The study further found low socioeconomic status, low level of education, low intelligence, life stress, lack of social support, trauma severity, adverse childhood and previous trauma to be consistently but to a differing degree related to an increased risk for PTSD. While protective effects of higher levels of intelligence have also been shown in a large prospective study in a cohort of adolescents independent of social and educational status, no explanatory model has yet been established (Breslau 2009).

While many risk factors will be independent of the fact if a person belongs to a specific population, such as immigrant groups or military personnel, a few risk factors may be more commonly found in certain populations. So have, to some extent, studies on risk factors for PTSD in military samples and in civilian samples found different risk profiles for PTSD (Brewin et al. 2000). Among these more group-specific factors, torture probably is one of the most widely discussed factors and has been shown to be related to an increased rate of PTSD in refugee populations as mentioned above (Steel et al. 2009). A meta-analysis by Porter and Haslam (2005) examined the impact of predisplacement and postdisplacement factors on overall mental health (Porter and Haslam 2005). While the study does not specifically differentiate between studies focused on PTSD and other mental disorders, the factors examined may to some degree also play a role for the development of PTSD in refugee populations. Among the predisplacement characteristics, region of origin, higher levels of education, higher age, higher socioeconomic status, being from a rural area and, to a lesser extent, female gender were associated with lower levels of mental health. The factors showing lower levels of mental health after flight and displacement were low levels of economic opportunity (work permit, access to employment, retaining socioeconomic status), living in institutional or temporary private accommodations, being internally displaced, being repatriated and coming from a region with an ongoing conflict.

Despite of the great variability in study findings on rates and risks for PTSD in general, PTSD has to be considered as a possible diagnosis in refugees and asylum seekers with suspected psychiatric symptoms, since these populations are particularly vulnerable groups which are more commonly and often repeatedly exposed to life's adversities preflight, while on flight and even after resettlement in another country, or when internally displaced in a stable part of the home country.

References

American Psychiatric Association (1980) Diagnostic and statistical manual of mental disorders, 3rd edn. American Psychiatric Association, Washington, DC

American Psychiatric Association (2013) Diagnostic and statistical manual of mental disorders, 5th edn. American Psychiatric Publishing, Arlington

Breslau N (2009) The epidemiology of trauma, PTSD, and other posttrauma disorders. Trauma Violence Abuse 10(3):198–210

Brewin CR, Andrews B, Valentine JD (2000) Meta-analysis of risk factors for posttraumatic stress disorder in trauma-exposed adults. J Consult Clin Psychol 68(5):748–766

Fazel M, Wheeler J, Danesh J (2005) Prevalence of serious mental disorder in 7000 refugees resettled in western countries: a systematic review. Lancet 365(9467):1309–1314

Goenjian AK, Najarian LM, Pynoos RS, Steinberg AM, Petrosian P, Setrakyan S et al (1994) Posttraumatic stress reactions after single and double trauma. Acta Psychiatr Scand 90(3):214–221

Keane TM, Marshall AD, Taft CT (2006) Posttraumatic stress disorder: etiology, epidemiology, and treatment outcome. Annu Rev Clin Psychol 2:161–197

Kessler RC, Sonnega A, Bromet E, Hughes M, Nelson CB (1995) Posttraumatic stress disorder in the National Comorbidity Survey. Arch Gen Psychiatry 52(12):1048–1060

Kessler RC, Berglund P, Demler O, Jin R, Merikangas KR, Walters EE (2005) Lifetime prevalence and age-of-onset distributions of DSM-IV disorders in the National Comorbidity Survey Replication. Arch Gen Psychiatry 62(6):593–602

Lindert J, Ehrenstein OS, Priebe S, Mielck A, Brahler E (2009) Depression and anxiety in labor migrants and refugees – a systematic review and meta-analysis. Soc Sci Med 69(2):246–257

Lopes Cardozo B, Vergara A, Agani F, Gotway CA (2000) Mental health, social functioning, and attitudes of Kosovar Albanians following the war in Kosovo. JAMA 284(5):569–577

Porter M, Haslam N (2005) Predisplacement and postdisplacement factors associated with mental health of refugees and internally displaced persons: a meta-analysis. JAMA 294(5):602–612

Silove D, Sinnerbrink I, Field A, Manicavasagar V, Steel Z (1997) Anxiety, depression and PTSD in asylum-seekers: associations with pre-migration trauma and post-migration stressors. Br J Psychiatry 170:351–357

Steel Z, Chey T, Silove D, Marnane C, Bryant RA, van Ommeren M (2009) Association of torture and other potentially traumatic events with mental health outcomes among populations exposed to mass conflict and displacement: a systematic review and meta-analysis. JAMA 302(5):537–549

Turnbull GJ (1998) A review of post-traumatic stress disorder. Part I: historical development and classification. Injury 29(2):87–91

World Health Organisation (1992) International statistical classification of diseases and related health problems, 10th revision (ICD-10). WHO, Geneva

Cross-Cultural Communication with Traumatised Immigrants

4

Sofie Bäärnhielm and Mike Mösko

Introduction

Culture affects communication of trauma, coping, help-seeking, and expectations of treatment. Expressions of symptoms of post-traumatic stress may vary according to cultural and contextual factors. Culture affects how people make sense of post-traumatic distress. In this chapter, we discuss cross-cultural communication in clinical settings with patients having an immigrant and refugee background as well as symptoms of post-traumatic stress. Cultural aspects of communication related to language, idioms of distress, discourse systems, help-seeking, and identification of signs of trauma and assessment and treatment will be considered. Barriers to communication and support for overcoming barriers in cross-cultural communication will be discussed. Consideration will also be given to how to create a trustful relationship and therapeutic alliance. Theoretical aspects will be presented together with a case illustrating communication and interaction with health care.

Traumatic experiences can lead to the development of post-traumatic stress disorder (PTSD) but also to major depression and several other psychiatric disorders, such as specific phobias, disorder of extreme stress not otherwise specified (DESNOS), personality disorders, and panic disorders (Foa et al. 2000). Depression is common, especially after personal loss (Silove 2007). The prevalence of post-traumatic stress symptoms varies among refugees. In a systematic review of surveys about

S. Bäärnhielm, MD, PhD (✉)
Department of Clinical Neuroscience, Transcultural Centre, Stockholm County Council &
Karolinska Institutet, Stockholm, Sweden
e-mail: sofie.baarnhielm@sll.se

M. Mösko, PhD
Department of Medical Psychology, University Medical Center Hamburg-Eppendorf, Study
Group on Psychosocial Migration Research, Hamburg, Germany
e-mail: mmoesko@uke.de

© Springer International Publishing Switzerland 2015
M. Schouler-Ocak (ed.), *Trauma and Migration:*
Cultural Factors in the Diagnosis and Treatment of Traumatised Immigrants,
DOI 10.1007/978-3-319-17335-1_4

post-traumatic stress disorders in general refugee populations in western countries, Fazel et al. (2005) found 9 % diagnosed with PTSD, 5 % with depression, and evidence of much psychiatric comorbidity. Refugees who have had severe exposure to violence often have chronic pain or other somatic syndromes (Kirmayer et al. 2011). PTSD is associated with ill-defined or medically unexplained somatic syndromes, such as dizziness, tinnitus, and somatoform syndromes, and several medical conditions such as cardiovascular, respiratory, musculoskeletal, neurological, gastrointestinal, endocrine, pain, sleep problems, and immune-mediated disorders (Gupta 2013).

Refugees often do not have experience of just one single trauma, but of multiple traumas, and hardship related to premigration and migration experiences, and additional acculturation difficulties in the new host society. Most people experiencing trauma recover in socially safe situations. Also, a majority of those having acute stress reactions or PTSD improve, but for some the symptoms may remain for a long time (Pottie et al. 2011). To identify patients in need of help, it is important to recognise that signs of post-traumatic stress can vary and be combined with psychiatric and somatic comorbidity. For immigrants and refugees living in exile, this can be of special concern as people in their new context might have poor knowledge about harsh conditions in their countries of origin and on migration routes.

It is often the case that immigrants and refugees, especially newly settled, have poor knowledge about how the health-care system works, what help they can obtain, and how to communicate their suffering and need for help and support in an understandable way in the new context. It is therefore necessary for health and mental health services and professionals to be sensitive to cultural and contextual aspects of communication.

Cross-Cultural Communication

The term cross-cultural communication refers to situations of communication between two persons of different cultural backgrounds. Most clinical encounters are in a sense cross-cultural as a layperson's perspective on health and illness often differs from the medical understanding. In the literature, the concepts of intercultural communication are more commonly used than cross-cultural communication. Ting-Toomey (1999/2001) relates intercultural to communicating meaning. One person tries to convey meaning and the other tries to interpret it. Both verbal and nonverbal information are important for conveying meaning. When conveying and interpreting are confirmed, a shared meaning is constructed. Also, culture, age gender, and social reference group may all contribute to diversity in styles of communication.

Cross-cultural communication often includes trying to penetrate the immediate surface of words in order to understand the meaning of the other. The anthropologist Ulf Hannerz (1992) discusses communication in culturally complex versus small-scale societies in terms of communication in social situations of greater or smaller cultural asymmetry. He compares communication in situations of small asymmetry with the tip of an iceberg. What is explicitly communicated can be largely tacit as much is known and already shared. In situations of greater asymmetry, more needs to be explained and contextualised in order to attain a shared understanding.

Hannerz argues for taking the perspective of the other in order to create a shared meaning. This view is also emphasised by Scollon and Wong Scollon (2001) who define successful communication as based on sharing as much as possible the assumptions we make about what each other means. They state, 'When we are communicating with people who are very different from us, it is very difficult to know how to draw inferences about what they mean, and so it is impossible to depend on shared knowledge and background for confidence in our interpretations' (p. 22).

When health professionals encounter patients with an immigrant and refugee background, much often needs to be asked and explained. What is under the tip of the iceberg needs to be visualised and verbalised. The clinician may only have scanty knowledge of the patient's context and social background leaving much to be discussed and explained. Vice versa, the patient might have poor knowledge about how the mental health-care system works and what sort of help is available. Trust and confidence are central to good-quality cross-cultural communication. A trustful relation in which the patient and the clinician want to convey and understand the meaning of the other is the basis for overcoming communication barriers.

Language

Language is central to clinical communication and affects patients' experience and expression of distress. Language provides both possibilities for expression and limits for communication. It is hard to communicate what we lack words for. With language, we can approach and distance ourselves from memories and experiences. Words and phrases do not just have cognitive meaning but also emotional and symbolic meanings (Westermeyer 1990). Language has also a dialogical character, and the meaning of words and concepts are partly influenced by interaction (Bot and Wadensjö 2004).

Cross-cultural communication often involves communication in a second language, translations, and working with interpreters. Westermeyer and Janca (1997) suggest that symptoms are subjectively experiences that are often not easily translated into numerous languages. They exemplify this with words for sadness, anger, anxiety, pain, boredom, weakness, and fatigue that may require more lengthy explanations. The capacity for using a second language may deteriorate due to age, stress, illness, and crisis.

For example, in psychotherapy as a verbal treatment approach, language can also be overrated in cases. If, for instance, a patient with a recurrent depressive disorder (current episode severe without psychotic symptoms) seeks for help in an inpatient mental health-care setting and speaks a different language than the professionals, it happened that the institutions refused to treat the patient with the argument that 'due to the communication barriers he is not able to take part in the [fundamental treatment component] group therapy'. As a consequence, the patient was refused in different institutions until one offered a treatment focussing in the nonverbal treatment components in terms of building up activities and daily structure.

Health Literacy

Health literacy is regarded as the 'degree to which individuals have the capacity to obtain, process, and understand basic health information and services needed to make appropriate health decisions' (National Institute of Health 2000, p. iv). Patients with a lower literacy level can have problems reading prescriptions or following medical recommendations. Lower health literacy can lead to poorer knowledge of the patient's disease and worse clinical outcomes (Rothman et al. 2004). There are specific vulnerable groups that have higher proportions of limited health literacy than the general population in Europe. This includes older people, members of ethnic minorities and recent immigrants, people with lower levels of education and/or low proficiency in the national language, and those who depend on public transfer payments (WHO Regional Office for Europe 2013).

Idioms of Distress

People may use different 'idioms of distress' for communicating suffering. The concept, idiom of distress, was coined by Mark Nichter (1981). He defines it as a socially and culturally resonant means of experiencing and expressing distress in local worlds (Nichter 2010). Idioms of distress may convey signals and information about past traumatic events, memories, and present stressors. The concept of cultural idioms of distress was introduced in the American psychiatric Diagnostic and Statistical Manual of Mental Disorders, DSM-5, in 2013. There it refers to linguistic terms, phrases, or ways of talking about suffering among individuals of a cultural group using shared concepts of pathology and ways of expressing, communicating, or naming essential aspects of distress.

In cross-cultural communication, it may be useful to be sensitive to patients' use of different idioms of distress when communicating experiences of trauma and sequel of trauma. DSM-5 emphasises that idioms of distress may influence expression of distress of PTSD and comorbid disorders. Examples of this are given, e.g. that panic attacks may be prominent in PTSD among Cambodian and Latin American patients due to the association of traumatic exposure with panic-like 'khyâl' (Cambodians) attacks (wind-related panic attacks including symptoms of panic attacks and other symptoms) and 'ataque de nervios' (Latin Americans characterised by symptoms of intense emotional upset and panic attacks).

In an overview of trauma survivors, Hinton and Lewis-Fernández (2010) discuss the clinical utility of the concept of idioms of distress. They suggest that idioms of distress may influence the personal meaning of trauma-related disorder, shape the course of the disorder, determine the pattern of help-seeking and self-treatment, but also help clinicians understand the patient's view of distress. Rasmussen et al. (2011) studied refugees from Darfur and identified the trauma-related idioms of distress, 'hozun' and 'majnun'. These concepts shared symptoms with both PTSD and depression but were not identical.

Studying social representation of trauma among Palestinians in the Gaza Strip, Afana et al. (2010) identified three types of concepts communicating post-traumatic distress: the concept 'sadma' referring to trauma as a sudden blow with immediate impact, 'faji'ah' meaning tragedy, and 'musiba' referring to calamity. The authors describe the meaning of the concepts in terms of how they function in communicating the meaning of suffering to others, the context of suffering, and how to mobilise social support.

Various somatic symptoms, for example, headache, pain, and sleeping problems, are common triggers for seeking care for post-traumatic stress. Kirmayer and Young (1998) suggest that somatic symptoms may be a culturally salient idiom of distress. Not only PTSD, but also depression and other mental disorders and illnesses, and conditions of distress can be expressed by culturally patterned idioms of distress. Depression is a major post-traumatic response, especially after loss. Migration often includes several and important losses for immigrants and refugees. In a Dutch study of depressive disorders among female Turkish immigrant patients, depression was characterised by a wide range of somatic complaints with anxiety and agitation (Borra 2011). DSM-5 (2013) points out that there are substantial differences in expressions of major depressive disorders. At the same time, it is emphasised that there is no simple linkage between cultures and symptoms and that clinicians should be aware that in most cultures most cases go unrecognised.

Communicative Style and Discourse Systems

Groups of people can have different cognitive styles and ways of communicating. Analysing intercultural communication, Scollon and Wong Scollon (2001) use the concept of discourse systems. They suggest that discourse systems might differ according to culture, as well as also being related to other factors such as age, generation, gender, and professional affiliation. The concept of discourse system refers to groups having a kind of self-contained system of communication with a shared language or jargon. Scollon and Wong Scollon characterise discourse systems according to the following: (1) ideology, (2) socialisation, (3) forms of discourse, and (4) face systems.

Ideology refers to holding a common ideological position and recognising a set of extra-discourse features defending the group. Socialisation is accomplished especially through the preferred form of discourse. Forms of discourse are performing models for identification and in- and out-group markers. Views about hierarchies and about who is the correct person to talk with might differ between discourse systems. People are members of many different discourse systems simultaneously. Differences in communicative style, and discourse system, between patient and clinician may lead to misunderstandings and prejudice evaluation. Differences can also be a way to manifest group belonging and identity.

With regard to trauma, different discourse systems can be manifested in, for example, different views about when to talk about trauma and who to talk about it with, or even whether or not it should be talked about. In clinical situations, a shared communicative style and discourse system can become a fast track for an in-group communication and relation. In-group communication can, for example, include situations of encountering patients with one's own social and cultural background. For the in-group member, small signals can convey information about communicating likelihood of traumatic experiences. On the other hand, in-group communication may entail a risk of false understandings and of a shared unformulated agreement to avoid sensitive areas.

Culture, Trauma, Emotional Reactions

Communication is both a cognitive and an emotional process in which both patients' and clinicians' emotional reactions affect communication. The clinician's encounter with immigrant and refugee patients with a different cultural background may touch deep unconscious feelings. Comas-Díaz and Jacobsen (1991) use the concept of ethnocultural transference in discussing how culture and ethnicity may be played out in emotional responses. Transference refers to the patient's emotional reactions and countertransference to the clinician's emotional reactions in psychodynamic psychotherapy. The concepts have relevance also outside psychotherapy and show how easy it is to involve one's own stereotypes about the other in communication. Stereotypes can play an important role in the manifestations of transference and countertransference.

Comas-Díaz and Jacobsen exemplify reactions of ethnocultural transference, for example, how ethnicity and culture can be denied to the extent of obscuring and avoiding any issues related to culture and ethnicity. Mistrust, suspicion, and hostility may be reactions to unacknowledged ethnocultural differences. Denial of ethnocultural differences may lead to countertransference reactions of thinking that one is above the cultural or political influence of the society. They also describe the opposite reaction of turning into a clinical anthropologist overly curious about the patient's ethnocultural background.

The encounter with patients who have experienced severe trauma can also evoke strong feelings affecting interpersonal communication. Clinicians may experience, for example, countertransference feelings such as despair and hopelessness but also feelings such as mistrust and denial. If the feelings are not identified by the clinician, they may easily be played out in actions. For example, feelings of despair can lead to avoiding listening to the patient and hopelessness to not trying to help the person, as no way of helping seems possible. Mistrust and denial may lead to not taking seriously information given by the patient.

David Kinzie (1994) discusses countertransference from his experience of treating Southeast Asian refugees. Although Kinzie refers to psychotherapeutic treatment, this has relevance also for other clinical encounters. Kinzie addresses a broad range of possible reactions and emotions such as sadness and depression. He suggests that these reactions may spring from both empathy and a realisation that what happened to the refugees could have happened to anyone. From his experience, anger and irritability to an unknown perpetrator can last for a long time after a patient has left and spill over into other activities and the private life of the therapist. As a frequent side effect for therapists working with traumatised refugees, Kinzie points to the risk of finding it difficult to work with non-traumatised patients, whose problems may appear trivial. In cross-cultural communication with traumatised patients, identifying one's own reactions and feelings may be a way to understand and improve the communication with the patient.

Cross-Cultural Communication Barriers

There are often several barriers facing immigrants and refugees when communicating post-traumatic distress to health professionals. Patients usually do not spontaneously talk about experiences of trauma, not even to health professionals (Westermeyer and Wahmenholm 1989; Norström 2004). Health professionals seldom ask patients with an immigrant and refugee background about previous trauma and signs of post-traumatic stress (Al-Saffar et al. 2004; Shannon 2012). Lack of trust in the health-care system can be a barrier for communication. Patients with a refugee background can even have experiences of health care being a part of a repressive state and of health professionals participating in torture. The lack of communication about trauma means that there is a risk that experiences of severe trauma and signs of post-traumatic stress are not identified.

A study of patients at a psychiatric outpatient clinic in an exposed suburban area in Stockholm with many immigrant and refugee patients showed that patients who had their trauma sufficiently addressed had a better self-related outcome with fewer symptoms of PTSD, were less depressed, and had greater confidence in staff compared to those who had trauma insufficiently addressed (Al-Saffar et al. 2004). The study found that being an ethnic Swede was related to having trauma sufficiently addressed while the opposite was true for immigrant groups. This study points to the importance of asking about trauma.

People can make sense of distress in many different ways. How individuals make sense of post-traumatic stress symptoms influences communication of distress and help-seeking. The distressed person might not connect post-traumatic symptoms such as flashbacks, nightmares, and concentration difficulties with previous traumatic experiences. Symptoms can be seen, for example, as signs of going mad and losing one's mind and be interpreted as stigmatising signs of severe mental illness. This type of meaning making can restrict an open communication about distress and experiences with friends and family members as well as health providers.

Another potential communication barrier is that patients and laypersons often do not have the knowledge that experience of trauma can have an impact on their health. Primary care is often the first contact with health care. In an American primary care study, the refugees' perspective on communication barriers regarding trauma was explored (Shannon et al. 2012). It was found that the refugees hesitated to initiate a conversation about trauma due to cultural norms requiring deference to the doctor's authority and that the patients lacked knowledge about how trauma affected health. From the patients' perspective, two key communication barriers were identified. One was that the doctors did not raise the topic. Another barrier was that the patients had a sense that a discussion of personal experiences and related health problems was not appropriate for a primary care visit. However, most of the refugees wanted to learn more about the impact of trauma on their health and discuss this with their doctors.

Bridging Barriers in Cross-Cultural Communication

There are several ways for overcoming barriers in cross-cultural communication within health and mental health care. Some relate to add additional competence into the health-care system by working with interpreters, culture brokers, cultural mediators, and health advisors and collaborating with local community organisations. These examples of innovative work may facilitate understanding, trust, and communication between the professional and the patient. For immigrants and refugees seeking care, knowledge about how the health-care system functions and confidence in it can be important components for establishing a trustful cross-cultural communication with individual professionals.

For clinicians, next to self-reflection and supervision, literature, travelling, and personal experiences of socialising in other social and cultural milieus can contribute with new knowledge and perspectives that facilitate interpretation of meaning in cross-cultural communication. Approaches that bridge perspectives and facilitate cross-cultural communication for patients can contribute to a sense of coherence between their own frames of meaning and medical perspectives.

The Narrative

Giving time to, and showing interest in, the patient's illness narrative can facilitate cross-cultural communication and understanding. Social science research has stressed the value of narratives for communicating distress in a meaningful way. In the book 'The Illness Narratives', Kleinman (1988) emphasised how the patient's story is central to clinical work and for understanding the particular patient. Kleinman's work has been followed by extensive research on how narratives can contribute to communicative meaning and contextualised information in clinical care. Through the illness narrative, the patient can communicate information about distress from her or his own perspective.

The narrative captures central aspects of the patient's illness experience and social context and serves as a forum for presenting, discussing, and negotiating illness and how we relate to it (Hydén 1997). Good (1997) argues that narratives are central to the understanding of the experience of illness and that the narrative can locate suffering in history and help to place events in a meaningful order in time. For clinicians, patients' narratives may facilitate the formulation of concrete and contextualised probing questions that are a link to both the patients' experiences and their understanding. Questions linked to the patient's context are easier to understand than abstract questions (Scarpinati Rosso and Bäärnhielm 2012). Abstract and decontextualised questions work when there is an underlying shared understanding of meaning (Bäärnhielm and Scarpinati Rosso 2009). Contextual information is of particular importance to clinical communication with patients in cross-cultural situations where clinicians can have poor understanding of the patient's milieu.

The usefulness of patients' narratives for communication of post-traumatic distress was shown in a study of psychiatric diagnosing where the ethnographic approach of the Outline for a Cultural Formulation in DSM-IV was utilised. The patient's narratives facilitated identifying traumatic events and post-traumatic symptoms (Bäärnhielm et al. 2014). While narratives can contribute to communicating meaning in cross-cultural situations, there are limitations for understanding. Kirmayer (2003) draws attention to the importance of a shared world of assumptions and values for understanding a patient's narrative. The clinician's response to trauma is influenced by how the world is imagined. Kirmayer also suggests that refugee patients' narratives of trauma may involve life circumstances outside the experience and imagination of the clinician.

Interpreters

When patient and clinician do not have a shared language, it is essential to have the support of an interpreter, if possible, a qualified interpreter with specialist training in mental health-care interpreting. Westermeyer (1990) differentiates between translating and interpreting; translating refers to the ability to exchange words from one language to another while retaining the same meaning. He sees interpreting as a more subtle skill which includes transmission of emotional and symbolic meaning. The quality of communication with an interpreter depends upon the capacity and training of the interpreter but also on the skills of the clinician as well as how well the patient is familiar with the situation of working with an interpreter.

As clinicians, we need to learn how to ask translatable questions. Wadensjö (1987) points out that an interpreter has to record the meaning of what is said and that this is facilitated by the clinicians not using too long phrases. When the clinician uses long phrases, it becomes difficult for the interpreter to remember, and there is a risk that only a summary is transmitted and communicated. Bradford and Munoz (1993) formulate some key points for psychotherapy and interpretation and stress the importance of interpreting in the first person, with the 'I' pronoun. This is important also in other clinical situations as talking about the patient in a third person can be both confusing and create a distance.

It is important for the patient that he or she understands the role of the interpreter and how the interpreter works. Especially, in the first clinical contact, it is important that the patient is informed about how communication works with the support of an interpreter and that the interpreter is bound by rules of confidentiality. For clinicians, it is important to learn to ask translatable questions. Discussing the need for culturally sensitive diagnostic procedures among Moroccan patients, Zandi et al.

(2008) argue that it is of value to formulate questions using concrete words (e.g. sad, tired, happy) and avoiding abstractions as much as possible (e.g. depression, shame, guilt). Abstract questions can have an unclear meaning.

Cultural Brokers

Cultural brokers, and other forms of cultural mediators, are helpful for bridging gaps of meaning. They function as a resource in helping interpret the cultural meaning of illness and healing, and this transcends linguistic interpretation (Miklavcic and LeBlanc 2014). Information from cultural brokers about cultural milieus, traditions, and meaning of communication can broaden the clinician's framework of knowledge for interpreting a patient's communication. Exactly how cultural brokers or mediators work varies between different settings.

A community-based model with health advisors or health communicators has been implemented in some parts of Sweden (Bäärnhielm et al. 2013). The health advisors meet groups of newly arrived refugees and immigrants and discuss health promotion and how the complex Swedish health-care system works. These issues are discussed in a dialogue form, in the mother tongues of the refugees and immigrants, in local municipalities. The health advisors meet the groups several times and address different topics: acculturative stress, post-traumatic stress, and where and how to obtain help, among others. This type of health promotion work makes it easier for laypersons to recognise post-traumatic symptoms and to know where and how to get help and how to communicate with health-care professionals in an understandable way.

Self-Reflection and Supervision

A self-reflexive stance is a basic element to improve quality of cross-cultural communication. A reflexive stance, or reflexivity, means trying to see oneself through the eyes of the other and is a method used in anthropology (Hylland Eriksen 2004). In situations of cross-cultural clinical communication, self-reflection over one's own communicative style, ways of using language, and reactions of countertransference can be helpful in getting an idea of the perspective of the patient. Professional supervision and peer consulting can be helpful in identifying one's own reactions and contribute to improve quality of communication. Also specific continuing education may trigger self-reflection.

Assessment and the Cultural Formulation Interview

For overcoming barriers in cross-cultural communication in assessment situations, the Cultural Formulation Interview (CFI) in DSM-5 is a new and helpful tool. With a 16-question interview based on the Outline for a Cultural Formulation in DSM-5, the CFI supports a narrative, person-centred communication in psychiatric assessment. This includes exploring the meaning of the other and an interest for idioms of distress, resilience factors, and expectations of help. The CFI includes open questions and is intended to be used with all patients in the initial assessment. For a further exploration, there are an interview directed towards informants' family members and 12 supplementary modules for a deeper exploration of different areas. Some of the modules have been developed for specific groups (e.g. immigrants and refugees, older adults) and topics (e.g. cultural identity; spirituality, religion, and moral traditions; coping and help-seeking). The module on immigrants and refugees includes questions about hardship, violence, and loss.

Adeponle et al. (2012) studied the impact of systematic use of the cultural formulation on patients, referred to a cultural consultation service, with a psychosis diagnosis in Canada. Misdiagnosis of psychotic patients occurred with patients from all ethnocultural groups, especially recently settled immigrants. Overdiagnosis of psychotic disorders was frequent. After using the CFI, 49 % of the patients with an intake diagnosis of psychotic disorder were re-diagnosed as nonpsychotic, and PTSD was among the common disorders diagnosed after the CF interview. Twenty percent of those who had a change from intake diagnosis of psychotic disorder were re-diagnosed as having PTSD.

Diagnostic Categories and Sense of Coherence

The concept of sense of coherence (SOC) may have relevance to how patients can make meaning out of the clinical cross-cultural communication in assessment situations. The SOC concept was developed by Antonovsky (1988) in order to understand how people successfully cope with stress. SOC includes three core components: comprehensibility, manageability, and meaningfulness. Comprehensibility refers to the extent to which one perceives the stimuli confronting one to make cognitive sense. Manageability refers to the extent to which one perceives that the resources at one's disposal are adequate to meet the demands. Meaningfulness refers to the extent to which one feels that life makes sense emotionally.

For patients, some form of coherence between psychiatric diagnostic evaluations and own perspective may contribute to an improved sense of coherence regarding illness understanding (Bäärnhielm 2004). A meaningful communication about medical information, for example, conveying psychiatric diagnostic categories of post-traumatic stress and suggestions for treatment, is facilitated by knowledge about the patient's perspective on illness and meanings given to post-traumatic symptoms. In a review about PTSD, Johnson and Thompson (2008) emphasise the importance of paying attention to patients' expressions of disorder and distress, the meaning they ascribe to post-traumatic symptoms and experiences, rather than focussing on diagnostic categories.

Building Trust and a Therapeutic Alliance

Trust and a therapeutic alliance between patient and clinician are central to the quality of cross-cultural communication. Trust can be created in many ways, in the individual encounter as well as on a community level with information about health issues and how the health-care system works. For establishing a therapeutic alliance, Nussbaum (2013) addresses the importance of active listening in conveying respect for a patient and his or her concerns. He also emphasises that how questions are posed can contribute to establishing a therapeutic alliance and that expressing concern about a patient's well-being is essential.

Trust and a therapeutic alliance can be especially important in cases of sexual violence. In cross-cultural communication about trauma, clinicians have to ask about trauma but also have to be sensitive to when and how the patient wants to talk about it. The clinician has to respect the limits of what the patient wants to say and if he or she is prepared to talk openly about trauma, as this can be affected by cultural norms and traditions. Discussing resilience-oriented therapy with asylum seekers, Laban et al. (2009) stress the importance of the quality of the alliance and that patients feel that therapy is embedded in coherent, reliable, and predictable interactions.

Case, Soran

Some aspects of cross-cultural clinical communication will be illustrated with the case of Soran. Soran's contact with health care and some glimpses from verbal communication with health professionals in the small town of Mårlunda will be presented and discussed. Soran is a 43-year-old man living in Sweden and is originally from Iraq.

Soran telephones the primary care clinic and asks for an appointment. He wants help with fatigue, pain, and sleeping problems. He has not been in contact with the primary care clinic before. Soran speaks fairly good Swedish and does not ask for an interpreter.

At the primary care clinic, Soran meets a general practitioner (GP). The clinical consultation starts with the GP asking about Soran's health problems. Soran responds:

I have headaches, I have problems with sleeping, and I have pain in my left side. I have back pain and something is pressing on my neck. When it is cold outside, it gets worse. I wake up in the night and cannot go back to sleep.

Soran continues to talk about long-lasting sleeping problems that make him very tired. The GP asks about what help Soran has sought earlier.

Soran: I have been in contact with a private Arabic-speaking doctor working here in Mårlunda. He told me to call you here. He said that you could help me.
GP: Did you have any contact with a doctor in Iraq before you came here?
Soran: No, it was not possible; the war was going on. I got sleeping pills from my friends and relatives. Sometimes the pills made me very tired even during the day. But they were very good sleeping pills; they made me sleep at night. I would like to have good pills like those.

The GP asks Soran more about the condition of his health when he lived in Iraq. Soran talks about sleeping problems, self-medication, and lack of medical care. The GP gets the impression that Soran has lived under quite stressful conditions in Iraq and wants to know more about this.

GP: Have you talked about this with your Arabic-speaking doctor?
Soran: No, I have not. He knows how it is in Iraq. I did not need to tell him.

While carrying out a physical exam, Soran asks the GP for some good sleeping pills. The GP becomes irritated and suspicious. Perhaps Soran is addicted to benzodiazepines and has just come for more drugs. Or has he just come for a medical certificate so he can stay away from his studies or work? The GP finds it meaningless to continue with a further examination and consultation without an interpreter.

GP: I think it is better if you come back when we have an Arabic interpreter here.
Soran: I do not want to have an Arabic interpreter. I can speak Swedish.
GP: The interpreter can help us when we do not understand each other.
Soran: I do not speak very good Arabic.

Soran explains that he does speak Arabic but does not understand it completely. Soran's mother tongue is Kurdish. The GP arranges for a new appointment with a Kurdish interpreter.

Soran returns 2 weeks later to the primary care clinic. The GP he met the first time is now on vacation, and Soran meets a female resident physician in family medicine. A male Kurdish interpreter is present. The resident asks Soran about his health problems. Her short questions about Soran's problems lead to a long discussion between the interpreter and Soran. The resident interrupts and asks if there is any problem with her questions.

Soran says in Swedish that he does not understand the interpreter. The interpreter explains that he speaks Kurdish with a Kurmanji dialect and Soran with a Sorani dialect. The interpreter understands Soran but Soran has difficulties understanding the interpreter. The interpreter says that it is important that they ask for a Kurdish-speaking interpreter who speaks the Sorani dialect.

A week later, Soran comes back to the primary clinic. He meets the resident physician and a male interpreter speaking the Sorani Kurdish dialect. The interpreter presents himself and explains that he is going to interpret everything that is said. He also informs the patient that everything said will be treated with confidentiality. Soran's problems have not improved, and the resident physician makes a comprehensive anamnesis about his symptoms as well as carrying out a physical examination. With the support of the interpreter, Soran understands her instructions and collaborates well.

The resident asks Soran to tell her about his background in Iraq and why he migrated. Soran narrates his life in Iraq and why he fled. He comes from the northern Kurdish part of Iraq. As a teenager, together with two cousins, he left his family and went up to the mountains and joined the Kurdish guerrilla; he became a peshmerga. He lived there for some years and participated in several armed conflicts with the Iraqi military. It was during this period that his sleeping problems and nightmares started. He obtained medication from his friends to help him sleep. Sometimes the medication made him so tired that he slept also during the day. After some years as a peshmerga, Soran was captured by the Iraqi military and imprisoned. After 18 months, he managed to escape with the help of some relatives.

The resident physician listens to Soran's narrative and asks what happened in the Iraqi prison. Soran looks at the resident and asks 'Do you really want me to tell you?' 'Yes' says the resident. Soran tells her how he was treated in prison. He was badly beaten and tortured in order to give information about the guerrillas and where they stored their weapons. Today he has recurrent nightmares about these interrogations, the torture, and also his own participation in the fighting. Certain situations, like bright light in a room, when he sees the police, or certain sounds, make him feel as if he is in the Iraqi prison again. He avoids public places as there is a risk of seeing the police. He also avoids political discussions with other Iraqi refugees as he then feels as if he is being interrogated and threatened.

The resident physician asks Soran how he managed to escape from the prison and Iraq. Soran responds 'I walked to Turkey, but I do not want to talk more about that, it is too hard for me'.

The resident respects what Soran says and does not ask any more questions about his journey through Turkey to Sweden. The resident continues to ask about symptoms of PTSD and depression.

In this case, communication between the patient Soran and the health-care professionals started with a discussion about somatic symptoms, fatigue, pain, and in particular sleeping problems. Initially, it was unclear whether Soran was sufficiently proficient in Swedish or if he needed an interpreter. The resident physician started a communication without checking if the interpreter and Soran spoke the same language and without informing and acclimatising Soran regarding how to work with an interpreter. The GP's decision to end the consultation and give Soran a new appointment could have been affected by countertransference feelings of irritation and mistrust.

When Soran was given space and time and someone showed interest in his story, he gave information that shed new light on his nightmares, pain, and problems. However, he was also very clear about how much he wanted to communicate in the present situation. His illness narratives made it easier for the resident physician to formulate probing questions that contributed to clarifying that Soran suffered from PTSD. He previously had periods of depression with high alcohol consumption. When the resident physician discussed treatment, Soran said that he often thought about his own participation in armed conflicts and what he had done to others.

Summary of Key Points for a Successful Intercultural Communication with Traumatised Immigrants

In interaction with the patient

- Listen actively to the patient and his or her concerns.
- Show your concern about the patient's well-being.

- If possible, be generous with the use of qualified interpreters (in Sweden, interpreters are usually free of charge in health care).
- Ask about previous trauma and post-traumatic symptoms.
- Be sensitive to what, when, and if the patient wants to talk about trauma.
- Try to share as much as possible with the patient assumptions about what each of you mean.
- Pay attention to patients' expressions of distress and meanings ascribed to post-traumatic symptoms and experiences.

In interaction with one's own thoughts and emotions

- Be aware that working with this target group requires more time for communication and arrangement.
- Find space and time to reflect about communication irritations.
- Try to find words or expressions to communicate with yourself the emotional challenges of working with this vulnerable patient group.

References

Adeponle AB, Thombs BD, Groleau D, Jarvis E, Kirmayer LJ (2012) Using the cultural formulation to resolve uncertainty in diagnoses of psychosis among ethnoculturally diverse patients. Psychiatr Serv 63(2):147–153

Afana A-H, Pedersen D, Rønsbo H, Kirmayer L (2010) Endurance is to be shown at the first blow: social representations and reactions to traumatic experiences in the Gaza Strip. Traumatology 16(2):43–54

Al Saffar S, Borgå P, Lawoko G, Edman G, Hällström T (2004) The significance of addressing trauma in outpatient psychiatry. Nord J Psychiatry 58:305–312

Antonovsky A (1988) Unraveling the mystery of health. How people manage stress and stay well. Jossey-Bass Publishers, San Francisco

Bäärnhielm S (2004) Restructuring illness meaning through the clinical encounter: a process of disruption and coherence. Cult Med Psychiatry 28:41–65

Bäärnhielm S, Hussein H, Baker U, Allebeck (2013) Hälsokommunikatörer: Kan de öka medvetenhet om hälsa, levnadsvanor och svensk hälso-och sjukvård? Läkartidningen 110:CAZZ (in Swedish, Swedish Medical Journal)

Bäärnhielm S, Åberg Wistedt A, Scarpinati Rosso M (2014) Revising psychiatric diagnostic categorization of immigrant patients after using the cultural formulation in DSM-IV. Transcult Psychiatry. 2014 Dec 9. pii: 1363461514560657. [Epub ahead of print]

Bäärnhielm S, Scarpinati Rosso M (2009). The cultural formulation: a model to combine nosology and patients' life context in psychiatric diagnostic practice. Transcultural Psychiatry, 46(3):406–428

Borra R (2011) Depressive disorder among Turkish women in the Netherlands: a clinical challenge. A qualitative study. Transcult Psychiatry 48(5):660–674

Bot H, Wadensjö C (2004) The presence of a third party: a dialogical view on interpreter-assisted treatment. In: Wilson JP, Drodzek B (eds) Broken spirits: the treatment of traumatized asylum seekers, refugees, war and torture victims. Brunner-Routledge, New York

Bradford D, Munoz A (1993) Translation in bilingual psychotherapy. Professional psychology. Res Pract 24:5252–5261

Comas-Díaz L, Jacobsen FM (1991) Ethnocultural transference and countertransference in the therapeutic dyad. Am J Orthopsychiatry 61(3):392–402

Fazel M, Wheeler J, Danesh J (2005) Prevalence of serious mental disorders in 7000 refugees resettled in western countries: a systematic review. Lancet 365:1309–1314

Foa EB, Keane TM, Friedman MJ (2000) Guidelines for treatment of PTSD. J Trauma Stress 13(4):539–588

Good BJ (1997) Medicine, rationality, and experience. An anthropological perspective. Cambridge University Press, Cambridge, UK

Gupta M (2013) Review of somatic symptoms in post-traumatic stress disorder. Int Rev Psychiatry 25(1):86–99

Hannerz U (1992) Cultural complexity. Studies in the social organisation of meaning. Columbia University Press, New York

Hinton DE, Lewis-Fernández R (2010) The cross-cultural validity of posttraumatic stress disorder: implications for DSM-5. Depress Anxiety 0:1–19

Hydén L-C (1997) Illness and narrative. Sociol Health Illn 1(19):48–69

Hylland Eriksen T (2004) What is anthropology? Pluto Press, England

Johnson H, Thompson A (2008) The development and maintenance of post-traumatic stress disorder (PTSD) in civilian adult survivors of trauma of war and torture: a review. Clin Psychol Rev 28:36–47

Kinzie DJ (1994) Countertransference in the treatment of southeast Asian refugees. In: Wilson JP, Lindy JD (eds) Countertransference in the treatment of PTSD. The Guilford Press, New York, pp 249–262

Kirmayer L (2003) Failures of imagination: the refugee's narrative in psychiatry. Anthropol Med 10(2):167–185

Kirmayer LJ, Young A (1998) Culture and somatization: clinical, epidemiological, and ethnographic perspectives. Psychosom Med 60:420–430

Kirmayer LJ, Narasiah L, Munoz M et al (2011) Common mental health problems in immigrants and refugees: general approaches in primary care. Can Med Assoc 183(12):E959–E967

Kleinman A (1988) Illness narratives. Suffering, healing and the human condition. Basic Books, New York

Laban CJ, Hurulean E, Attia A (2009) Treatment of asylum seekers: resilience-oriented therapy and strategies (ROTS): implications of study results into clinical practice. In: de Joop J, Coljin S (eds) Handboek, culturele psychiatrie. De Tijdstroom, Utrecht, pp 129–146

Miklavcic A, LeBlanc MN (2014) Cultural brokers, clinically applied ethnography, and cultural mediation. In: Kirmayer LJ, Guzder J, Cécile R (eds) Cultural consultation. Encountering the other in mental health care. Springer, New York, pp 115–137

National Institute of Health (2000) Current bibliographies in medicine – health literacy (1990–1997)

Nichter M (1981) Idioms of distress: alternatives in the expression of psychosocial distress: a case study from South India. Cult Med Psychiatry 5:379–408

Nichter M (2010) Idioms of distress revisited. Cult Med Psychiatry 34:401–416

Norström E (2004) I väntan på asyl. Retorik och praktik i svensk flyktingpolitik. Umeå: Boréa förlag (Dissertation in Swedish)

Nussbaum AM (2013) The pocket guide to the DSM-5 diagnostic exam. APA, Arlington

Pottie K, Greenaway C, Feighter J et al (2011) Evidence-based clinical guidelines for immigrants and refugees. Can Med Assoc 183(12):E824–E925

Rasmussen A, Katoni B, Keller AS, Wilkinsson (2011) Posttraumatic idioms of distress among Darfur refugees: Hozun and Majnun. Transcult Psychiatry 48(4):392–415

Rothman RL, DeWalt AD, Malone R, Bryant B, Shintani A, Crigler B, Weinberger M, Pignone M (2004) Influence of patient literacy on the effectiveness of a primary care–based diabetes disease management program. JAMA 292(14):1711–1716

Scarpinati Rosso M, Bäärnhielm S (2012) The use of cultural formulation in Stockholm: a qualitative study on mental illness experiences among migrants. Transcult Psychiatry 49(2):283–301

Scollon R, Wong Scollon S. (2001). Intercultural Communication, 2 ed, UK: Blackwell Publishing.

Shannon P, O'Dougherty M, Mehta E (2012) Refugees' perspectives on barriers to communication about trauma histories in primary care. Mental Health Fam Med 9:47–55

Silove D (2007) Adaption, ecosocial safety signals and the trajectory of PTSD. In: Kirmayer ILJ, Lemelson R, Barad M (eds) Understanding trauma. Integrating biological, clinical, and cultural perspectives. Cambridge University Press, New York, pp 242–258

Wadensjö C (1987) Tema kommunikation. Kontakt genom tolk. Linköpings universitet. 10:4–40. [in Swedish]

Westermeyer J (1990) Working with an interpreter in psychiatric assessment and treatment. J Nerv Ment Dis 178:745–749

Westermeyer J, Janca A (1997) Language, culture and psychopathology: conceptual and methodological issues. Transcult Psychiatry 34(3):291–311

Westermeyer J, Wahmenholm K (1989) Assessing the victimized psychiatric patient. Hosp Community Psychiatry 40(3):245–249

WHO Regional Office for Europe (2013) Health literacy – the solid facts. WHO Regional Office for Europe: Copenhagen

Zandi T, Havenaar JM, Limburg-Okken AG, van Es H, Sidali S, Kadri N, van der Brink W, Kahn RS (2008) The need for culture sensitive diagnostic procedures. A study among psychotic patients in Morocco. Soc Psychiatr Epidemiol 43:244–250

Trauma and Migration: The Role of Stigma

5

Levent Küey

Migration has been a collective experience for humankind throughout history. There has almost never been a society which has not experienced migration in some form or the other, and currently no such society exists. Some societies have sent many immigrants abroad, some have received or hosted, and still others have been in transit along paths of migration; almost all have experienced migration, though to varying degrees and in varying forms. Humankind does in fact owe its current existence to a combination of migration and evolution.

Migration is thus a universal and historical fact. One could list a vast variety of historical samples: migration of early human beings out of Africa; migration of European peoples to the east coast of North America in the nineteenth century; further migration of many of them to the west of North America; migration of people from South America and Central America and Mexico via the US border to the north; migration of workforces from southern and eastern European countries to northern and western European countries in the twentieth century; migration of war refugees during and after world wars; migrations of post-colonial and post-cold war periods; migration of highly educated professionals from developing countries to more developed countries (the so-called brain drain or gain); and recent migration of refugees and asylum seekers from conflict areas, especially from Africa and the Middle East, to more stable and developed countries.

Although these events have their own historical, socio-economic and political reasons and dynamics, migration is used as an umbrella term to signify a wide variety of facts and processes including 'forced migration', 'voluntary migration', 'migration of the work force', 'economic migration' and so on. Furthermore, the groups of people taking part in migration are also defined under similar umbrella

L. Küey, MD
Department of Psychology, Faculty of Social Sciences and
Humanities, Istanbul Bilgi University, Istanbul, Turkey
e-mail: kueyl@superonline.com

© Springer International Publishing Switzerland 2015
M. Schouler-Ocak (ed.), *Trauma and Migration:
Cultural Factors in the Diagnosis and Treatment of Traumatised Immigrants*,
DOI 10.1007/978-3-319-17335-1_5

terms (e.g. immigrants, refugees, asylum seekers, guest workers, etc.). On the other hand, it should be kept in mind that groups of people referred to under such umbrella terms, while sharing some commonalities, also show some distinctive features.

In general, migration is defined as the geographical movement of people from one place to another, but every instance of migration needs to be assessed in its singularity. Such an approach helps to discuss certain special aspects of migration, such as where the demarcation line between voluntary migration and forced migration should be drawn or what the legal and health conditions of refugees and asylum seekers are in different parts of the world at different times and how these could be improved. In fact, the definition and features of migration and the related phenomenon are not consistent in every geographical and historical context (Bartram et al. 2014).

Since there is no 'one uniform migration', reviewing its impact on mental health by taking it as an independent variable and examining its effects on the people who had migrated or hosted the immigrants would be misleading. This 'geographical move' involves a complex web of cultural, economic, social, psychological and political reasons, motives and implications, including the ones relevant to the mental well-being and mental ill health of the peoples involved. Immigrants do not all prepare in the same way and their reasons for migration are varied. The process of migration and subsequent cultural and social adjustments also play key roles in the mental health of the individual. Clinicians must take these ranging factors into account when assessing and planning unique intervention strategies aimed at the individual in his or her social context.

These mental health implications and traumatic consequences of migration, especially on refugees and asylum seekers, are the subject matter of the other chapters of this book; this chapter, meanwhile, focuses more on the traumatising effects of stigma and discrimination.

The Issue of 'the Other'

In order to understand the traumatising effect of stigma and discrimination on immigrants, the issue of 'the Other' should be briefly reviewed from a historical and conceptual perspective. Different human social groupings are commonly seen as 'others' by members of other groups. Mercier (2013), philosopher and novelist, captured it precisely as follows: 'Others are really others. Others'. We human beings need to set up social networks with our fellows for existence and survival, which inevitably sets the basis for social groupings and, in turn, generates the categorisation of 'in-groups' and 'out-groups', 'me' and 'others' or 'us' and 'them'.

To obtain an overview of the roots of the issue of 'the Other', some of the works by scientists of the humanities were reviewed (see, e.g. Şenel 1982, 2003, 2014; Ilin and Segal 1942; Leakey 1994; Engels [1884] 2010; Hirs 2010; Mayor 2012). Historically, during the hunter-gatherer period of humanity, the main categorisation which was used as a crucial tool for survival was the distinction between 'harmful/poisonous (food)' and 'edible/nutritious (food)'. Any obstacle in reaching necessary aliments was to be removed or killed including the other human beings or animals. These 'others', however, were not categorically conceptualised as 'the Other'; they were merely obstacles to be eliminated in order to ensure survival. The establishment of such categorisations (i.e. 'in-groups' vs. 'out-groups', 'me' vs. 'others' or 'us' vs. 'them') has their roots in the historical period in which people were shifting from the hunter-gatherer lifestyle to the period of the first settlements. The first settlements developed near to the big rivers. The Nile, Yellow River, Euphrates-Tigris (i.e. Mesopotamia) and Amazon, with their continuous flow of water, provided the preconditions for the earliest agricultural production. The first horticultural and agricultural societies were formed, and farming offered the inhabitants of these first settlements more sustainable means of nutrition such as wheat, corn and rice. Furthermore, shelters and housing, mainly made of mud and agricultural leftovers such as straw, became the living area; these new homes were obviously more protective than caves had been and were to form protection against the attacks of others. These processes also forced people to create more elaborate social groupings and organisations in these first cities. Göbekli Tepe, in southeastern Turkey, has been shown to be a good example of such a process in modern day (Benedict 1980). This development, in turn, gave way to more clearly defined social strata and the division of labour into categories such as social leaders, priests and workforces. The emerging social classes and hierarchy set the basis for sharing the surplus value and production as well as fulfilling people's spiritual needs, especially in face of overwhelming natural changes and disasters. These social organisations were established through cooperation, collaboration and solidarity among the members of the 'in-groups'. Moreover, they were an effective means of defending the group against 'out-groups'. These modes of production and sharing were also reflected in their corresponding modes of thinking and mindsets. Conceptual categories of 'members of my city' or 'my citizens' or 'my civilisation' and 'members of other cities' or 'non-citizens' or 'other civilisations' or 'foreigners' had become a paradigmatic fact of the human condition. The *zeitgeist* of the city states had developed, and conceptualisations of 'us/friends' vs. 'them/enemies' had emerged and been established along with the formation of city states and city walls.

The conflicts of interest between members of 'in-groups' were solved through the use of inner regulations based on shared goals, ideals, values and rules, while conflicts with 'out-groups' were solved either by armed confrontations and wars or negotiations and treaties. Not only socio-economical life itself but also the psychological mindsets and mental structure of humanity gave birth to the categorisation of 'us' vs. 'others'; hence, such categorisation has also been the source of discrimination and stigmatisation in the centuries that followed. This is a reality of human history/existence which cannot be ignored and should not be seen from a romantic idealistic perspective, but rather from a realistic humanistic perspective.

Accordingly, the crucial question is not whether the categorisations of 'us' vs. 'others' exist, but rather *how* and *by whom* these categorisations are determined. In any given society, the 'social power relations' determine the stratification of 'us' vs. 'them' groupings. This stratification works both for intergroup relations and for intragroup relations. Whether a group is to be designated as 'the Other' and labelled with prejudice and discrimination will depend heavily on the *zeitgeist* of the current dominant social power.

Throughout history, the *zeitgeist* of any social power has evolved alongside socio-economic changes. In the era of empires, the social power was in the hands of a dynasty which also owned the armed forces and land in the name of 'the holy'. The majority acknowledged the existence of minorities, a sort of 'parallel existence', unless these minorities or 'others' expressed a will to take over the power. Discrimination against marginalised people, for example, people with mental illness or so-called witches, was an unquestioned exercise like all the other discrimination in the name of 'the holy and the king'. Moreover, other empires or their immigrants, named barbarians, were considered to be real threats, i.e. 'the Other'.

In the era of nation states, the social power seems to be in the hands of the state, run by the 'elected or selected powers'. Nation states, independent of their sociopolitical administrative regimes, relied heavily on the motto of 'one nation, one flag, one language'; in some cases, 'one religion and/or one leader' is also added to this motto. The *zeitgeist* of the current dominant 'social power' and the majority in general do not acknowledge the existence of minorities. Minorities are either exterminated or assimilated. They are defined and discriminated as 'the Others', people who have different ethnic origins, belong to other cultures and talk other languages (as their mother tongue). 'The Other' is discriminated against in the name of national identity and uniformity. The borders of these states are strictly controlled, and border crossing is regulated by national regulations and international treaties. Travelling documents and working and residence permits are also strictly controlled by national authorities. Other than tourists, anyone geographically moving from one national state to another, either legally or illegally, becomes an immigrant, refugee or asylum seeker and is open to discrimination.

Although some sociologists consider the current historical period as the 'postnational' era (Soysal 1994), immigration and refugee policies are mainly controlled by national states and to some extent by international organisations founded through treaties signed by these national authorities. According to the *zeitgeist* of the current times, 'us' denotes productive human resources while 'the Other' is anyone outside of this group, such as the disabled. Of course, humanity has also developed policies and taken humanistic steps against such discrimination. The human rights of various minorities, including disabled and disadvantaged groups, immigrants, refugees and asylum seekers are protected by many international laws and treaties (see some of the relevant United Nations documents listed at the end of 'References'), at least *de jure*, if not *de facto*.

Here, as far as the focus of our discussion is concerned, it is important to add that each era had inherited 'the Other' of the preceding era. Hence, in today's societies, all the historical 'Others' could be and frequently are designated as 'the Other'. This explains, why in various parts of the world, many people are still discriminated on the basis of their 'in-group' features, i.e. on the basis of race, nation, ethnicity, religion, sex, sexual orientation, gender identity, skin colour, health condition or abilities and mostly socio-economic class and inequalities.

Prejudice and discrimination based on such designations have been causing devastating trauma due to personal cruelty and mass violence and consequently human suffering on a vast scale in almost all societies. Human history is full of violent acts which are examples of specific discrimination of people with migration backgrounds. Today, the challenge seems to be to confront all the discriminative practices which have built up over the course of human history and have been inherited by our current societies. The solutions in such a process of confrontation do not lie in the challenges and solutions of previous eras; modern challenges cannot be resolved by referring to the means of premodern times. Tackling the discrimination of populations with migration backgrounds, whether it is based on nationality, ethnicity or religious belief, should therefore not be based on the values and *zeitgeist* of previous eras of national states or emperorships. Fundamentalism based on religious beliefs and national identities are premodern suggestions to postmodern challenges and the ones which lead to deepening suffering rather than furthering human collaboration. Our current task is to develop new postmodern ways of overcoming discrimination, thus leading to a more humane cosmopolitanism (Appiah 2006) by enjoying our intergroup diversities and differences. As stated elsewhere (Bartram et al. 2014), national identity is not the focus of attention in cosmopolitanism; people are considered equal as individuals, as global citizens. In today's world, migration is considered as a key component of social transformation in general. The salience of national identity is a matter of great regret for many people, in part because of its consequences on how immigrants are sometimes treated by host societies. 'Nationalism is something to be resisted or suppressed, particularly when one considers its consequences. Modern nationalism had fed vicious violence and wars ranging from individual acts of cruelty to genocide' (Bartram et al. 2014).

Migration and Mental Health

According to Parla (1997), while 'Self is constructed through confrontation with the mirroring effect of the Other, the Other is discovered through self-confrontation'. The construction of the self-identity is an ongoing joint reconstruction process in which we need Each Other. Migration is a process by which the immigrant and the host meet Each Other. The complexity of migration and related processes, including various modes of acculturation, marginalisation, integration, assimilation, stigmatisation, hybrid identities or multi-identities and multiculturalism or cosmopolitanism, all attract the interest of scholars from various disciplines.

Vulnerability caused by factors related to migration and its effects on the psychological well-being of immigrants, refugees and asylum seekers have been widely revealed in many pieces of research as well as in the other chapters of this book. Three stages of the migratory process and possible vulnerability factors have been defined respectively, revealing a clear picture of the process (Bhugra and Jones 2001). The first stage is the 'pre-migration period' where the individuals decide to migrate and plan the move. Immigrants create a network of relations, both in the host and origin societies. The decision to migrate is not usually made in isolation by the individual, but in the context of these relational networks (Hinze 2013). The second stage is the 'process of migration' itself and the physical transition from one place to another, involving all the necessary psychological, social and economical steps. Finally, the third stage is the 'post-migration stage', when the individuals deal with the social and cultural frameworks of the new society to adapt to new roles and become interested in transforming their group. At these stages, possible factors affecting vulnerability include the individual personality features of the immigrants and experiences of loss, bereavement, depression, post-traumatic stress disorder and cultural shock. Besides this, the attitudes and behaviours of the members of the host society towards the people with an immigration background constitute another domain of vulnerability factors determining mental health outcomes at the post-migration stage. These outcomes could be summarised by a spectrum between the dimensions of assimilation/integration and marginalisation/rejection, depending on the degree to which contact is made with the host culture on one hand and the degree to which the culture of origin is maintained and relations with the home culture are sustained on the other. In fact, most immigrants show a combination of these processes and outcomes.

The migration process is inevitably stressful and stress can lead to mental illness, but does not necessarily do so. Such stress may not be related to an increase in all types of mental illness or to the same extent across all immigrant groups. On the other hand, for many immigrants, migration can bring new opportunities leading to higher living standards and improved quality of life and personal satisfaction.

Migration forces the immigrant to reconstruct himself/herself along with his/her life story or the answers to the questions 'who am I, where am I coming from and where am I going?'. What happens when one migrates, or as it is phrased in a Turkish song 'Bir yiğit gurbete düşse gör başına neler gelir?' (translated as 'what happens when one faces homesickness?'). One of the first reactions of the immigrant is a strong desire to return home or at least a dream of doing so; this homesickness characterises the foreigner. The fear of losing one's affiliations and belongings triggers a phantasised and idealised reconstruction of the lost home. The conflict is between the real (not romanticised) host country that the migrant is living in and the idealised lost homeland that is kept alive in the mind of the migrant; this conflict asks for 'a dual existence'. This conflictual state is described very well by a Turkish-German writer, Emine Sevgi Özdamar (2000). It is a state of 'living in between' (Oren 1987) or a craving to create a new way of living in a 'third new space', one which contains both rather than either or Existing in a third space is a process where we meet Each Other. That is exactly why immigrants are not a distinctive group; they are a key part of the whole society, with far-reaching implications for how the people of the host country understand important aspects of themselves. Migration has also been a progressive factor: an opportunity for maturation for the many involved.

Trauma and Mental Health

Various psychological traumas, particularly those experienced in early years, have been widely shown to have detrimental effects on the mental well-being of humans. Such early traumas have been considered as part of the explanatory models for mental disorders which occur in later years, e.g. early loss of a mother connected to depressive states in adulthood. Furthermore, traumas experienced during adulthood also have a crucial impact on the development of post-traumatic stress disorder. When migration is recognised as a traumatic life event for immigrants, the intermediate variables which increase or decrease the traumatic effects of migration and vulnerability become an important focus of attention. We consider stigmatisation and discrimination, among other variables, to have the highest traumatising impacts on the lives of immigrants. Furthermore, we consider stigmatisation and discrimination to be closely and negatively related to the working and living conditions of the immigrants and their psychosocial status in the society. This could lead to a vicious cycle, lower social status causing higher discrimination and vice versa. Discriminative behaviours put the immigrant in a double-bind situation: they must either reject the host society and become marginalised or accept being assimilated. In other words, it creates ghettos on one side or loss of identities on the other. Neither of these alternatives leads to better mental health.

A part of the story that is often neglected is that discrimination and stigmatisation of social groups with a migration background are also harmful for the host societies. Discriminative acts prevent the members of the host societies from finding creative solutions which lead to new possibilities of enrichment via confrontation with different cultural backgrounds. The possibility of reaching 'transnational citizenship' (Balibar 2003) is lost due to stigmatisation and discrimination. For all of these reasons, enhancing our understanding of the re-traumatisation of immigrants through stigmatisation is an issue of concern.

Stigma and Stigmatisation

One of the factors mediating the stressful effects of migration on mental ill health is the degree of discrimination and stigmatisation that immigrants are facing. Stigma is considered to be an amalgam of ignorance and stereotypes, prejudices and discrimination (Rose et al. 2007). Here, ignorance could be defined as a lack of knowledge and interest, while stereotypes refers to the cognitive aspect of the social categorisation of people into 'in-groups' and 'out-groups'. Prejudices or negative attitudes towards 'out-groups' reflect the emotional aspect of this categorisation, while discrimination, i.e. excluding and avoiding behaviours, refers to the behavioural patterns of the host society towards perceived 'out-groups', inevitably harming them (Hinshaw 2007).

From a more sociological point of view, the process which ends with discriminative acts starts with the phenomenon of labelling (Link and Phelan 2001). Any group which is labelled on the basis of their differences stimulates stereotypes towards members of that group and strengthens the categorisation of 'us' vs. 'them'. Such categorisation, whether factual or illusionary, creates emotional responses such as fear, anxiety, anger, pity, shame, alienation, embarrassment, and prejudices which can lead to discriminative acts.

Discrimination of the immigrant in the host society has a crucial role in converting the experience of migration into a traumatic life event. Discrimination against immigrants originates primarily from the categorisations of 'in-group' vs. 'out-group' or 'us' vs. 'them', designated by the dominant paradigms in that society. The cycle of stigmatisation and exclusion (Sartorius 2006) starts with the labelling of immigrants, both as a group and individually, as 'the Other'; this causes alienation and mobilises stereotypes related to that group, in turn leading to ignorance and prejudice and thus causing discrimination and stigmatisation not only against that specific group but also against all immigrants. Immigrants, as a minority group in the host country and culture, are frequently open to accusations by the majority pertaining to any issue which emerges and which is perceived to be related to the minority's situation. The result of such stigmatisation is policies which demand that minority groups are assimilated and behave, feel, work and live as the majority group do.

It has been clearly shown that the discrimination of immigrants is reinforced by expressed signs of difference (Hinze 2013). When differences in race, ethnicity, cultural habits and religious beliefs and rituals are not taken as a basis for enrichment but rather as a basis for prejudice and discrimination, they serve as stress factors which predispose a person to or trigger mental ill health. Furthermore, prejudice and discrimination originating from a single feature of the members of a minority group are usually generalised to the whole person and all of their features. For example, members of a minority group who are discriminated against due to their ethnic or national origins could also be discriminated against on the basis of assumptions about their intellectual performance. This generalisation of stigma leads to the reinforcement of stereotypes and exclusion. Even factual differences such as language and non-verbal communication style differences could become the basis for such generalisations. Moreover, stigmatisation disregards the heterogeneity of various within any one group, instead considering any stigmatised group as homogenous (Mok 1998). In fact, such discrimination has caused vast human suffering in almost all societies across the world, throughout history. Many human-made disasters and acts of mass violence have been executed in the name of such group differences and diversities.

Responses to Stigma

In almost all societies, multiple sources of stigmatisation and discrimination have led to the creation of the society's own 'scapegoats', its very own 'Others'. In a given society, immigrants, refugees and asylum seekers are one of the most readily available groups of 'Others' to be stigmatised. Stigma against people with migration background puts a heavy and complex burden on the lives of immigrants. The difficulties of daily life such as working conditions, social relations and so on, can be wounding enough in themselves, but the extra burden of discriminative attitudes and behaviours can have a deeply traumatic impact on the immigrant's psychological well-being and social relations. While on one hand aiming to overcome the task of adaptation and integration in the host society and facing the related distress and possible disabling effects of this process, immigrants also often face the traumatisation caused by stigma and exclusion.

Richman and Leary (2009) have described three forms of response to this discrimination. One form of response is to experience the limiting consequences of stigma via the internalisation, i.e. through self-stigma or 'self-oppression' (David and Derthick 2014); this involves the devaluation and inferiorisation of oneself and one's group and diminished self-esteem and self-efficacy. A second response is righteous anger and more active attitudes towards discriminating prejudices, while the third form is indifference. Many immigrants show a combination of these responses to varying degrees, depending on the stage of their migration process and the interaction of their subjectivity with the objectivity of the sociocultural contexts they are living in.

Internalised stigma or self-stigma can be regarded as consisting of three dimensions: self-stereotyping, self-prejudice and consequently self-discrimination (inspired by Hinshaw 2007). Self-stereotyping reflects the cognitive aspects of social categorisation (i.e. 'I am a member of a disadvantaged, inferior group'); self-prejudices reflect the emotional aspects of differentiation ('I am different and rejected and deserve this situation'); lastly, self-discrimination refers to internalised behavioural patterns ('I do not have the same rights; I cannot do what they can do'). Internalised stigma stimulates a vicious cycle of traumatisation via lowered self-esteem and expectations, mixed emotions of anger and shame and frequently learned helplessness and a decrease in personal capacity and coping skills, in turn leading to an increase in the stigmatisation faced in the external environment.

Internalised stigma and oppression are both heavily traumatising and hidden. Furthermore, it is often ignored in scientific circles and theory (David and Derthick 2014). Hence, the voices, concerns and real-life experiences of many devalued and marginalised groups, including refugees and asylum seekers, often remain unheard (David and Derthick 2014). A further consequence of internalised oppression is that the victim of the trauma could very quickly become a perpetrator himself/herself as an act of survival, as illustrated in the case of Stockholm syndrome or analysed and described as identification with the aggressor (Duran 2014).

The Issue of 'Roots'

On our way to conclusions and discussions of how to overcome the stigma and traumatisation related to migration, the issue of roots deserves to be mentioned briefly, from a sociological perspective (Yumul 2006). Describing people according to their roots and identifying them with their homelands and nationalities have been a characteristic of our *zeitgeist*. Roots not only feed a tree but also fix the tree to the land. This makes it impossible to belong to different lands at the same time. When the nations and nationalities are '*fixed*' *in homelands*, culture and nationalities are strongly linked with that land. In this *zeitgeist*, culture is not linked with the life journey itself but with roots fixed in a specific country. The migrant is therefore considered to be 'rootless', suffering from pathological cultural identities. Along these lines, the words of Deleuze and Guattari further clarify our position: 'We are tired of trees. We have to give up believing in trees and roots. They have been the reasons for severe human suffering' (Deleuze and Guattari 1987).

One may ask whether this is possible in real life; are there real people experiencing this position? The film director Fatih Akın and his filmography is a good example of being in the 'third transnational space' (Balibar 2003), enjoying 'rootless' multi-identities or *multiculturalism*. In one interview (2007), Akın initially hesitated for a while when he was asked the following: 'Where do you belong? If you were a tree, where would your roots be?'. Then he answered: 'Tree? Tree? Hmmm… Well, I would prefer to be a rose. No, no, not even a rose. Do I need to be a plant? If I am a plant, then I would be stuck in one land. In fact, I am a human being; I would prefer to feed myself from different lands/cultures'. It was as if he was describing how all his multicultural experiences belonged to him, but he did not belong or was not rooted in any one singular 'in-group' or land.

A novelist with a multicultural background, Amin Maalouf, is another real example of someone who has internalised a similar approach, enjoying his multi-identity. In the words of his protagonist, Leo Africanus, 'I come from no country, from no city, no tribe. I am the son of the road… all tongues and all prayers belong to me, but I belong to none of them' (Maalouf 1988).

Conclusions

We are living in a world of diversity in many facets of life. The challenge is not this diversity itself, but how we maintain and handle it. Is diversity taken as grounds for segregation and discrimination, power exercise and oppression; group terror or state terror; increasing inequalities and injustice? Does diversity form a basis for traumatising the minorities? Isn't discrimination, based on being from this or that group, the oldest and most severe psychosocial trauma for the discriminated groups, including immigrants, refugees and asylum seekers? Or, on the other hand, could diversity be used as a more solid ground from which to reap the rewards of richness and multiculturalism as part of human coexistence?

Such questions lead us to a new set of questions: What could happen when a human meets a fellow human currently designated 'the Other' in that society? Are stigmatisation and discrimination inevitable? Could meeting 'the Other' alternatively lead to human enrichment motivated by a hospitality-based acknowledgement? On the other hand, most importantly, what are the opportunities that migration offers, both to migrants and to host populations?

We do not accept the idea of cultural hierarchy; thus there is no 'pure' culture that is superior to other cultures. This is also why a movement of purification imposed within a cultural area cannot be legitimate. Eventually, the recognition of multicultural identity is a new dimension of human rights, in other words the right to choose one's culture and to respect the cultural choice of others.

The focus must be on creating and improving ways of living with diversity for the unity of humanity. Living in diversity is the fact; a uniform society, free of diversity, is the illusion or the wishful thinking of some oppressors and is in its very essence pathetic. How could diversities in human existence be orchestrated *de facto* for the benefit of us all?

Humankind is in need of developing an integrated self; this, in turn, depends on meeting and accepting the existence of 'the Otherness' in 'the Other'. We need the mirroring of Each Other.

For the immigrant, the need to develop an integrative self-image and to reconstruct an identity in order to safeguard mental health can be thwarted by stigmatisation. Stigmatisation lashes out at 'the Other', and in so doing, it breaks down our own mirrors. A world without mirrors is a world without selves.

References

Akın F (2007) An interview during the 6th. Turkish-German psychiatry congress, "Diagnosis and Identity(ies)". University of Boğaziçi, İstanbul

Appiah KA (2006) Cosmopolitanism: ethics in a world of strangers. W. W. Norton & Company, New York

Balibar E (2003) We, the people of Europe?: reflections on transnational citizenship (trans: Swenson J). Princeton University Press, Princeton

Bartram D, Poros M, Monforte P (2014) Key concepts in migration. SAGE Publications Ltd, New York

Benedict P (1980) Survey work in Southeastern Anatolia. In: Çambel H, Braidwood RJ (eds) Prehistoric research in Southeastern Anatolia I. Edebiyat Fakültesi Basimevi, Istanbul

Bhugra D, Jones P (2001) Migration and mental illness. Adv Psychiatr Treat 7:216–223

David EJR, Derthick AO (2014) What is internalized oppression, and so what? In: David EJR (ed) Internalized oppression: the psychology of marginalized groups. Springer Publishing Company LLC, New York

Deleuze G, Guattari F (1987) A thousand plateaus: capitalism and Schizophrenia (trans: Massumi B). University of Minnesota Press, Minneapolis

Duran E (2014) Forward. In: David EJR (ed) Internalized oppression: the psychology of marginalized groups. Springer Publishing Company LLC, New York

Engels F ([1884] 2010) The origin of the family, private property, and the state. Penguin Classics, London

Hinshaw SP (2007) The mark of shame: stigma of mental illness and an agenda for change. OUP, Oxford

Hinze AM (2013) Turkish Berlin: integration policy and urban space. Globalization and community, 21st edn. University of Minnesota Press, Minneapolis

Hirs PQ (2010) Social evolution and sociological categories. Routledge Revivals, New York

Ilin M, Segal E (1942) How man became a giant. Kamarov A. (Illustr.), (trans: Kinkead B). JB Lippincott, Philadelphia

Leakey R (1994) The origin of humankind. Basic Books, New York

Link BG, Phelan JC (2001) Conceptualizing stigma. Annu Rev Sociol 27:363–385

Maalouf A (1988) Leo Africanus (trans: Sluglett P) New Amsterdam, Chicago. Available at http://www.brainyquote.com/quotes/quotes/a/aminmaalou570117.html. Accessed 22 Jan 2015

Mayor FT (2012) Hunter-gatherers-the original libertarians. Indep Rev 16(4):485–500

Mercier P (2013) Perlmann's silence (trans: Whiteside S). Grove Press, New York

Mok TA (1998) Getting the message: media images and stereotypes and their effect on Asian Americans. Cult Divers Ment Health 4(3):185–202

Ören A (1987) Arada, Şiirler. Dağyeli Verlag, Frankfurt (in Turkish)

Özdamar ES (2000) Life is a caravanserai: has two doors I came in one I went out the other (trans: Floton LV). Middlesex University Press, London

Parla J (1997) The fugitive glance at the TV: presentifications. In: Kuran Burçoğlu N (ed) Multiculturalism: identity and otherness. Boğaziçi University Press, İstanbul

Richman LS, Leary MR (2009) Reactions to discrimination, stigmatization, ostracism, and other forms of interpersonal rejection-a multimotive model. Psychol Rev 116(2):365–383

Rose D, Thornicroft G, Pinfold V, Kassam A (2007) 250 labels used to stigmatise people with mental illness. BMC Health Serv Res 7:97

Sartorius N (2006) Lessons from a 10-year global programme against stigma and discrimination because of an illness. Psychol Health Med 11:383–388

Şenel A (1982) İlkel Topluluktan Uygar Topluma Geçiş Aşamasında Ekonomik Toplumsal Düşünsel Yapıların Etkileşimi. A.Ü. Siyasal Bilgiler Fakültesi Yayınları, Ankara

Şenel A (2003) İnsan ve Evrim Gerçeği. Özgür Üniversite Kitaplığı, Ankara

Şenel A (2014) İnsanlık Tarihi/Kemirgenlerden Sömürgenlere, 3rd edn. Imge Kitabevi Yayinlari, Ankara

Soysal YN (1994) Limits of citizenship: migrants and postnational membership in Europe. University of Chicago Press, Chicago

Yumul A (2006) Melez Kimlikler. In: Yumul A, Dikkaya F (eds) Avrupalı mı, Levanten mi? Bağlam Yayınları, İstanbul

Some of the Relevant United Nations Documents

International convention on the protection of the rights of all migrant workers and members of their families. Adopted by General Assembly resolution 45/158 of 18 December 1990. Available at http://www2.ohchr.org/english/bodies/cmw/cmw.htm. Accessed 8 Jan 2015

UNHCR convention and protocol relating to the status of refugees, available at http://www.unhcr.org/protect/PROTECTION/3b66c2aa10.pdf. Accessed 8 Jan 2015

United Nations General Assembly, International convention on the elimination of all forms of racial discrimination, 21 December 1965, United Nations, Treaty Series, vol 660, p 195, available at: http://www.refworld.org/docid/3ae6b3940.html. Accessed 8 Jan 2015

United Nations convention on the rights of persons with disabilities, available at http://www.un.org/disabilities/default.asp?id=259. Accessed 8 Jan 2015

United Nations General Assembly resolution 429(V) of 14 December 1950, available at http://www.unhcr.org/refworld/docid/3b00f08a27.html. Accessed 8 Jan 2015

Migration, Trauma and Resilience

Antonio Ventriglio and Dinesh Bhugra

Introduction

In these days of globalisation, there is massive movement of people across the globe. Migration across the world has always been present, but perhaps the speed of migration has changed rapidly in the previous hundred years. Migration can be due to any number of reasons – from economic betterment to educational opportunities which may act as attraction and pull factors. On the other hand, political changes, disasters and strife may act as push factors where people may have to leave. Recent tragedies in the waters of Italy have raised specific issues about the processes of asylum seeking and refugees. The trafficking of women and children adds another dimension to the whole process. These examples illustrate that migrants as well as the process of migration are not homogenous, so clinicians must remain aware of individual experiences. The stages of migration can be roughly divided into three: pre-migration, actual process of migration and settlement post-migration, which may take several years. Pre-migration may be a few days or a few years. In the former case, the migrant may not have any or limited opportunities to prepare for the process. When migration is planned, for example, for those who may choose to study abroad, preparing for admission may itself take years. The framework for migration and its sequelae will vary.

A. Ventriglio (✉)
Department of Clinical and Experimental Medicine, University of Foggia, Foggia, Italy
e-mail: a.ventriglio@libero.it

D. Bhugra
Tavistock and Portman NHS Trust, London, UK

President, World Psychiatric Association, Geneva, Switzerland
e-mail: Dinesh.bhugra@kcl.ac.uk

© Springer International Publishing Switzerland 2015
M. Schouler-Ocak (ed.), *Trauma and Migration:*
Cultural Factors in the Diagnosis and Treatment of Traumatised Immigrants,
DOI 10.1007/978-3-319-17335-1_6

Definitions

It is helpful to understand what is meant by different terms. Migration itself can be permanent or temporary. In the latter case, it may vary from a few months to a number of years. It may also take years for individuals to become acculturated to the new country. Migration is the physical process of moving from one geographical area to another. This may be within the same country or from one country to another. The actual process of migration may be planned or sudden. The individual may migrate by themselves or with their family or in a group. The reasons for migration have been defined as pull or push factors (for details see below).

Trauma

Leaving a place of abode for whatever reasons may well be a life event which may be interpreted as positive or negative by the migrant, as well as by those who are left behind. Trauma of arrival may also be painful. It depends upon a number of factors how the migration is viewed and dealt with, both internally and externally, as to how an individual deals with the trauma.

Resilience

Resilience is the ability to cope with and manage stress and trauma. It is defined as adaptive responding to stressful or traumatic circumstances or events (Elliott et al. 2010).

Some of the resilience depends upon the personality of the individual, their world view, support systems and other factors.

Types of Migration

It is very rare that two people migrating at the same time from the same setting to another will have the same experiences. The expectations of the new place and the sense of loss at leaving one place can be extremely brutal. The patterns of migration are many and are strongly influenced by push or pull factors (Rack 1982). Push factors are related to war, violence, poverty and trauma. Pull factors include educational, personal or economic improvement and the two may work in tandem. For example, extreme poverty may lead to both push and pull factors. Furthermore, whether there is time to plan and arrange for migration, or whether it is sudden, may ill prepare the individual. The three stages described as part of the migration process are pre-migration, migration and post-migration. These three stages may overlap and are not always very distinct (Bhugra 2004a).

Pre-migration may last from a few years to a few days. For example, a woman who has married may be waiting in anticipation for the visa and other formalities to be completed, whereas during times of war or other disasters, individuals may have a very short time to prepare and migrate. The heterogeneity of reasons for migration and the actual experiences may determine the results in the post-migration stage. Actual migration may be traumatic, as seen in trafficked women and children, or may be relatively straightforward, especially if the individual is migrating for educational or economic reasons and the migration papers are in place. The process of illegal immigration itself can be very traumatic. The process of settling down after migration depends upon a number of factors. Most important of these are the personality of the individual and the social support expected and available. It is quite likely that the attitudes displayed by the new country (in international migration) will affect the settling down.

The post-migration period in settling down may be a few weeks or months or rarely may take years. In addition, the interaction between individualistic (egocentric) or collectivist (sociocentric) countries and individuals is worth noting. We will very briefly look at the model described by Hofstede (2000) and then describe in some detail the responses to trauma in the post-migration phase.

Stress related to migration can be dealt with in a number of ways. The individual migrant's personality, coping strategies, antecedent factors and peer migration circumstances, social support and other factors will affect adjustment. These stressors can be both acute (due to the impact of migration itself) or chronic or ongoing (which are more likely to be related to post-migration processes). Smith (1985) has described these (see below). Furnham and Bochner (1986) and Ruiz et al. (2011) identify eight theoretical constructs of loss, fatalism (which may also have a cultural bias but may be embedded in a sense of loss of control), expectations of and from the new society, negative life events and social support along with loss of or clash of values and skills deficit (in dealing with the new culture).

Gender, education, age, social class, access to reasonable housing and employment will influence adjustment as well as dealing with stress. These factors are well known for aetiological impact on depression (Chandra 2011). Other vulnerable groups, such as the elderly, those with a learning disability and lesbians, gay, bisexual, and transgender (LGBT) individuals will have specific issues that clinicians and policymakers must take into account. Feelings of persecution may further add to a sense of vulnerability.

Cultural Bereavement

While studying the experiences of refugees, Eisenbruch (1990, 1991) noted the presence of cultural bereavement. He describes this experience as a profound sense of grief and loss as a result of leaving one culture behind (especially) due to suddenness and disasters. This grief and loss can manifest itself in a number of ways. Apart from the loss of belongings, friends, family and possessions, migration also brings with it a sense of loss of belonging. This loss is related to a sense of rootlessness, especially if the migration is forced or traumatic.

The psychoanalytic model explaining loss may be pertinent here. Bowlby (1961, 1980) described four stages of response in children who had experienced loss.

These were numbness or protest, yearning and searching, disorganisation and despair and reorganisation. The violent push factors may lead to levels of numbness and protest which, in spite of the safety of the new place, may lead to isolation and withdrawal, or another pathological sequel such as fanaticism may produce revision in the internal world view of the migrant. Bowlby (1961) postulated that the processes of mourning in response to loss are complex and may carry with them not only the impact related to healthy mourning but also the identification with the lost object. For migrants especially related to experiences of trauma, there can be multiple lost objects. The main focus of loss is the resulting disappointment, persistent separation anxiety and grief with strenuous and angry efforts to recover it. Under these circumstances, traumatised migrants may either have unrealistic expectations or may well accept their fate passively.

Culture Conflict

Culture conflict may be external, whereas individuals brought up and seeped in one culture may find it difficult to accept certain norms of the new culture, creating internal conflict which may present as an external conflict. It is hypothesised that such a conflict may further lead to alienation and the individual may respond in a pathological way.

Another form of culture conflict is within the family or kinship, where different individuals and members of the family may be in conflict with one another. This is often seen as a conflict between individuals who may be at different levels of acculturation. For example, the younger generation may feel that they have more in common with the modern attitudes of majority culture, whereas the older generation may see their traditional attitudes as paramount. It has been argued that south Asian females may feel trapped under these circumstances and use deliberate self-harm as a way out (Bhugra 2004b).

Culture conflict describes these tensions in attitudes and resulting behaviours, which may lead to difficulties in integration within the family and within the individuals themselves. Clinicians need to be sensitive to explore these values and degree of conflict.

Culture Shock

Many migrants, once arriving in the new country, may experience shock at the structures and the values of the new culture. These responses are defined as emotional reaction, with both negative and positive aspects to it (Oberg 1960; Bock 1981). It is inevitable that not only will culture shock affect adjustment and acculturation, but it will influence the way migrants settle down and may cause dysphoria (Pantelidou and Craig 2006). It is quite likely that this sense of detachment and dysphoria may lead to an element of poor self-esteem.

These experiences, combined with a degree of alienation and poor self-esteem, may affect their sense of achievement. A perceived discrepancy between aspiration and achievement may further lead to depressive cognition, which may be dealt with either by withdrawal or by aggression and need to be assessed.

Racism and Ethnic Identity

Racism is a particular kind of discrimination which is seen as based on a belief that people can be differentiated mainly or entirely on the basis of their heritage or ancestral lineage (Cochrane 2001). Racism then leads to an assumption that people are to treated differently because some groups are seen as inferior and also because other groups see themselves as superior and worthy of certain privileges. This needs to be differentiated from prejudice, which leads to negative attitudes based on general stereotypes. Harding et al. (1969) and Sherif and Sherif (1956) suggest that racial discrimination and minority status can be stressful for a number of reasons. Harding et al. (1969) propose that racial discrimination has the net effect of producing two types of group membership. Inevitably, one will be an inside-of-group and the other will be an outside-of-group distinction. Thus, those who are in one group and excluded from the other will experience stress. The external attacks in either of the group settings will rekindle the previous effects of trauma and rejection.

Cochrane (2001) suggests that prejudice finds many forms of expression. The most extreme example is genocide, but it can also lead to discrimination embedded in legal and political systems which may treat migrants as second-class citizens. There are various types of prejudice and racism. Clinicians must be aware that, in spite of personal resilience, migrants may find it difficult to deal with systematised, systematic or institution racism.

A key aspect of understanding and dealing with prejudice and racism concerns the subjective interpretation of racial events, which is said to be worse than the actual experience.

Hofstede (2000) describes that cultures have five dimensions. Although most of his work has been carried out in multinational companies, the dimensions are equally applicable to broader cultures. It is worth looking at these because individuals born and brought up in one culture may carry some of the cultural characteristics, cultural values and attitudes with them wherever they go. It is important that clinicians are aware of these differences. Hofstede (2000) describes cultural dimensions as egocentric versus sociocentric, masculine or feminine, distance or closeness from culture of power and a long-term or short-term orientation and uncertainty avoidance. Of these, perhaps it is worth noting the distinguishing characteristics of egocentric and sociocentric societies and masculine versus feminine cultures, as these are likely to be significant areas of potential clash. These are illustrated, respectively, in Tables 6.1 and 6.2. It is worth emphasising here that not all individuals from a masculine or feminine culture will have those characteristics, in the same way that those coming from sociocentric societies will not all be sociocentric individuals.

Table 6.1 Broad typology of cultures

Sociocentric	Egocentric
Extended/joint family	Nuclear family
Status predetermined	Status oriented
Strong social links	Weak social links
Little or no choice	Choice of partner
Interdependent	Independent
Group advance	Individual advance
Tradition	Modern

Modified from Hofstede (2000)

Table 6.2 Traits of masculinity/femininity

	High masculine	Low masculine (feminine)
Social norms	Ego oriented	Relationship oriented
	Money and things are important	Quality of life and people are important
	Live in order to work	Work in order to live
Politics and economics	Economic growth high priority	Environment protection high priority
	Conflict solved through force	Conflict solved through negotiation
Religion	Most important in life	Less important in life
	Only men can be priests	Both men and women as priests
Work	Larger gender wage gap	Smaller gender wage gap
	Fewer women in management	More women in management
	Preference for higher pay	Preference for fewer working hours
Family and school	Traditional family structure	Flexible family structure
	Girls cry, boys don't; boys fight, girls don't	Both boys and girls cry; neither fight
	Failing is a disaster	Failing is a minor accident

Cultural identity thus plays a major role in settling down in a new setting. Berry (2007) defines cultural identity as a sense of attachment or commitment to a cultural group which has both cultural and psychological components. Berry (2007) observes that thus it is crucial that, in a cultural group, negative and positive experiences, attachment patterns, gender roles, nutrition and genetic vulnerability will play a role. Perception of the trauma, quality of life and appraisal of the stress will be some of the factors that are likely to influence the traumascape. At collective level, political factors, governance and power, economic factors including social inequalities and group support will affect responses to trauma. Furthermore, schemes held up by the community on trauma, suffering and religious and political fanaticism and conviction and access to care and reconciliation will also play a role in managing and dealing with stress.

Berry and Anniss (1974) put forward a model suggesting that cultural groups and individuals who have high psychological differentiation are less likely to show acculturative stress. They describe high psychological differentiation as behaviour in the perceptual, cognitive, social and affective domains (as based on Witkin et al. 1962 and Witkin 1967). The ecological links are related to primary needs in specific physical environments including economic possibilities (Berry and Annis 1974). Thus, it is inevitable that pre-migration experiences may well affect post-migration adjustment and acculturative stress (see below), especially if these are affected by trauma. Smith (1985) proposes that individuals from ethnic minorities may feel victimised and may thus be exposed to stress. Another possibility is that they may feel vulnerable or see the process of discrimination and stress as additive burden – both acute and chronic. These hypotheses also provide a suitable framework for intervention (see below).

De Jong (2007) highlights that cultural factors influence both problem-focused and emotion-focused coping. In trauma, grief is an important response, but cultural variations will play a major role in managing grief and trauma. The presentation, help-seeking and health care systems themselves are strongly influenced by cultural factors. Internal conflict within the individuals and communities and external conflict have to be taken into account while planning interventions dealing with trauma and grief. Depending upon the individual resilience, social support, material resources and other factors may need to be explored.

Traumascape, as what De Jong (2007) argues, means the systemic dynamics of local and international representations and actions around extreme stress. It is based on the notions of a framework used for examining the 'new' cultural economy as a complex model. Traumascape, according to Tumarkin (2005), is a location of tragedies and trauma. De Jong (2007) emphasises that in a post-war or post-disaster setting, stakeholders will have divergent perceptions of the traumascape, which may lead to identifying the needs and concerns of the local population. However, it is quite possible that many local models may need to be taken into account.

De Jong (2007) proposes an ecological-cultural-historical model for extreme stress. When looking at the ecology and history, De Jong (2007) suggests that these are at individual and collectivist levels. These at individual level indicate that the life history of an individual is embedded in the traumascape of a collective history in a specific era. Both the individual and the collective histories play a role in understanding the experience related to trauma. These histories have a reciprocal role to play. At individual level, coping strategies, family support and previous experiences exist, and the individual has a sense of belonging. Dealing across cultures or with cultures which may not be well known to the individual, other strategies may need to be employed. These include the processes of assimilation, acculturation or deculturation. A major part of assimilation process is to take into account how individuals see their inner 'self'. In egocentric individuals, it may be easier to settle down in new cultures which are egocentric. They tend to move more easily between cultures and form friends easily. Sociocentric individuals, on migrating to egocentric cultures, may find it difficult to settle down if they are not surrounded by individuals from their own culture – a model described as cultural congruity (see Bhugra 2005).

Thus, a very complex picture starts to emerge about the individual, their migration experience and their post-migration experience, especially in the context of acculturation or assimilation in the face of their own stressors and social support.

Berry (1992, 2007) suggests that there are three ways of conceptualising outcomes of acculturation. The first conception is that of behavioural shifts – changes which are generally not difficult and which include dress, food and language. This has what Berry (2007) describes as culture shedding, culture learning and culture conflict. However, in these days of social media and internationalisation of the media, some culture learning and culture shedding may already take place before the individual has migrated. Adjustment to the newer culture and its values may or may not be straightforward. Berry (1970, 2007) and Berry et al. (1987) describe acculturative stress, when the individual faces change events in their lives that challenge their cultural understanding and values on how to live (in this case, survive). Acculturative stress put simply is the stress faced by the individual in a different culture in managing adjustment and is akin to stress reaction. In a previous paper, Berry and Annis (1974) had suggested that acculturative stress that cultural groups undergoing social and cultural change experienced will experience a certain amount of psychological discomfort. They argue that acculturative stress is related to various psychological variables. Furthermore, it can be argued that an unaware feeling of the new culture (which may be called cultural deficiency) may well contribute both to culture shock and acculturative stress. Berry (2007) prefers the term 'acculturative stress' rather than 'culture shock', though it can be argued that the latter may reflect a sudden, acute and perhaps more disruptive response. Each of these stress experiences can be managed by strategies which individuals may adapt to in other circumstances. Taking cognisance of what they are experiencing and what they are feeling is an important way of managing what is going on.

Dressler (2007) raises the significant issue of cultural consonance. This is particularly helpful in assessing migrants who may have experienced violence or loss. He points out that even migrants (without a history of trauma) who move to more modern societies show an increase in their blood pressure levels, possibly attributed to conflict between tradition and modernity (Dressler 1999). Dressler (2007) argues that moving from one culture to another can lead to stressor and stress-induced psychiatric disorders, but individual and cultural variables have to be taken into account. Cultural consonance refers to the observation that culture is both shared and learnt, and the focus of the culture is both within the individual and the society at large. Cultural consensus has four facets, which include sharing, quantification of consensus within the culture, examination of intra-cultural diversity and, lastly, the cultural set of responses. Cultural consonance therefore is embedded in the cognitive schema of the population. Dressler (2007) defines cultural consonance as 'the degree to which individuals in their own beliefs and behaviours, approximate the shared expectations encoded in cultural models'. Thus, cultural consonance not only shapes the world view of the individual but can also express links between individual values and group values.

Carta et al. (2013) demonstrated that in a refugee camp in Burkina Faso, one in five individuals demonstrated signs of post-traumatic stress disorder (PTSD) and 60 %

met the criteria for trauma and stressor-related disorders, especially in women aged over 40. Trauma-related deaths in the family were reported by 83 % of 408 individuals interviewed. Nearly 90 % of individuals reported problems related to food and housing, thus confirming Smith's (1985) stress-inducing life events and chronic difficulties. These authors conclude that acute and chronic stressors play a role in the adjustment post-migration. An interesting finding is the high rates among women, which is useful to know as women are often the carers. Similar findings among youngsters may indicate suffering due to stress but not related to PTSD (Montgomery 2011).

The role racism plays in the genesis and perpetuation of stress in refugees and asylum seekers and in other migrants is worth noting. It is unlikely that rich migrants will face institutional racism in these days of rapid globalisation, but poor migrants, refugees and asylum seekers may well do so. Racism can work at many levels and is of many varieties. People may feel that all migrants are the same, but once they know one individual, they may believe that are exceptions. The impact of racism can be at individual level and at institutional level. It is important that clinicians be aware of the role institutional racism may play in preventing people from seeking help from health care systems and also in therapeutic engagement.

In an interesting overview, Bethencourt (2013) notes that racism is relational and changes over time. He points out that 'the prejudice concerning ethnic descent coupled with discriminatory actions existed in various periods of history (p 1), but the scientific framework provided by the theory of races gave it further impact. The notion and existence of racism date back to antiquity. This indicates that, although there may have been racism, this was perhaps to do with notions of creating 'the other'. Such a creation is critical in validating one's own identity. 'The other', whether it is related to gender, religion, ethnicity, culture, mentally ill or migrant status, allows one to see themselves in contrast. In Europe, racial supremacy was opposed by working class virtue in the clash between the two totalitarian regimes (fascist-Nazi and Communist) in the Second World War (Bethencourt 2013, p 335). Desegregation was a form of institutional racism, as was apartheid. The caste system in India also reflects a type of institutional racism. Once a migrant enters another cultural system, then there is the issue of traversing these institutional barriers.

Resilience

Resilience has already been defined above, but it has to be looked at various levels too. For example, there will be resilience at an individual level, which will be dependent upon a developmental understanding of what the individual has gone through. At the same time, resilience also depends upon social resilience embedded in the social networks and support systems. As has been mentioned earlier, if a sociocentric individual from a sociocentric society migrates to an egocentric society, they may find it difficult to settle down, especially if they are isolated and may not have access to other sociocentric individuals from their own culture – a concept described as cultural congruity (Bhugra 2005). Social resilience depends upon a number of factors. First and foremost is the acknowledgement and recognition by the majority culture or society. Then, social identity at the group level is helpful in providing a 'sense of belonging' to the individual migrant. Understanding and, more important, believing in the migrant who has been traumatised will provide a degree of support, whether it is from the community itself or from the majority community. This allows an individual to move forward in dealing with the trauma. Other informal support networks are important, and these may include community leaders, religious leaders, professionals from the same community and others.

Smith (1985) provides a helpful framework in managing stress experienced by migrants. She notes that race and stress are interlinked and stress-resistant delivery model as expressed takes race into account in any intervention model. Identifying the individual's chief sources of stress, whether trauma related or ethnicity related, is the first step. Then a clear outlining of stress-resistant forces and strengthening these becomes important using common reference points. Following this are the educative and instillation of hope phases. In the uncovering phase, the individual is encouraged to locate the injury to the self which can then lead to helping the traumatised individual to be re-parented in therapy. This can then be used to rework the impact of trauma. The last two phases include self-development and ideal self-stage and completion. The therapist needs to be aware of cultural issues and history of trauma and should utilise these in a culturally sensitive and culturally appropriate manner.

Conclusions

In this necessarily brief overview, we have attempted to bring together factors which may affect the post-migration experience. We have not looked at pre-migration experiences and individual development and the nature of trauma or post-trauma reactions. It is inevitable that the experiences of migrants will be heterogenous, and responses to the actual process of migration will also be varying. Clinicians therefore need to focus on the individual with whom they are interacting and explore individual factors, proximal factors such as family and kinship and distal factors such as employment, social group, etc. It is essential that normal human experiences are not medicalised or pathologised. A human understanding of the trauma which migrants may have experienced of their own responses and an understanding of what may have gone on and assessing external support factors will play a major role in helping individuals to adjust and overcome their experience.

References

Berry JW (1970) Marginality stress and ethnic identification in an acculturated aboriginal community. J Cross-Cult Psychol 1:239–252

Berry JW (1992) Acculturation and adaptation in a new society. Int Migr 30:69–85

Berry JW (2007) Acculturation and identity. In: Bhugra D, Bhui KS (eds) Textbook of cultural psychiatry. Cambridge University Press, Cambridge, pp 169–178

Berry JW, Annis RC (1974) Acculturative stress: the role of ecology, culture and differentiation. J Cross-Cult Psychol 5:382–406

Berry JW, Kim U, Minde T, Mok D (1987) Comparative studies acculturative stress. Int Migr Rev 21:491–511

Bethencourt F (2013) Racism: from the crusades to the twentieth century. Princeton University Press, Princeton

Bhugra D (2004a) Migration and mental health. Acta Psychiatr Scand 109(4):243–258

Bhugra D (2004b) Culture and self-harm: attempted suicide in South Asians in London, Maudsley monographs 46. Psychology Press, London

Bhugra D (2005) Cultural identities and cultural congruency: a new model for evaluating mental distress in immigrants. Acta Psychiatr Scand 111(2):84–93

Bock P (1981) Culture shock. Knopf, New York

Bowlby J (1961) Processes of mourning. Int J Psychoanal 42:317–339

Bowlby J (1980) Attachment and loss, vol 3. Basic Books, New York

Carta MG, Oumar FW, Moro MF, Moro D, Preti A, Mereu A, Bhugra D (2013) Trauma and stressor related disorders in the Tuareg refugees of a camp in Burkina Faso. Clin Pract Epidemiol Ment Health 9:189–195

Chandra P (2011) Mental health issues related to migration in women. In: Bhugra D, Gupta S (eds) Migration and mental health. Cambridge University Press, Cambridge, pp 209–219

Cochrane R (2001) Race, prejudice and ethnic identity. In: Bhugra D, Cochrane R (eds) Psychiatry in multi-cultural Britain. Gaskell, London, pp 75–90

De Jong J (2007) Traumascape: an ecological-cultural-historical model for extreme stress. In: Bhugra D, Bhui KS (eds) Textbook of cultural psychiatry. Cambridge University Press, Cambridge, pp 347–363

Dressler WW (1999) Modernization, stress and blood pressure: new directions in research. Hum Biol 71:583–605

Dressler WW (2007) Cultural consonance. In: Bhugra D, Bhui KS (eds) Textbook of cultural psychiatry. Cambridge University Press, Cambridge, pp 179–190

Eisenbruch M (1990) The cultural bereavement interview: a new clinical research approach for refugees. Psychiatr Clin N Am 13:715–735

Eisenbruch M (1991) From post-traumatic stress disorder to cultural bereavement: diagnosis of Southeast Asian refugees. Soc Sci Med 33:673–680

Elliott R, Sahakian B, Charney D (2010) The neural basis of resilience. In: Cooper C, Field J, Gorwami U, Jenkins R, Sahakian B (eds) Mental capital and well-being. Wiley-Blackwell, Chichester, pp 111–118

Furnham A, Bochner S (1986) Culture shock. Routledge, London

Harding J, Proshansky H, Kutner B, Chen I (1969) Prejudice and ethnic relations. In: Lindsey G, Aronson E (eds) The handbook of social psychology, vol 5. Addison-Wesley, Reading

Hofstede G (2000) Culture consequences. Sage, Thousand Oaks

Montgomery E (2011) Trauma, exile and mental health in young refugees. Acta Psychiatr Scand 440(Supp 1):1–44

Oberg K (1960) Culture shock, adjustment to new culture environments. Pract Anthropol 7:177–182

Pantelidou S, Craig TKJ (2006) Culture shock and social support: a survey of Greek migrant students. Soc Psychiatry Psychiatr Epidemiol 41(10):771–781

Rack P (1982) Race, culture and mental disorder. Tavistock, London

Ruiz P, Maggi C, Yusim A (2011) The impact of acculturative stress on the mental health of migrants. In: Bhugra D, Gupta S (eds) Migration and mental health. Cambridge University Press, Cambridge, pp 159–171

Sherif M, Sherif C (1956) An outline of social psychology. Harper & Row, New York

Smith EMJ (1985) Ethnic minorities: life stress, social support, and mental health issues. Couns Psychol 13:537–579

Tumarkin M (2005) Traumascapes: the power and fate of places transformed by tragedy. Melbourne University Press, Carlton

Witkin HA (1967) A cognitive-style approach to cross-cultural research. Int J Psychol 2:233–250

Witkin HA, Dyk RB, Faterson HF, Goodenough DR, Karp SA (1962) Psychological differentiation. Wiley, New York

Part II

Trauma and Migration: Diagnostic Issues

Clinical Diagnosis of Traumatised Immigrants

7

Ibrahim Özkan and Maria Belz

The effects of the multicultural reality of our society also appear in our work as clinical psychologists, psychotherapists and psychiatrists. The encounter with migrants seeking psychosocial help presents challenges not only during the treatment itself; even before therapy has begun, we may have to adjust our approach during the diagnostic process. The following chapter will discuss the challenges and particularities of diagnosing migrants with mental disorders.

Migratory Phenomena Affecting Mental Health

In order to understand the genesis and course of a mental health problem, it is essential to have a look at the biography of every patient. So-called "life events" are known to be a causal factor and as such, are crucial in the understanding of mental illness: "[…] it has been established that a cluster of social events requiring change in ongoing life adjustment is significantly associated with the time of illness onset" (Holmes and Rahe 1967, p. 213). Migration requires a pronounced ability to cope with these changes in daily life. Describing this phenomenon, Berry (2006, p. 294) introduces the term "acculturative stress": "[…] individuals experience change events in their lives that challenge their cultural understandings about how to live. […] In these situations, they come to understand that they are facing problems resulting from intercultural contact that cannot be dealt with easily or quickly by simply adjusting or assimilating to them". Sluzki (2001, cited in Czycholl 2009, p. 28) differentiates this concept by dividing migration into five different phases, each with their typical strains. Every phase contains specific tasks of adjustment

I. Özkan (✉) • M. Belz
Department for Cultures, Migration and Mental Disorders, Asklepios Fachklinikum Göttingen,
Rosdorfer Weg 70, Göttingen 37081, Germany
e-mail: i.oezkan@asklepios.com

© Springer International Publishing Switzerland 2015
M. Schouler-Ocak (ed.), *Trauma and Migration:*
Cultural Factors in the Diagnosis and Treatment of Traumatised Immigrants,
DOI 10.1007/978-3-319-17335-1_7

which the migrating person has to cope with. If the person has sufficient resources, he or she can pass through these without experiencing permanent, subjectively negative stress: "[…] most people deal with stressors and re-establish their lives rather well, with health, psychological and social outcomes that approximate those individuals in the larger society" (Berry 2006, p. 294). However, when these resources are missing (such as through pre-migratory mental health problems, a lack of social support, or unstable identity, i.e. of adolescents), migratory stress can cause mental health problems. Especially in the second phase after the overcompensation of one's nativity phase after arriving in the new host society (the "phase of decompensation"), the person's identity is challenged. This is the time when immigrants are highly vulnerable (Machleidt 2010), as the immigrant, and also future generations, is likely to experience ongoing rejection or discrimination regardless of his or her actual social integration, which is associated with mental health problems (Leong et al. 2013; Tummala-Narra and Claudius 2013). These findings point out the importance of migratory phenomena as two sided: social realities such as popular political currents, media reporting about immigrants or structural discrimination has a huge impact on the quantity of acculturative stress the individual experiences and therefore in the long run on his or her will to integrate into the host society. Berry (2006) makes a connection between a person's desire to have contact with the host society and/or his/her wish to conserve ties with his/her native cultural origins with the amount of acculturative stress the person experiences, describing integration (simultaneously having contact with the host society and maintaining links with their cultural origins) as the less stressful acculturation strategy.

When taking a person's history, migration, as a major life event, should be taken account of. Having insufficient possibilities to cope with acculturative stress can be a risk factor for mental health problems. Experiences of discrimination should be considered in particular.

Differences in Socialisation

When working with immigrants, professionals may encounter patients who seem to have been socialised in a different way. Several differences are reported in the literature, as discussed below (see also Özkan and Belz 2013). These descriptions should not be used as fixed, nation- or ethnicity-specific facts which apply to all members of the labelled group. Stereotypes should be avoided, as national or ethnic groups also show a high heterogeneity (Ebner 2010).

Parenting and Family Structure

Family structure and the role of different family members seem to be culturally influenced (Gün et al. 2010). The authors report that families from collectivistic contexts place more emphasis on the cohesion of the family than on individuals needs, while having clearly structured (hierarchic, paternalistic, gender- and generation-related) relationships between the family members. We observe these roles to be challenged by migration: children acquiring the host language and adapting more quickly to the new society gain more powerful positions in the family than their parents depending on how much help they receive. This loss of control can be a factor in the genesis of mental health problems in the parents. In other cases, this threat to the former role models can lead to the rigid conservation of the family structure, which can also impact on the children's health. We also observe extreme forms of parentification as being harmful for children as well as for parents. Von Wogau (2003, p. 69) describes the challenges to gender roles as being "impacted, for example, when spouses who work acquire power which may be contradictory to former family roles". Other authors describe differences in parenting behaviour, for example, self-control and social behaviour (Julian et al. 1994, cited in Rodriguez et al. 2006) or orientation to culture (Harrison et al. 1990 cited in Rodriguez et al. 2006). De Haan (2011) reports the interesting finding that after migration, the parenting behaviour of the culture of origin is neither preserved nor is it totally adapted to the parenting of the host society, indicating that a perspective fixed on nationality or ethnicity is not helpful in working with immigrants. Instead of stereotyped assumptions, we should have a closer look at the context of each family: "Each individual family has its own culture, spoken and unspoken rules, norms of behaviour, ideologies and myths – families have been construed as interpretive communities" (von Wogau 2003, p. 67). From this view, it is not surprising that studies looking for ethnic differences in parenting behaviour find more similarities than differences and observe other factors (maternal age, marriage status, socio-economic status) as being influential (Rodriguez et al. 2006). Earner and Rivera (2005, p. 532) give advice for our diagnostic praxis: "While newcomers tend to share many significant challenges, each family has unique needs depending on where they come from, how long they have been here, or what resources they can count on, among others. Generalisations and assumptions should be avoided in working with immigrant and refugee families".

Tradition

Brzoska and Razum (2009) see differences of rites, traditions and values compared to the majority population as influencing health behaviour. Few patients tell us about the use of traditional healers (i.e. Hoca). More often they report more common religious practices such as fasting (i.e. in Ramadan). This aspect should be considered during medical treatment by adapting the intake time of medicine if possible and needed.

Talking about tradition in the context of immigrants, we often observe negative connotations (i.e. by focussing on the way in which interethnic partnerships or divorce are dealt with, as well as on honour killings). Here there are two important aspects to be considered. First, tradition can mean an infinity of behavioural patterns and values. Traditions (i.e. religious practices, social support) can form an important resource to help the person cope with strain (Brzoska and Razum 2009).

Fassaert et al. (2011, p. 132) emphasise that "allowing migrants to preserve their traditions, might be effective measures in improving the mental well-being of migrants". Second, it is not possible to make generalisations. Regarding immigrants or single national or ethnic groups as homogeneous is inappropriate and causes false assumptions about the individual. Brzoska and Razum (2009) summarise that clinicians should not seek a fixed recipe, but rather a flexible approach which is detached from stereotypes and orientated towards individual needs.

Sense of Shame

The affects of shame and guilt are described as being culture specific. A distinction between shame cultures and guilt cultures is made (Benthien 2011). Güç (2010) postulates that these affects are used to regulate interpersonal relationships, with shame observed more commonly in Islamic cultures, expressing the collectivistic imprint.

Regarding the willingness to report traumatic experiences, shame seems to be a relevant factor. Ebner (2010) describes greater difficulty reporting intimate details among people with a heightened sense of shame when the experiences are connected to the honour or reputation of the family. According to Wenk-Ansohn (2004), such avoidance of disclosure increases with the extent of humiliation and shame associated with the event, while the definition of sexual abuse differs between traditions. In the case of woman who has been raped, she might conceal the event in order to avoid social exclusion due to a loss of honour. During diagnosis, this can result in the patient only reporting unspecific symptoms such as pain and a fragmentary biographical description.

Concepts of Illness

The understanding of the causes, appropriate treatment and prognosis of mental illness is culturally influenced (Dogan et al. 2009). Özkan (2010, p. 116) lists different types of causality beliefs:

- Magical religious causality: punishment by god and being bewitched
- Natural causality: illness caused by weather conditions
- Organic/medical causality: experiencing symptoms (pain)
- Relational causality: environmental problems like strain at work
- Emotional causality: affective conditions (loneliness, grief, lack of pleasure)
- Somatic causality: emotional events causing physical conditions, e.g. "my heart stopped"

Other authors also describe somatic (Ebner 2010) and magical religious causality (Brzoska and Razum 2009; Ebner 2010; Yildirim-Fahlbusch 2003). In this context it is important to remind the reader that differing concepts of illness are not migrant or culture specific. Concepts such as those listed by Özkan (2010) can also be observed in native patients. We recommend asking the patient about his or her concept of illness in the diagnostic phase, as illness-related beliefs have an enormous impact on their coping and compliance during therapy (Brzoska and Razum 2009). Knowledge about the patient's concept of illness also helps in interpreting the presented symptoms and in avoiding misinterpretations. According to Ebner (2010), a holistic concept (avoiding a perceived separation of body and soul or mind) results in somatic complaints being understood as being linked to psychosocial conflicts. Also, magical, religious causality beliefs could be misinterpreted as psychotic symptoms.

Somatisation

Somatisation is a phenomenon which is often reported as being specific to non-western cultures (Aichberger et al. 2008; Aragona et al. 2010; Lin et al. 1985). In practice, terms like "morbus mediterraneus", "morbus bosphorus" or "mamma mia syndrome" are still used. Kizilhan (2009) describes how a lack of knowledge about the human body and lower tolerance to psychological strain can result in somatic complaints such as widespread pain. He also lists culture-specific syndromes with their own aetiology and culture-specific way of treatment. In actual fact, the distinction between somatising and non-somatising cultures is outdated: "Contrary to the claim that non-Westerners are prone to somatise their distress, recent research confirms that somatisation is ubiquitous" (Kirmayer 2001, p. 22). Hausotter and Schouler-Ocak (2007, p.93) explain the reported somatic complaints as a "preverbal, body-related way of conflict resolution" due to interaction problems between patient and professional. These misunderstandings may result in diagnostic and therapeutic errors (Brucks and Wahl 2003; Kirmayer 2001). Kirmayer (2001) also reports that most patients who express their distress through a somatic complaint are nonetheless able to express psychosocial aspects when asked. He postulates: "Clinicians must learn to decode the meaning of somatic and dissociative symptoms, which are not simply indices of disease or disorder but part of a language of distress with interpersonal and wider social meanings" (p. 22). The consideration of psychological factors within the diagnostic process helps to avoid these errors. In cases of low language skills, the use of translators can help the patient to express their psychosocial strain. Overall, the assumption of somatising cultures and culture-specific syndromes is an inappropriate generalisation which should be avoided in order to ensure a qualitative, individualised diagnosis and treatment.

Expectations Towards the Professional

Due to different concepts of illness and region-specific experiences with mental health care, patients can approach therapy with differing expectations of the professional. Hausotter and Schouler-Ocak (2007) report that migrants often expect a focus on somatic complaints. Consequently, these patients may emphasise their somatic symptoms during diagnosis and neglect psychosocial complaints. In such case, it is crucial to give the patients a basic understanding of psychotherapy in order to enlarge the focus.

Franz et al. (2007) found higher rates of passiveness and delegation of personal responsibility to the professional among Turkish patients. In order to build a constructive therapeutic alliance, we recommend that such aspects are considered already early on in the diagnostic phase by asking the patients what they think could help them and what already does help them. These resources can be used later on in order to activate the patient.

Interaction with the Sick

The role of relatives and their interaction with the patient may also differ between cultures. Peseschkian (1998) notes a contrast between cultures where the patient is at the centre and many people pay visits in order to show solicitousness and cultures where the patient is told to rest and therefore receives few visits. Endrawes et al. (2007) find "a high sense of duty and obligation to maintain family ties and keep the family together despite the difficulties imposed by the illness of their relative" among Egyptian families. The role of relatives can be more important in working with migrants. In practice, patients are often accompanied by relatives who want to participate more actively in the consultations compared to the relatives of native patients. Colleagues often describe this as annoying. In our experience, however, the presence of a relative can also be used as a resource. In the diagnostic phase especially, relatives can be an important source of information. This third-party history can complete our diagnostic impression.

Refugees: Relevance of Trauma and Legal Issues

As well as experiencing acculturative stress, refugees are more likely to suffer other stressful life events. Before or during fleeing, they often experience situations of objectively or subjectively life-threatening stress such as war, torture, persecution or other forms of physical or sexual violence (Özkan 2004). Because of the "building block effect" (Neuner et al. 2004), which describes a highly positive correlation between the number of traumatic events and the development of PTSD, an increased prevalence of PTSD (Gaebel et al. 2005) and also of other mental health problems such as depression (Steel et al. 2009) is found among refugees. Many traumatised refugees suffer from more than one psychiatric disorder (Kessler et al. 1995). Some authors claim the need for extra categories of illness to describe the higher complexity and severity of symptoms (i.e. DESNOS, Teodorescu et al. 2012). Due to the ongoing stress while fleeing which can delay post-traumatic symptoms and destabilising factors in the host country, some refugees experience post-traumatic symptoms long after the initial traumatic event. The delayed onset of PTSD after months or years is not rare (Ziegenbein et al. 2008). Legal and political issues within the host country affect the patient's ability to recover and represent one of the main factors leading to chronification.

The length and the development of the asylum procedure particularly can have a harmful effect. The ongoing situation of insecurity hinders the possibility of recovery processes, preventing the person from distinguishing between the past insecurity which they might be re-experiencing in their flashbacks and the current, ideally secure situation. Symptoms of hyperarousal are also heightened by this ongoing psychosocial stress. Repeated forced confrontation in nontherapeutic situations (i.e. during interviews or trials during the asylum procedure) can induce dissociative symptoms leading to statements which are incomplete, lacking in detail or contradictory. The experience of not being believed (when a person has experienced "unbelievable things") can also have a tremendously negative impact on the person's ability to recover (i.e. by enforcing the avoidance).

Furthermore, the living conditions of asylum seekers have a large psychosocial impact. The accommodation in asylum centres means isolation from society. Persons without secure residential status are not allowed to visit a language course, reinforcing their isolation. Not having permission to work leads to a lack of daily structure, promoting depressive symptoms. All of these factors enhance a person's vulnerability to experiencing discrimination.

Many refugees suffer traumatisation in their country of origin and while fleeing. Psychosocial factors in the host country (e.g. living conditions and the asylum procedure) can have a harmful effect on the course of the disease.

Problems Related to Reduced Language Proficiency

Working with immigrants in Germany, we often encounter patients with no or very reduced knowledge of the German language. Of course, while treatment by a therapist speaking the same language as the patient would be the best choice in many cases, it is rarely available. Too often, this group of patients consequently stays without any psychiatric or psychotherapeutic treatment, while others are treated with medication only because a "talking therapy" is not possible due to the missing common language. Reduced possibilities for communication increase the risk of diagnostic errors such as under-diagnosing neurological symptoms: Searight and Armock (2013), for example, reported visual and acoustic flashbacks being interpreted as schizophrenic symptoms; such a situation can lead to medical malpractice (e.g. administering antipsychotics instead of trauma therapy). Drennan and Swartz (2002, cited in Searight and Armock 2013) report that less attention is paid in diagnostic settings to patients who do not speak the language of the professional. The use of translators, on the other hand, enables us to communicate with patients who do not speak our language – an option which is rarely used for multiple reasons.

Working with interpreters changes the therapeutic context. If he or she has little experience with it, the therapist can be unsettled by changes in the familiar therapist-patient setting due to the presence of a third party. Not understanding what is said in the other language or inexact translation of own words (Pugh and Vetere 2009) can mean a loss of control not only for therapists but also for patients. The loss of important information due to selective translation can also lead to under-diagnosing (such as of psychotic symptoms: see Abdallah-Steinkopff 1999; Marcos 1979, cited in

Searight and Armock 2013). Professionals can also feel observed and judged by the third person and thus unable to act as he or she would do in other therapist-patient interactions. The presence of translators can change the dynamics between professional and patient (Pugh and Vetere 2009). When a strong relationship is observed between patient and translator, the therapist can perceive the translator as competition (Abdallah-Steinkopff 1999).

These difficulties can be prevented through the use of translators who are trained for and experienced in the psychotherapeutic setting. Searight and Armock (2013, p. 9) reason in their review that "mental health interpretation can be reasonably accurate with adequate interpreter training". When translators are trained to be accurate (Searight and Armock 2013) and know about their role within the diagnostic context (Trivasse 2006; Wright 2014), their involvement enables us to communicate in a trouble-free manner with the patient and to make good diagnostic decisions: "The interview, itself, is the main diagnostic tool for mental health assessment, which makes accurate interpretation particularly important in this context" (Searight and Armock 2013; p. 23).

Reduced language proficiency is often an obstacle in the mental health care of immigrants. The use of translators can enable communication between professional and patients. The translator should be trained for the psychotherapeutic setting.

Use of Psychometric Measures

Psychometric measures are frequently used in psychological diagnostics. Being standardised, they can improve the quality of the diagnostic process. Because of the need of objectivity, however, they should never be used in isolation without taking a proper history. Self-assessment tools give the patient the opportunity to report symptoms without having to announce them out loud. This can be helpful when dealing with shame-related experiences and symptoms (e.g. traumatic events, sexual matters, psychotic symptoms, substance abuse, self-injury).

Despite the reported advantages, the use of psycho-diagnostic instruments is disputed. Given that they are often based on western concepts and categories (i.e. DSM-IV or ICD-10), their validity for other cultures is often doubtful (Denis 2004). Also, the translations of these instruments are rarely validated for the specific population regarding linguistic and epidemiologic factors (Ebner 2010). Standard values are often only available for western populations (Denis 2004). Especially for migrants who have already been living abroad for decades, the applicability of instruments which are translated and validated for the current population of their country of origin should not be assumed.

Professionals should always bear in mind that depending on the social background of the patient, the likelihood of illiteracy may be increased. Since this can be a shame-associated subject, the patient may not report their illiteracy when asked to fill out a questionnaire and may answer the items in a random way.

The use of psychometric measures is a helpful addition to the exploration and formation of a clinical impression. However, a lack of validation often limits their benefit in diagnostics with immigrants.

What Do Professionals Need? A Critical View of the Term "Intercultural Competence"

When working with immigrants, professionals often see themselves as being faced with specific challenges. If they focus more on differences and have stereotyped assumptions about the immigrant, their own uncertainty increases and they may recommend that they are treated by professionals who are "competent" to work with "this kind of patient". Due to the lack of transculturally specialised professionals, however, these patients often remain untreated. Even if they are able to access transcultural treatment, this means yet another segregation.

In order to address this conflict, we must examine the term of cultural or intercultural competence further. Although the literature contains far-reaching definitions (see, e.g. Betancourt et al. 2002; Chen and Starosta 2003) including aspects of knowledge, awareness, motivation and behavioural skills, in practice, the widespread concept of competence focuses only on knowledge about cultural specificities and behavioural skills. Also, language competency is often assumed to be crucial. The essence of this lay understanding is that a "competent" professional knows how to treat "the immigrant". The utopian essence of this assumption is rarely conscious.

Immigrants as well as single national or ethnic groups are heterogeneous. The diversity approach (e.g. van Keuk et al. 2011) names criteria under which individuals can differ, including age, gender, sexual orientation, disability, religion and sociocultural background. The idea of "competence" as defined above is based upon the culturalised assumption of the homogeneity of an in-group as well as strong cultural differences between the patient and the professional. The "competent" professional is supposed to have canned knowledge about the right treatment for the patient based on his or her culture of origin, while the individuality of the patient stays disregarded.

The ability to provide treatment of an equal standard to immigrants and natives requires more than formalised knowledge. Professionals need to possess an attitude of awareness about possible differences without using stereotyped and culturalised assumptions. Own cultural imprints should be reflected upon in order to avoid ethnocentric attitudes. Reducing one's own perception of the other as being strange helps to minimise uncertainty and stress which may occur on the part of the professional within the treatment interaction.

References

Abdallah-Steinkopff B (1999) Psychotherapie bei Posttraumatischer Belastungsstörung unter Mitwirkung von Dolmetschern. Verhaltenstherapie 9:211–220

Aichberger MC, Schouler-Ocak M, Rapp MA, Heinz A (2008) Transkulturelle Aspekte der Depression. Bundesgesundheitsbl Gesundheitsforsch Gesundheitsschutz 51:436–442

Aragona M, Catino E, Pucci D, Carrer S, Colosimo F, Lafuente M, Mazzetti M, Maisano B, Geraci S (2010) The relationship between somatization and posttraumatic symptoms among immigrants receiving primary care services. J Trauma Stress 23:615–622

Benthien C (2011) Tribunal der Blicke. Kulturtheorien von Scham und Schuld und die Tragödie um 1800. Böhlau, Köln

Berry JW (2006) Acculturative stress. In: Wong PTP, Wong LCJ (eds) Handbook of multicultural perspectives on stress and coping. Springer, Dallas, pp 287–298

Betancourt J, Green A, Carrillo E (2002) Cultural competence in health care: emerging frameworks and practical approaches. The Commonwealth Fund. Available at: http://www.commonwealthfund.org/~/media/Files/Publications/Fund%20Report/2002/Oct/Cultural%20Competence%20in%20Health%20Care%20%20Emerging%20Frameworks%20and%20Practical%20Approaches/betancourt_culturalcompetence_576%20pdf.pdf. Accessed 15 Apr 2014

Brucks U, Wahl WB (2003) Über-, Unter Fehlversorgung? Bedarfslücken und Strukturprobleme in der ambulanten Gesundheitsversorgung von Migrantinnen und Migranten. In: Borde T, Matthias D (eds) Gut versorgt? Mabuse-Verlag, Frankfurt am Main, pp 15–33

Brzoska P, Razum O (2009) Krankheitsbewältigung bei Menschen mit Migrationshintergrund im Kontext von Kultur und Religion. Z Med Psychol 18(3–4):151–161

Chen G-M, Starosta WJ (2003) Intercultural awareness. In: Samovar LA, Porter RE (eds) Intercultural communication: a reader. Wadsworth, Belmont, pp 344–354

Czycholl D (2009) Chapter 6. Prozesse interkultureller Öffnung in der Altenhilfe. In: Schaefer J-E (ed) Alter und Migration. Mabuse Verlag, Tübingen

De Haan M (2011) The reconstruction of parenting after migration: a perspective from cultural translation. Hum Dev 54(6):376–399

Denis D (2004) Standardisierte Diagnostik bei der Begutachtung psychisch reaktiver Traumafolgen in aufenthaltsrechtlichen Verfahren. In: Haenel F, Wenk-Ansohn M (eds) Begutachtung psychisch reaktiver Traumafolgen in aufenthaltsrechtlichen Verfahren. Beltz, Weinheim, pp 98–126

Dogan D, Tschudin V, Hot I, Özkan I (2009) Patients' transcultural needs and carers' ethical responses. Nurs Ethics 16(6):683–696

Earner I, Rivera H (2005) What do we know about immigrant and refugee families and children? Child Welf: J Policy Pract Program 84(5):532–536

Ebner G (2010) Psychiatrische Begutachtung von Migrantinnen und Migranten. In: Hegemann T, Salman R (eds) Handbuch Transkulturelle Psychiatrie. Psychiatrie Verlag, Bonn, pp 216–241

Endrawes G, O'Brien L, Wilkes L (2007) Egyptian families caring for a relative with mental illness: a hermeneutic study. Int J Ment Health Nurs 16(6):431–440

Fassaert T, de Wit MS, Tuinebreijer WC, Knipscheer JW, Verhoeff AP, Beekman AF, Dekker J (2011) Acculturation and psychological distress among non-western Muslim migrants—a population-based survey. Int J Soc Psychiatry 57(2):132–143

Franz M, Liujić C, Koch E, Wüsten B, Yürük N, Gallhofer B (2007) Subjektive Krankheitskonzepte türkischer Migranten mit psychischen Störungen – Besonderheiten im Vergleich zu deutschen Patienten. Psychiatr Prax 34:332–338

Gaebel U, Ruf M, Schauer M, Odenwald M, Neuner F (2005) Prävalenz der Posttraumatischen Belastungsstörung (PTSD) und Möglichkeiten der Ermittlung in der Asylverfahrenspraxis. Z Klin Psychol Psychiatr Psychother 35:12–20

Güç F (2010) Dissoziation und Schuld-Scham-Affekte in der Behandlung von Migranten aus islamischen Ländern. Psychother Dialog 4:313–318

Gün AK, Toker M, Senf W (2010) … keine Lust, meinem deutschen Therapeuten zu erklären, dass ich kein Pascha bin. … Ali Kemal Gün und Mehmet Toker im Gespräch mit Wolfgang Senf. Psychother Dialog 4:352–356

Hausotter W, Schouler-Ocak M (2007) Begutachtung bei Menschen mit Migrationshintergrund. Elsevier, München

Holmes TH, Rahe RH (1967) The social readjustment rating scale. J Psychosom Res 11(2):213–218

Kessler RC, Sonnega A, Bromet E, Hughes M, Nelson CB (1995) Posttraumatic stress disorder in the National Comorbidity Survey. Arch Gen Psychiatry 52:1048–1060

Kirmayer LJ (2001) Cultural variations in the clinical presentation of depression and anxiety: implications for diagnosis and treatment. J Clin Psychiatry 62:22–28

Kizilhan J (2009) Interkulturelle Aspekte bei der Behandlung somatoformer Störungen. Psychotherapeut 54(4):281–288

Leong F, Park Y, Kalibatseva Z (2013) Disentangling immigrant status in mental health: psychological protective and risk factors among Latino and Asian American immigrants. Am J Orthopsychiatry 83(2,3):361–371

Lin E, Carter W, Kleinman A (1985) An exploration of somatization among Asian refugees and immigrants in primary care. Am J Public Health 75(9):1080–1084

Machleidt W (2010) Theoretische Modelle der Migration. Sozialpsychiatrische Informationen 40(4):17–20

Neuner F, Schauer M, Karunakara U, Klaschik C, Robert C, Elbert T (2004) Psychological trauma and evidence for enhanced vulnerability for PTSD through previous trauma in West Nile refugees. BMC Psychiatry 4(1):34

Özkan I (2004) Praxisansätze und Grenzen der traumazentrierten Arbeit mit ethnischen Minoritäten. In: Sachsse U (ed) Traumazentrierte Psychotherapie: Theorie, Klinik und Praxis. Schattauer, Stuttgart, pp 394–400

Özkan I (2010) Krebs und Migration: Interkulturelle Sensibilisierung für die psychoonkologische Arbeit. In: Diegelmann C, Isermann M (eds) Ressourcenorientierte Psychoonkologie. Kohlhammer, Stuttgart, pp 113–120

Özkan I, Belz M (2013) Kultursensibles Vorgehen in der Diagnostik. In: Sack M, Sachsse U, Schellong J (eds) Komplexe Traumafolgestörungen. Schattauer, Stuttgart, pp 144–148

Peseschkian N (1998) Die Notwendigkeit eines transkulturellen Austausches. Dargestellt am transkulturellen Aspekt der Positiven Psychotherapie. In: Heise T (ed) Transkulturelle Psychotherapie. Hilfen im ärztlichen und therapeutischen Umgang mit ausländischen Mitbürgern. VWB – Verlag für Wissenschaft und Bildung, Berlin, pp 195–210

Pugh M, Vetere A (2009) Lost in translation: an interpretative phenomenological analysis of mental health professionals' experiences of empathy in clinical work with an interpreter. Psychol Psychother Theory Res Pract 82(3):305–321

Rodríguez MC, Davis M, Rodriguez J, Bates S (2006) Observed parenting practices of first-generation Latino families. J Community Psychol 34(2):133–148

Searight H, Armock JA (2013) Foreign language interpreters in mental health: a literature review and research agenda. N Am J Psychol 15(1):17–38

Steel Z, Chey T, Silove D, Marnane C, Bryant RA, van Ommeren M (2009) Association of torture and other potentially traumatic events with mental health outcomes among populations exposed to mass conflict and displacement: a systematic review and meta-analysis. JAMA 302(5):537–549

Teodorescu DS, Heir T, Hauff E, Wentzel-Larsen T, Lien L (2012) Mental health problems and post-migration stress among multi-traumatized refugees attending outpatient clinics upon resettlement to Norway. Scand J Psychol 53(4):316–332

Trivasse M (2006) A question of interpretation. Healthc Couns Psychother J 6(3):15–17

Tummala-Narra P, Claudius M (2013) Perceived discrimination and depressive symptoms among immigrant-origin adolescents. Cult Divers Ethn Minor Psychol 19(3):257–269

van Keuk, E., Ghaderi, C. Joksimovic, L. & David, D.M. (eds.) (2010) Diversity-Transkulturelle Kompetenz in klinischen und sozialen Arbeitsfeldern. Stuttgart: Kohlhammer

Von Wogau JR (2003) Looking through a cultural lens: Interkulturelle Kompetenz in den verschiedenen Phasen der Therapie. Systeme 17:66–83

Wenk-Ansohn M (2004) Frauenspezifische Aspekte in der interkulturellen Begutachtung. In: Haenel F, Wenk-Ansohn M (eds) Begutachtung psychisch reaktiver Traumafolgen in aufenthaltsrechtlichen Verfahren. Beltz, Weinheim, pp 160–183

Wright CL (2014) Ethical issues and potential solutions surrounding the use of spoken language interpreters in psychology. Ethics Behav 24(3):215–228

Yildirim-Fahlbusch Y (2003) Türkische Migranten: Kulturelle Missverständnisse. Deut Ärzteblatt 18:993–995

Ziegenbein M, Machleidt W, Calliess IT (2008) Psychiatrische Begutachtung im interkulturellen Feld. In: Golsabahi S, Heise T (eds) Von Gemeinsamkeiten und Unterschieden. VWB, Berlin, pp 213–224

Special Problems in the Assessment of Psychological Sequelae of Torture and Incarceration

8

Ferdinand Haenel

Introduction

Since the diagnosis of the event-related post-traumatic mental disorder – so-called traumatic neurosis – was introduced by Berlin neurologist Hermann Oppenheim in 1889, a great dispute divided German neurologists into two groups. One of these groups was of the opinion that the symptoms of the traumatic neurosis were being misused in order to gain advantages, while the neurologists of the opposing opinion believed it to be a real disease caused by life-threatening events such as train accidents or wartime experiences (Oppenheim 1889; Fischer-Homberger 2004).

From 1883 onwards, the gradual adoption of Otto von Bismarck's social laws that included work accident and invalidity insurances, coupled with growing militarisation and the tense political situation in Europe on the verge of World War I, formed the historical and sociopolitical background of this debate which at times was conducted extremely fiercely and polemically and which seems to continue even today.

Concerning the practice of psychiatric assessment of survivors of National Socialist concentration camps due to the *Bundesentschädigungsgesetz,*[1] for instance, it was revealed that a great amount of German psychiatrists, some of whom were involved themselves in the crimes committed within German psychiatry in the Third Reich, assessed event-caused mental sequelae among concentration camp prisoners as inherited or as a result of circumstances that dated back to before their internment (Pross 1993; Goltermann 2009). In return, however, there were numerous

---

[1] Federal compensation law for Jewish holocaust survivors.

F. Haenel
Facharzt für Psychiatrie und Psychotherapie, Leiter der Tagesklinik, Behandlungszentrum für Folteropfer, Klinik für Psychiatrie und Psychotherapie, Charité – Campus Mitte, Turmstr. 21, 10559 Berlin, Germany
e-mail: f.haenel@bzfo.de
http://www.bzfo.de

© Springer International Publishing Switzerland 2015
M. Schouler-Ocak (ed.), *Trauma and Migration:*
Cultural Factors in the Diagnosis and Treatment of Traumatised Immigrants,
DOI 10.1007/978-3-319-17335-1_8

psychiatrists of the opposite opinion, including W. G. Niederland, U. Venzlaff, W. v. Baeyer, H. Häfner, K. Kisker, K. Hoppe and K. Eissler; research by these scientists has made crucial contributions to our present knowledge about the sequelae of event-caused mental traumata (v. Baeyer et al. 1964; Hoppe 1967; Niederland 1968; Venzlaff 1963). At that time, too, a polemical and extremely polarised dispute had arisen between the colleagues. The title that Kurt Eissler chose for a publication in the magazine "Psyche" concerning this topic speaks volumes: "Die Ermordung von wievielen seiner Kinder muß ein Mensch symptomfrei ertragen können, um eine normale psychische Konstitution zu haben?"[2] (Eissler 1958).

In the practice of assessment in the 1990s, there was particularly strong divergence concerning the clinical psychotraumatological assessment of former political detainees of the German Democratic Republic due to the *Strafrechtliche Rehabilitierungsgesetz*[3] (Denis et al. 2000; Haenel 1998), as too was the case with the clinical assessment of Bosnian war refugees (Henningsen 2003).

The question arises as to what are the special causes that lead to such great divergence in psychotraumatological assessments. The following are decisive factors:

- Symptom-based causes
- Trauma-specific relational aspects
- Comorbidities that can superimpose specific symptoms of PTSD
- Difficulties resulting from the differentiation between damage-related and damage-unrelated disorders
- Linguistic and cultural difficulties in procedures on asylum and residence legislation
- Deficient knowledge in asylum and residence legislation

Symptom-Related Characteristics in the Assessment of Psychologically Reactive Sequelae of Trauma

The definitions of post-traumatic stress disorder (PTSD) and personality changes after extreme traumata as defined in DSM-IV (APA 1994) and ICD-10 (WHO 1992) include aspects that can essentially influence the assessor's exploration of symptoms. Accordingly, intense strain on the psyche culminating in physical vegetative reactions is typical for people suffering from PTSD when being confronted with inner or outer stimuli that symbolise an aspect or association of the traumatic experience. As a result, thoughts, feelings or conversations related to the trauma as well as activities, places or persons that evoke traumatic memories are purposely avoided. This avoidance can lead to an inability to recall certain aspects of the trauma.

---

[2] "How many murders of his own children does a man have to bear without showing any symptoms in order to have a normal mental constitution?"

[3] Reparation of SED Injustices Act.

Further symptoms of a similar type that interfere with the assessor's exploration are listed in the table below. They are additionally listed as partial symptoms in the definition of PTSD in the American Psychiatric Association's DSM-IV:

C-1 efforts to avoid thoughts, feelings or conversations associated with the trauma
C-2 efforts to avoid activities, places or people that arouse recollections of the trauma
C-3 inability to recall an important aspect of the trauma
C-4 markedly diminished interest or participation in significant activities
C-5 feelings of detachment or estrangement from others
C-6 restricted range of affect (e.g. unable to have loving feelings)
D-2 irritability or outbursts of anger
D-3 difficulty concentrating

In addition to these partial symptoms of PTSD in DSM-IV, feelings of shame, blame, guilt, fear, horror and anger, all of which can also serve as obstacles to the exploration, are listed as partial symptoms of PTSD in DSM-5 (APA 2014).

It becomes clear (even from the non-medical perspective) that these symptoms are an obstacle to medical exploration and diagnosis. The assessment of victims of torture with psychological sequelae differs radically from the assessment of patients who suffer from other psychiatric disorders. The decisive difference between the assessment of survivors of torture with mental sequelae and the assessment of persons with other mental disorders is that in survivors of torture, it is the symptomatology itself which can hinder exploration and thus lead to errors. This is by no means a new discovery, but a phenomenon known from studies on the reactive mental sequelae seen in victims of the National Socialist concentration camps ("Abkapselung extremtraumatischer Erfahrungen von der Umwelt, weil sie nicht kommunizierbar sind", "Widerstand gegen die Exploration"[4] (von Baeyer et al. 1964)).

The clinical pictures of this latter group of traumatised victims would – following the present diagnostic classification in ICD-10 – most likely be defined as "Enduring personality change after catastrophic experience" as F62.0. Here as well one can find symptoms that oppose the exploration:

Hostile or distrustful attitude towards the world
Social withdrawal
Feelings of emptiness or hopelessness
A chronic feeling of "being on edge" as if constantly threatened
Estrangement

Feelings of shame and guilt are not represented as partial symptoms in the definitions of the diagnoses of PTSD in DSM-IV and personality change, but are now included in DSM-5. In our context they must be especially accentuated, for

---

[4] Splitting off of extremely traumatic experiences from the environment because they cannot be communicated; resistance to exploration.

we will never come to know the real number of victims who choose to remain silent for this reason – consider especially the victims of sexual abuse (Wenk-Ansohn 2002).

Case 1 of Mr. C. from South-East Anatolia/Turkey[5] Mr. C. is a Kurdish farmer from Turkey. He comes from south-east Anatolia and has been living for 2 years in Germany as an asylum seeker. He complained about having trouble sleeping and concentrating, as well as about anxiety, nightmares, general anhedonia and a lack of vitality. He reported that he had fled to Germany in the early summer of 1995 after having been detained, interrogated and tortured by the Turkish police for about 20 days over each of the previous 2 years and that it was likely that he would have been arrested and tortured again in the future. As the owner of an isolated farmhouse 4 km from the nearest village, he had been suspected of providing members of the PKK with food. The first time he was arrested, the military police had burned down his house and forced the whole family to move to the next village.

When I asked him what form of torture he had undergone, Mr. C. answered that he had been beaten with clubs over his whole body, had the soles of his feet beaten (Falanga), had been hosed down with pressurised cold water while naked, had been subjected to electric shocks and had been kept in solitary confinement without sufficient food.

At 44, Mr. C. had aged prematurely. His manner at the interview was pleasant. Initially somewhat reserved and speaking quietly but hurriedly, he modestly did his best to answer all questions as quickly as possible. However, at the same time he appeared breathless and agitated, and this became worse when he began to tell the story of his persecution. He was sweating profusely. He started to mix up details and the chronological order of events, which confused the interpreter; as an examiner, I began to doubt the authenticity of his story. When I asked him to repeat the contradictory information, at the same time assuring him that we had plenty of time for the interview, he was able to rectify the jumbled order of events in his report, reassembling them into a more plausible and comprehensible whole. His basic mood was depressed. He showed evidence of emotional rigidity. Outwardly his drive appeared reduced, while inwardly he showed clear signs of increased arousal. When I made a hand movement that he had evidently not expected during the physical examination, he started and involuntarily shrank back. At the physical examination I noticed a large number of small scars spread across his back for which he was unable to account. He also had a roughly 2.5-in.-long, sickle-shaped scar on his left shoulder. He reported that this had been caused by a blow with the butt of a gun during his first term of imprisonment. It had been treated in a makeshift manner with a few large stitches. A second, very obvious scar that ran across the inside of his right thigh, around 2 in. long and 1 in. wide, was below the surface of the skin and showed no signs of surgical stitches; this he

---

[5] The abbreviations of names and places in this, as in the following case history, have been changed. When not affecting the political context, locations and time specifications have been left out completely.

attributed to an untreated stabbing during his second period of imprisonment. He reported that from time to time the soles of his feet became painful after he had been walking for some time. The balls of his feet were soft and could be easily depressed onto the underlying bones. When he walked, he placed his feet flat on the ground, failing to place his heels down first and roll forward on to his toes. This is an indication that he was subjected to torture by "Falanga", i.e. blows to the feet (Skylv 1993).

At the second and third case history interviews, the dissociation of events and their chronological sequencing were repeated in the same way as during the first interview, and again, like during the first interview, Mr. C. was able to piece them together again and add further details when I took time to put my questions patiently and calmly. Despite the fact that Mr. C. shifted his perspective on the events and actions several times, in the end his report was free of contradictions.

Towards the end of the third interview, when Mr. C. was persuaded to describe an aspect of a certain event in greater detail and to tell me at what time of the day he had been arrested the second time and which family members had been present, he broke down in tears.

All sources of information on the political situation in eastern Anatolia (Amnesty International, the German Foreign Office, press reports and coinciding reports from other persons subject to persecution in the same region) are in agreement that in the civil war between Turkey and the PKK, pressure is being exerted on the rural population either to join the so-called village guard system organised by the Turkish authorities or to provide the PKK with medical aid, food and logistic support. It is not possible for people living in rural areas to retain a neutral position between these two strongly opposed forces. "Attacks carried out against uninvolved parties by the security forces in the form of destruction of property, detention, physical or psychological abuse or homicide are widespread in this region" (German Foreign Office 1994, 1995).

Together with what we know about the political situation in this region, Mr. C.'s history and his mental and physical status indicated with almost absolute certainty that the information he had given in his application for asylum was correct. However, this clarity was only apparent to us, evidently to the Federal Office for the Recognition of Asylum – Mr. C.'s application was rejected. According to the minutes of the hearing, an event which torture victims often associate emotionally with the interrogations to which they have been subjected under torture in their own countries, Mr. C. had been given exactly 1 h to present his reasons for applying for asylum, with the aid of an interpreter.

This was a requirement with which Mr. C. was unable to comply in his current mental condition.[6]

---

[6] By the time of the examination, Mr. C's application for asylum had already been rejected by the Administrative Court. The described diagnostic findings of the author were then declared as new findings and so far unconsidered evidence by another Administrative Court of Appeal that justifies a subsequent asylum procedure.

Dissociative Symptoms of Complex PTSD

Mental sequelae of torture and incarceration are usually connected with dissociative symptoms of differing severity. By definition, the main characteristic of dissociation is the disruption of the integrative functions of consciousness, memory, identity or perception of environment (APA 1994; WHO 1992). Accordingly the intrusive symptomatology – including uncontrollable, sequential reliving of extreme traumatic events experienced in the past, either by day or by night in the form of nightmares, as well as acting or feeling as if the traumatic event was recurring in the presence with flashback episodes – can be regarded as a dissociative symptomatology. Likewise, the inability to recall an important aspect of the trauma (symptom C3 in DSM-IV or D1 in DSM-5) is seen as dissociative amnesia.

Dissociative phenomena are widespread; even mentally healthy people can be affected. The phenomena are to be viewed as concomitant symptoms in the entire psychopathological spectrum, similar to fever with somatic diseases. Severe, complex and chronic PTSD with a distinct degree of dissociative symptoms can cause complaints similar to a chronic schizophrenia (Haenel et al. 2000).

According to the definitions of DSM and ICD, an existing, partly dissociative disease such as schizophrenia or PTSD excludes the diagnosis of a dissociative disorder. Nevertheless, especially for complex sequelae of traumata, dissociative symptoms can exceed the degree of PTSD by far and create special difficulties during assessment, as shown in the following example.

Case 2 of Mr. Z. Kurdish, Male, from Turkey Mr. Z., a bright, conscious man who appeared rather young for his 27 years, arrived for the assessment accompanied by a fellow countryman. During the examination, it was revealed that he had not been fully informed about the assessment's purpose. He had merely been told that there was a doctor he was supposed to go to.

As regards this person, he showed normal awareness, but concerning the time, however, he appeared disorientated. He falsely believed the current date to be 1 day in the future. Initially Mr. Z. seemed cautious, somewhat sceptical, reserved, tense and self-controlled. He asked the interpreter spontaneously to repeat every question from the assessor twice, and when asked about this, he explained that he was tremendously excited and "fear was coming up". Every time when he was asked about his past, he stated, memories of his incarceration in Karakol (police prison) would come up. At first, Mr. Z. focused his eyes predominantly on the interpreter and only addressed the assessor indirectly, e.g. by starting his answers with "Please tell him…" or "Ask him if he knows the feeling of leaving his parents and siblings".

Mr. Z. behaved in a self-controlled manner and appeared somewhat helpless and anxious, distrustful and limited in emotions. At some points of his story however, such as when he was talking about his mother, he was temporarily unable to control his emotions and burst into tears. Throughout the assessment, Mr. Z. repeatedly asked to be questioned as little as possible about his antecedent family as well as his persecution and incarceration in Karakol because he would "lose" himself in the memories it triggered, as he stated.

Moreover, some questions had to be repeated because of Mr. Z.'s occasional mental absence. Later, when he had finally exposed many chapters of his story of persecution, he absent-mindedly stared into space for minutes and was retracted through being addressing continually.

His syntax and formal chain of thoughts were structured in a simple way, as the interpreter stated.

Sometimes, however, he said seemingly incomprehensible sentences that were only to be understood from the context, e.g. "I am after my bread" which meant that he was only living in the mountains for financial and not for political reasons.

Cognitive dysfunction, delusion and hallucination as signs of a psychotic genesis were not to be found, neither in the case history nor the present. Consistently, a light subliminal agitation and increased vegetative arousal could be observed.

What is significant in Mr. Z.'s case history is the difficulty of the assessment because of his dissociative states that occurred as soon as the examination was focused on possible traumatic experiences. As a result, the assessor was repeatedly forced to return to the exploration of less burdensome and more positive aspects of his biography. Such dissociative phenomena which were accompanied by an agitation and affective tenseness recurred several times when Mr. Z. was questioned about experiences of his incarceration.

For the assessor, who needs as much information as possible in a limited time frame, these dissociative phenomena can lead to significant difficulties in carrying out the assessment: if assessors behave too cautiously towards the patient, they might not be able to get a complete idea of the patient's history, and the contracting authority might accuse him or her of a deficient examination. If he or she is too brisk, however, the patient might fall into a dissociative state which can last for an extended period of time. During such "flashbacks", patients can scenically relive the trauma of their torture, thereby, for instance, sliding from their chair onto the floor, covering their head with their arms and hands and crying and begging to stop beating them. In this case, when the patient apparently misjudges the assessor and interpreter to be torturers, a stabilising therapeutic intervention becomes necessary, and the assessment must be interrupted.

Assessors are held between these two extremes, as is every therapist who works with victims of civil war or torture. Nevertheless, they must conduct the exploration within a limited time frame and conclude on a clear and decided statement, which requires a high level of experience and expertise. Contrariwise, however, it often is the dissociative states reproduced during the examination which exceed the subjective information given by the victim and enable the assessor to make an objective diagnosis of PTSD (Herman 1994). Additionally, the thematic context in which such dissociative phenomena occur during the assessment can give evidence of the type of traumatic experience. Most importantly, these phenomena as well as any other symptoms that hinder the assessment should be documented precisely and in detail as examination findings and later be included in the discussion and evaluation in a comprehensible way.

Trauma-Specific Aspects of Transference and Countertransference

In addition to the difficulties in concentrating and the memory decline around fundamental aspects of the traumatic experiences, both of which frequently present themselves in victims of torture, it should be taken into account that asylum seekers who have been interrogated and tortured in their home country can emotionally connect past inquisitions under torture to the current hearing at the *Bundesamt für Anerkennung ausländischer Flüchtlinge*.[7] Expressed in psychoanalytic terms, the interviewer of the Federal Office would be in a specific transference, namely, in the transference of the perpetrator. According to the behavioural therapeutic model, the situation of the hearing would represent a stimulus that is associatively linked to an aspect of traumatic experiences and that can excite intensive psychological stress and even physically vegetative reactions. This can ostensibly cause two entirely contrary psychological manifestations: either anxious agitation, excitation and affective tension or lack of emotions, avolition and taciturnity. At such moments, which can occur during hearings and examinations conducted by the Federal Office, the traumatised applicants are usually unable to describe their history consistently, directly and accurately as demanded by the Federal Office.

While on the one hand the reactive mental symptoms themselves can be an obstacle to an objective medicolegal evaluation, on the other hand assessors' attitudes towards the survivor of torture and his or her history may also be a hindrance to objective appraisal and evaluation. As in psychotherapy with survivors of torture and persecuted persons (Lansen 1993; Wilson and Lindy 1994; Haenel 2000), widely divergent attitudes and countertransferences, from too great a distance and a lack of empathy to too little a distance and too much empathy and over-identification, and even personal empathic enmeshment with the survivor may all occur in the relationship between an assessor and the person under assessment (Hoppe 1967).

An assessor may thus show too great a distance and too little empathy if he or she is insufficiently informed about the psychological sequelae of trauma, the political and historical facts or the conditions of imprisonment in the survivor's country of origin. This may also occur if the assessors, based on their own experience of life and their image of a fundamentally harmonious world, consider the survivor's reports to be exaggerated and implausible (Wilson and Lindy 1994). From the perspective of the survivor, the assessor then assumes a characteristic of the past perpetrator when he or she also seems to deny or ignore what has happened. This kind of relationship is responsible for the frequently observed resignation and reserve of survivors in exploratory interviews, which frequently lead assessors incorrectly to assume that they have no trauma-induced mental symptoms at all or that these are only mild. This lack of recognition is a renewed injury to the survivor, and a time-consuming and expensive chain of appeals across all instances of the administrative system and courts may result.

---

[7] Federal Office for the Recognition of Foreign Refugees.

Conversely, too little distance and too much empathy may develop in an assessor as a defence against his or her own feelings of guilt and shame (Hoppe 1967). Assessors may also react in this way to the emotional shock and horror felt on hearing survivors' descriptions of their traumatic experiences or to an unconscious fear that the survivor will associate or even equate him or her with the perpetrator. This can lead to an exaggerated, overly involved, militant desire to help the survivor, which, if it remains unexamined, leads the assessor to submit non-objective, global and polemic arguments to colleagues and authorities.

Psychiatric expertise and knowledge of the political and historical background of survivors' countries of origin are therefore necessary but not sufficient requirements for the evaluation of their psychological sequelae. Assessors must, as in psychotherapy, possess the ability to assume a position midway between the extreme countertransference poles of too great and too little distance, which can be described as "the greatest possible empathy combined with the greatest possible distance" (Lansen 1996) or "controlled identification" (Hoppe 1967).

Assessors must also take into account the substantial resistance that posttraumatic psychological symptoms can present to assessment. Examiners must be prepared to take time and exercise patience to deal with disturbances in concentration and to sense intuitively when a person has buried memories of severe traumatic experiences. They must counter the survivors' withdrawal and isolation tendencies, their mistrust of the world and their frequent general attitude of passive resignation with an active willingness to engage in and interest for their stories and fate and for the specific meanings of the trauma in their lives as a whole.

Distinction from Other Psychiatric Disorders

The distinction of trauma-related disorders from disorders of other types, e.g. those with psychoneurotic genesis, poses a challenge for psychotraumatological assessment, especially since PTSD is only one specific psychological consequence of trauma, among many others. Anxiety, depressive, somatoform, dissociative, borderline and addictive disorders may all occur as non-specific sequelae of trauma disorders (Kessler et al. 1995; Flatten et al. 2004). Additionally, patients with existential life-threatening traumata are not only at risk of developing further psychological disorders, but also of experiencing a variety of other somatic disorders in old age (Glaesmer et al. 2011). In such cases, assessment can thereby be considerably complicated if the specific psychotraumatological symptom characteristics have declined or disappeared.

However, it must be noted that – possibly as a result of decades of ignorance and even denial of event-related disorders in medical history – traumatic experiences are sometimes overestimated in terms of their relevance for the occurrence of psychological sequelae of trauma by the expert community and affected people. The elicitation of a psychodynamic case history can be helpful in order to differentiate specific trauma-related symptoms from others with psychoneurotic genesis (Haenel 2002, 2006).

Moreover, the assessment provides reference points and evidence for the skilled clinician on whether the symptoms of a mental disorder are simulated (Resnick 1988; Birck 2002). While subjects with real disorders not only complain about severe troubles but also about slighter, more subtle ones that include a negative symptomatology with loss of experience and behaviour and which are described in a differentiated way, simulating patients focus mainly on dramatic, phantasmagoric and positive symptoms that occur in an unusual variety and combination and that are described to be consistently severe over a long period, in contrast to real disorders that are subject to fluctuations. A summarising tabular overview concerning this topic can be found in Birck (2002).

Additionally, in legal procedures on residency, it is important to distinguish posttraumatic disorders from other event-related disorders such as migration-related adaptive disorders or reactive depressive disorders. Concerning the Social Compensation Law, the extent to which an extremely traumatic event has contributed to a substantial aggravation of a pre-existing or latent mental disorder must also be taken into account.

Right to Asylum and Residence

In asylum procedures the assessor is usually asked whether and which health disorders are existent and to what extent these disorders can be attributed to specified torture or prison experiences. Here of course, from the existence of PTSD symptoms of criteria B to F (DSM-IV) or B to H (DSM-5), no conclusion can be made about the existence and type of traumatic experiences (criteria A). Instead, a careful exploration of case history with the aid of a qualified interpreter, a psychological diagnostic assessment, a physical examination possibly including documented scar findings and, where appropriate, additional psychological test diagnostics are to be expected in order to complete an accurate assessment. In the evaluation, a discussion must take place about the extent to which the results of the examination form an overall consistent body of evidence that the specific traumatic experiences reported by the patient are plausibly experience based.

Other residence legal questions are aimed at health-related hindrances to deportation. The expert is then asked whether there are mental or physical health disorders in the affected and to what extent they may worsen with profound and life-threatening consequences in case of repatriation.

Occasionally, a judge may ask how long a psychiatric treatment would need to be carried out in order to reach a health state in which the patient's repatriation would not be connected with any health-related risks. It should be noted that in patients with psychological post-traumatic sequelae, a lifelong vulnerability can exist, including the danger of symptoms being reinforced in case of current situations in their home countries connected with past traumatic experiences. Connections which are established a priori between the therapy and repatriation and which the patient perceives as a threat do not make therapeutic sense since they prevent trust and openness, prerequisites of a stable and predominantly positive therapeutic relationship with the therapist. Psychotherapy begun under such auspices offers little prospect of success.

Special Problems in Residence Legal Procedures Determined by Linguistic and Cultural Differences

In psychotraumatological assessment in asylum procedures, the examined patients are persons from other cultures than the host culture, with different traditions, religions, languages and possibly different understandings of illness and symptom manifestations (Haenel 2011). In most cases, interpreters are needed in order to conduct an assessment, and care must naturally be taken to gain a correct and literal linguistic translation. At the same time, what was said previously about the relationship between the patient and assessor is also applicable to the relationship between the patient and interpreter, leading to an enlarged assessment setting and a complex relational triad that is susceptible to interference. Hence, the patient's lack of trust in the interpreter may hinder the assessment or lead to its failure in the same way as a lack of confidence in the assessor. Like in the therapeutic context, all three involved parties form a relational system in the context of the assessment, and feelings, values, thoughts and fantasies occur towards each other both consciously and unconsciously. These may not only relate to the current situation but also – though to a smaller extent – to past relationship experiences in the manner of their transference and countertransference towards each other, thereby impairing the assessment (Haenel 1997). Respectively, clinical supervision might prove helpful for assessors in this field.

However, necessary prerequisites for the assessor include not only psychiatric and psychological expertise with knowledge and experience of the psychological reactive sequelae of trauma and exploration of the patient's history with the help of interpreters but also information about the political and cultural background of the country of origin.

> **Conclusion**
>
> Concerning the right to asylum and residence, psychotraumatological assessments often take place in the context of sociopolitical disputes. Consequently, the danger of attempted influence and instrumentalisation of medical or psychological experts by interested groups or authorities is particularly high (Henningsen 2003). This can be most safely prevented through broad knowledge and experience in general psychopathology on the part of the assessor, as well as the acquisition of further knowledge through advanced training. For this reason, the *Bundesärztekammer*[8] has been successfully offering the structured curricular training programme entitled "Begutachtung psychisch reaktiver Traumafolgen in aufenthaltsrechtlichen Verfahren"[9] for 10 years with the aim of enabling

---

[8] State Chamber of Physicians.

[9] Assessment of psychologically reactive sequelae of trauma in residence legal procedures.

medical and psychological colleagues to gather professional expertise in their area of psychotraumatology (Bundesärztekammer 2005, 2009).

References

APA/American Psychiatric Association (1994) Diagnostic and statistical manual of mental disorders, fourth edition (DSM IV). American Psychiatric Press, Washington, DC

APA/American Psychiatric Association (2014) Diagnostic and statistical manual of mental disorders, fifth edition (DSM 5). American Psychiatric Press, Washington, DC

Birck A (2002) Traumatisierte Flüchtlinge. Asanger, Heidelberg

Bundesärztekammer Curriculum: Begutachtung psychisch reaktiver Traumafolgen in aufenthaltsrechtlichen Verfahren bei Erwachsenen. http://www.bundesaerztekammer.de/downloads/currbegutpsychotrauma.pdf. 2005

Bundesärztekammer Fortbildungscurriculum: Begutachtung psychisch reaktiver Traumafolgen im Sozialen Entschädigungsrecht. http://www.bundesaerztekammer.de/downloads/curriculum_gutachten_23062011.pdf. 2009

Denis D, Kummer P, Priebe S (2000) Entschädigung und Begutachtung psychischer Störungen nach politischer Haft in der SBZ/DDR. Med Sachverstand 96:77–83

Eissler K (1958) Die Ermordung wie viel seiner Kinder muß ein Mensch ertragen können, um eine normale psychische Konstitution zu haben. Psyche 5(63):241–291

Fischer-Homberger E (2004) Die Traumatische Neurose. Psychosozialverlag, Gießen

Flatten G, Gast U, Hofmann A, Liebermann P, Reddemann L, Wöller W, Siol T, Petzold ER (2004) Posttraumatische Belastungsstörung, Leitlinie und Quellentext. Schattauer, Stuttgart

General Foreign Office (1994, 1995) Lageberichte Türkei

Glaesmer H, Brähler E, Gündel H, Riedel-Heller S (2011) The association of traumatic experiences and posttraumatic stress disorder with physical morbidity in old age, a German population-based study. Psychosom Med 73:401–406

Goltermann S (2009) Die Gesellschaft der Überlebenden. DVA, München

Haenel F (1997) Aspekte und Probleme in der Psychotherapie mit Folteropfern unter Beteiligung von Dolmetschern. Systhema 11:136–144

Haenel F (1998) Special problems in the assessment of the psychological sequelae of torture and incarceration. In: Oehmichen M (ed) Maltreatment and torture. Schmidt Roemhild Verlag, Lübeck

Haenel F (2000) Die Beziehung zwischen Gutachter und zu Untersuchenden und ihre Bedeutung bei der Begutachtung chronisch psychischer Traumafolgen. Med Sachverstand 96:84–87

Haenel F (2002) Zur Abgrenzung psychisch reaktiver Haft- und Folterfolgen von schädigungsunabhängigen neurotischen Störungen. Med Sachverstand 98:194–198

Haenel F (2006) Zu Problemen der Begutachtung psychischer Haft und Folterfolgen bei Personen mit Persönlichkeitsstörungen. Med Sach 102:S171–S174

Haenel F (2011) Die Posttraumatische Belastungsstörung – Psychiatrisch-psychotherapeutische Behandlung von Folter- und Bürgerkriegsüberlebenden. In: Machleidt W, Heinz A (eds) Praxis der Interkulturellen Psychiatrie und Psychotherapie. Urban & Fischer, München, pp 307–319

Henningsen F (2003) Traumatisierte Flüchtlinge und der Prozess der Begutachtung. Psyche 57:97–120

Herman JL (1994) Sequelae of prolonged and repeated trauma: evidence for a complex posttraumatic syndrome (DESNOS). In: Davidson JRT, Foa E (eds) Posttraumatic stress disorder: DSM-IV and beyond. American Psychiatric Press, Washington, DC

Hoppe K (1967) The emotional reactions of psychiatrists when confronting survivors of persecution. Psychoanalytic Forum 3:187–196

Kessler RC, Sonnega A, Bromet E, Hughes M, Nelson CB (1995) Posttraumatic stress disorder in the national comorbidity survey. Arch Gen Psychiatry 52:1048–1060

Lansen J (1993) Vicarious traumatization in therapists treating victims of torture and persecution. Torture 3:138–140

Lansen J (1996) Was tut "es" mit uns? In: Graessner S, Gurris N, Pross C (eds) Folter – an der Seite der Überlebenden. Beck Verlag, München

Niederland W (1968) Studies of concentration-camp survivors. In: Kristal H (ed) Massive psychic trauma. International University Press, New York

Oppenheim H (1889) Die traumatischen Neurosen nach den in der Nervenklinik der Charitè in den 8 Jahren 1883–1891 gesammelten Beobachtungen. Hirschwald, Berlin

Pross C (1993) Wiedergutmachung – Kleinkrieg gegen die Opfer. Athenaeum Verlag, Frankfurt

Resnick PJ (1988) Malingering of posttraumatic disorders. In: Rogers R (ed) Clinical assessment of malingering and deception. Gilford Press, New York, pp 84–103

Skylv G (1993) Falanga – diagnosis and treatment of late sequela. Torture 3:11–15

Venzlaff U (1963) Erlebnishintergrund und Dynamik seelischer Verfolgungsschäden. In: Paul H, Herberg H-J (eds) Psychische Spätschäden nach politischer Verfolgung. Karcher Verlag, Basel

von Baeyer W, Häfner H, Kisker K (1964) Psychiatrie der Verfolgten. Springer, Berlin

Wenk-Ansohn M (2002) Folgen sexualisierter Folter – Therapeutische Arbeit mit kurdische Patientinnen. In: Birck A, Pross C, Lansen J (eds) Das Unsagbare. Springer, Berlin, pp 57–78

Wilson J, Lindy J (1994) Countertransference in the treatment of PTSD. Guilford Press, New York

World Health Organisation (1992) The ICD-10 Classification of mental and behavioral disorders and diagnostic guidelines. WHO, Geneva

Gender and Trauma

9

İnci User

A review of the literature on gender and trauma reveals that in many studies the term gender is employed as if it were synonymous with the term sex. Gender is not a biological reality, but a sociocultural construct that enables researchers to distinguish constitutional characteristics from socially acquired ones. Gender ought to be used as an analytical tool to understand social interactions, inequalities and human experiences including suffering.

Sex and Gender

The terms sex and gender are not alternative nominations of the same phenomenon. While *sex* refers to fundamental biological differences reflected in the physical and psychological characteristics of men and women, *gender* refers to their socially constructed differences and their different locations within the social system. Every culture has different notions regarding masculinity and femininity, attributes different 'typical' characteristics and behaviours to men and women and imposes different role requirements and duties upon them. Everyday life, work, income and human relationships are shaped by norms and traditions that regard and treat the two sexes differently. The values and ideas that are at the basis of these norms and traditions are also reflected in laws, organisations and social structures.

İ. User
Department of Sociology, Marmara University, Istanbul, Turkey
e-mail: inciuser@gmail.com

© Springer International Publishing Switzerland 2015
M. Schouler-Ocak (ed.), *Trauma and Migration:*
Cultural Factors in the Diagnosis and Treatment of Traumatised Immigrants,
DOI 10.1007/978-3-319-17335-1_9

... historically specific patterns of gender relations within any culture and community shape
individual identity and social interaction, segregating, stratifying and symbolically engen-
dering key social institutions (...) The result is not uniformity in women's experiences but
rather diversity, both within any given society and among the world's cultures (Enarson and
Morrow 1998:3).

The meanings of being a man or a woman do not only vary from one society to
another, but also among different groups of men and women in a given society, at a
given time. Furthermore they vary within one culture over time, because the cultural
values and meanings that lead to the construction of genders are dynamic and open
to change. Femininity and masculinity mean different things to the single individual
in the course of her/his development (Kimmel 2000:2–3).

Individuals display their gender identities in varying ways, because gender identity does not have the same salience for everyone. Men in general tend to regard
themselves as if they were genderless, because they don't have as many gender-
related problems as women, for whom their gender is far more salient. This is very
similar to the fact that upper class people or members of a hegemonic ethnic group
tend to think less often about class or ethnicity than do members of subordinate
classes or ethnicities who are faced with the reality of discrimination. The salience or
accessibility of gender as an aspect of the self varies among individuals as well as for
the single individual in different contexts (Deaux and Major 2000; Kimmel 2000).

The different ways in which men and women participate in social institutions and
processes are shaped by prevailing constructions of gender, and this results in a
limited access by women to economic, political and social resources. Most of the
time, the treatment of the genders is not only different but also inequitable.
Contemporary sociology considers gender as an important dimension of social
inequality and stratification, because it is one of the factors that determine the
opportunities or obstacles faced by different individuals and groups in a society.
Gender is not a fixed category but varies in relation to age, race/ethnicity and class.
In a complex society that is stratified and that comprises different racial and/or ethnic groups, there is a hierarchy of genders. According to Connell (1987), men and
women have very different life trajectories related to their gender statuses. Even
though the dominant gender category in almost every society consists of men
belonging to the economically, politically and ethnically most powerful groups,
some groups of women also occupy higher places than many men along the gender
hierarchy. Such women may be enjoying the privileges of wealth, occupation or
social connection with powerful men. In other words, men or women do not experience life in well-defined, uniform ways depending on their sex, but rather in a much
more complicated way. Thus, any individual's gender status may change according
to her/his age and her/his own or collective experiences of mobility in the stratification system.

The concept of 'gender role' may appear to be similar to 'sex role', but the two
concepts belong to different theoretical traditions. In sociological terms, gender is
socially constructed, i.e. brought about as a result of human interactions and value
negotiations within a culture. The sex role theory proposes fixed and static role sets
for all men and women in a given society and implies that these role sets suit the

psychological make-ups of both sexes. The theory of social construction, however, observes that human beings are not passive and mechanic recipients of social roles. During social interaction people choose, interpret, negotiate, produce and reproduce their gender identities and roles.

From a social psychological perspective, gender-related behaviour can be explained by drawing upon two theoretical constructs: the first is the 'self-fulfilling prophecy', based on the observation that people behave to others in accordance with their expectations of them, thus forcing them to react in a certain way in order to fulfil these expectations. This concept refers to people's active role in maintaining and creating social reality. The other theoretical construct is 'self-presentation' and refers to people's choices to present their identities in such a way as to reflect what they think a given context is expecting from them. Both constructs imply that the social environment can channel our behaviours so that we act in accordance with socially constructed gender role expectations (Deaux and Major 2000:84).

Gender stereotypes are characteristics believed to be typical for men or women within a given culture. They shape our expectations regarding what is appropriate for men and women and our behaviours towards each gender. People are encouraged to conform to these stereotypes. Patterns of femininity and masculinity are thus produced, and they direct individuals' choices and behaviours. Across contemporary societies, gender norms tend to become increasingly similar due to the fast exchange of information across cultural boundaries and the resulting globalisation of beliefs and values, as well as fads and fashions. However, in the details, there are still many differences in how gender is constructed in different contexts.

Psychological and psychiatric perspectives that emphasise the personal impacts of trauma and suffering do not explain all aspects of the traumatic experience, because traumatic events always happen in a cultural and historical context that shapes and assigns significance to them. Individuals experience trauma and its aftermath in interaction with this context, and they respond in accordance with their personal as well as sociocultural backgrounds. Structural problems and inequalities prior to the traumatic events are reflected in the composition and characteristics of the victims. Neither is the resulting suffering merely a personal matter. Like every other psychiatric problem, it is identified, labelled and treated by social agents emphasising the restoration and continuity of the individual's functioning in social life.

> In reality, the events we call trauma are part of larger configurations of suffering that have their own social ecology and political economy. Discrete trauma and disasters occur against a backdrop of structural violence that renders some groups and individuals far more vulnerable; focusing exclusively on the trauma may deflect attention from these enduring forms of disadvantage. (Kirmayer et al. 2010:170)

As mentioned above, gender is an important dimension of structural inequality. Therefore, traumatic events and their impacts upon people have to be understood from a gender-sensitive and gender-informed perspective. A gender-sensitive approach to any problem will try to foster gender awareness and to improve gender equity in research, planning, and implementation.

Gender and Health

Gender is an important socio-demographic determinant of health (Lee 1998; Schambler 2008). At different stages of life, men and women have different risks due to their different social responsibilities and lifestyles. The most widely accepted gender difference in health is that women have higher levels of morbidity, whereas men have higher mortality rates. Regarding the facts that men in the USA have higher death rates for all 15 leading causes of death, and that their average longevity is 7 years below women's, Courtenay (2000) has suggested that health-related beliefs and behaviours are one of the many ways in which masculinities and femininities are demonstrated. Accordingly, men engage in a number of health-compromising behaviours in order to prove their masculine strength, whereas women are increasingly engaged in health-promoting behaviours. Obviously, the health statistics and the cultural explanations used in Courtenay's study concern the USA, and individual health behaviours are not the sole predictors of health. However, men's risk-taking behaviours are not specific to the USA, and the health-compromising and risky behaviours of men, as well as their tendency to under-report symptoms (especially those that have been identified as more typical for the female gender), should be studied cross-culturally.

Any health issue may be related to sex, to gender or to both. An example might be women's health problems during the reproductive years. Women's heightened vulnerability to physical and mental hazards in this period of life is not a simple matter of sex. Reproductive risks that are peculiar to the female sex vary in relation to level of education, economic status and marital status. Different groups of women do not only have different health risks, but they also enjoy very different levels of access to health care. Migrant or ethnic minority women may display additionally increased vulnerability due to cultural factors as well as to discrimination and institutionalised racism. Hence, not every woman's health will be compromised to the same degree in the reproductive years.

Gender, Mental Health and Trauma

The theoretical definitions of normality are various, and they tend to change over time (Davison and Neale 1998:6–23). Each of the different approaches to conceptualise normality can be disputed because they entail certain value judgements. The classification systems for mental illness are not universal, and they are also modified over time. From a gender-sensitive perspective, one might apprehend that the definition of normality may partly be based on widely held gender stereotypes. Since the 1980s numerous researchers have emphasised the importance of incorporating gender as an analytic variable into mental health research. Gender-blind theories and research have been criticised because they have reduced women's vulnerabilities to biological reasons, whereas in fact it is mostly social circumstances that increase vulnerability. The belief that women have a constitutional tendency to mental illness is very old and very deeply ingrained in medicine (Russell 1995:4–26; Schambler 2008:151–154). Gender bias extends from models of the human being which draw upon male behaviours and experiences only to clinical trials that exclude female subjects. For a long time this bias has prevented researchers from studying the gender-specific needs and problems of women. Even sexual abuse and violence as critical life events and stressors have been ignored until recently.

Three major problems have been identified, because of which the relationship between gender and mental health is poorly understood (Astbury 1999:8–9):

1. Evidence on gender is not collected. Even if it is collected, it is not presented in a gender-disaggregated form to inform researchers, clinicians and policy makers.
2. Evidence is lacking on how gender interacts with structural determinants including income, education, workplace and social position, roles related to family, unpaid work and caring and the experience of intimate, gender-based violence.
3. Conceptual remapping is required of all those explanatory models of emotional distress and disorder where large gender differences exist but have not yet been adequately explained due to an excessive focus on biological mechanisms. This is especially important given that gender differences in chronic life stressors, negative life events and violence have not been properly investigated.

Gender socialisation determines which problems men and women feel comfortable seeking assistance for and which conditions they will conceal because they consider them to be stigmatising. This may lead to the under-reporting of certain symptoms and the emphasising of others. Hence, women may be too anxious to report alcohol abuse and feel more comfortable discussing emotional problems, whereas men do the reverse. Therefore, both population screenings and clinical measurements should employ instruments that are sensitive to biases due to gender stereotyping (Astbury 1999:10).

About one third of the total number of injury-related deaths in the world are due to intentional violence (suicides, homicides, terrorism and armed conflicts). The number of both the victims and the survivors of violence and disasters increased considerably during the last hundred years (Kirmayer et al. 2010). There is a growing need to understand traumatic experiences, responses to trauma, trauma-related mental health problems and effective treatment strategies. Trauma has two components: the objective component is related to what has actually happened to the individual, and the subjective component is related with how the individual has perceived and experienced the event. The subjective evaluation of the event determines whether or not it is traumatic.

> What constitutes a trauma then is not entirely dependent on the nature of the event but also on the personal and social interpretation of the event and the responses of the affected person, their family and community, as well as the wider society. Culture influences the individual and collective experience of trauma at many levels: the perception and interpretation of events as threatening or traumatic; modes of expressing and explaining distress; coping responses and adaptation; patterns of help-seeking and treatment response. Most importantly, culture gives meaning to the traumatic event itself, allowing individuals, families and communities to make sense of violence and adversity in ways that may moderate or amplify their impact. (Kirmayer et al. 2010:156)

The gender dimension should be taken into consideration when trying to understand trauma. To begin with, different types of trauma may happen to both sexes at varying frequency, and there may be gender-specific sensitivities towards trauma. Gender-sensitive research can better inform primary and secondary prevention measures as well as therapeutic and rehabilitative models implemented for trauma victims.

Post-traumatic stress disorder (PTSD) is defined as an anxiety disorder 'that occurs when a person experiences an event during which he or she perceives a threat to his or her own life, the life of a significant other, or his or her physical integrity, and the person responds with intense fear, helplessness or horror. Symptoms of post-traumatic stress disorder include intrusive thoughts, such as flashbacks and nightmares, emotional numbing, avoidance of reminders of the event, and hyperarousal, such as increased startle response and irritability' (Ayers 2007:254). Earlier definitions of PTSD emphasised that the precipitating event should be objectively unusual and severe, 'outside the normal range of experience' (DSM III) and 'likely to cause pervasive distress in anyone' (WHO International Classification of Diseases, 10th revision). Until the early 1990s, these definitions were current. Inevitably, research most often focused on extremely stressful events and their negative psychological impacts. PTSD symptoms can occur after various events such as death or serious illness of a close person, parental divorce, family relationship problems, romantic relationship problems, arrest and incarceration or non-life-threatening illness (Gold et al. 2005). Now, such events are also considered to be traumatic if they are reported to have been very stressful for the person. Finally, in the DSM-IV, the event criterion was changed, and the individual's perception of threat was accepted to precipitate PTSD in some cases (Ayers and Pickering 2001). Life stress and lack of social support are among the strongest predictors of PTSD, showing that social factors determine risk of exposure and chances of recovery (Kirmayer et al. 2010). Starting in the mid-1990s, a growing emphasis was put upon resilience and upon the positive aspects of the traumatic experience because most people survive traumatic events without any symptoms of psychopathology, and some of them even report to have mentally benefitted from the experience.

About 1 in 12 adults experiences PTSD at some point in his/her lifetime (Stuber et al. 2006:55). Even though the post-trauma symptoms were initially defined based on the observation of war veterans, PTSD is not a man's or a soldiers' disorder. There is an enormous body of research about the victims of wars, terrorism, road accidents, natural or technological disasters on the one hand and about patients with cancer, HIV/AIDS, difficult delivery or heart attacks, as well as people who have experienced abuse in childhood, rape or assault, incarceration or being kidnapped on the other hand (Matsuoka et al. 2008; Kirmayer et al. 2010). A great part of this research indicates that PTSD is probably more prevalent among girls and women than among boys and men (Tolin and Foa 2006). Women appear to have a higher PTSD risk than men after individual as well as collective or mass experiences of traumatic events (Brewin et al. 2000; Stuber et al. 2006; Bleich et al. 2003; Ditlevsen and Elklit 2012).

One explanation of the gender difference in the prevalence of PTSD might be that women are more likely to experience traumatic events in the course of their lives. The epidemiological data regarding this possibility is mixed and inconclusive (Tolin and Foa 2006), but in fact, most studies point to an increased risk for men rather than women (Creamer et al. 2001; Ditlevsen and Elklit 2010). If the risk for men is actually larger, then women in general must either be faced with events that are more deeply traumatising or they must have a greater tendency to develop PTSD. Women's stronger tendency to develop PTSD may also be related to the fact that the types of traumas to which they are more frequently exposed (e.g. sexual assault and rape) are socially stigmatised, and therefore they do not receive sufficient social support (Nolen-Hoeksema 2011:122). Ideologies, which consider the family unit as sacred and do not approve of interference with domestic violence because it is regarded as an aspect of 'family privacy', also contribute to women being deprived of adequate support and to higher rates of trauma-related problems.

Women's apparently greater vulnerability may be due to differences in the gendered life experiences of the two sexes. This vulnerability is specifically high in relation to assaultive violence, and one might conclude that women's higher prevalence of PTSD may be related to the greater burden of rape. However, even when the rape factor is controlled, the gender disparity in vulnerability persists. What is more, when all types of assaultive violence are taken into account, men are far more frequently exposed to violence (Stuber et al. 2006:55).

Men's and women's experiences of physical trauma constitute a gender issue that is too complicated to be summarised as 'men experience greater physical trauma as compared to women'. This summary statement may be true, but it requires a more detailed analysis: all over the world, men are subjected too much greater physical violence in wars and armed disagreements. However, the age group which is affected is very specific. What is more, in many societies, recruitment to armed forces may be limited to particular strata rather than universal. Men's increased vulnerability to job-related accidents in the workplace is another well-known fact, but again, not all strata of an industrialised society are employed as blue-collar workers. Men's traumatic experiences may be overlooked or poorly understood, because it is difficult for people to comprehend how the 'tough and invulnerable' man can at the same time be a suffering victim. This is why some male survivors of sexual assault have been turned away by rape crisis centres, and one of them was told that the centre had no staff to treat perpetrators (Mejia 2005:31). There is relatively little evidence about the gender-specific experiences of men in relation to traumatic effects. Since men are socialised according to an ideology of masculinity, a core value of which is invulnerability, they are assumed to experience great conflict in cases of victimisation: on the one hand there is the burden of victimisation, and on the other hand, there is the message that they do not measure up to the standards of the masculine ideology (Mejia 2005:38).

The interaction between culture and gender also influences vulnerability. In a study comparing survivors of two very similar hurricanes in Florida and Mexico, women in both groups were found to have higher rates of trauma-related symptoms than men. However, the difference between Mexican women and men was much larger than the difference between American women and men (Norris et al. 2001). In cultures that segregate genders more strictly and keep women in very subordinate positions, gendered vulnerability to trauma increases.

There also appear to be gender differences in the lifespan distribution of PTSD. In a review of several studies on trauma and PTSD, the highest prevalence of the disorder was seen to be in men in their early 40s and women in their early 50s. The lowest prevalence for both genders was in their early 70s. Overall, the prevalence of PTSD among women was twice as high, but for some ages the female-male ratio approached 3:1. The highest female-male ratio was found for the age range 21–25. The conclusion of the researchers was that for a better understanding of the development of PTSD, reproductive factors and social responsibilities ought to be taken into consideration (Ditlevsen and Elklit 2010).

Reviewing research evidence collected over 25 years, Tolin and Foa (2006) concluded across studies that male participants were significantly more likely to report a potentially traumatic event than were female participants; the observed twofold risk of PTSD among females was therefore not related to higher exposure. A detailed study of the characteristics of the traumatic events revealed however that men were more exposed to specific types of trauma (e.g. motor vehicle accidents, combat, war, disaster or fire, non-sexual assault, serious illness or seeing somebody die), whereas women reported significantly more experiences of sexual assault and childhood sexual abuse. A possible interpretation might be that sexual traumas are more likely to cause PTSD. However, comparing men and women who reported the same trauma categories across studies, Tolin and Foa (2006) found that women had a greater frequency of PTSD in all these categories except for sexual assault as an adult, where the PTSD frequency did not show any significant gender difference. When other symptoms occurring after traumatic events were examined, men were found to tend towards more aggressive behaviours and substance abuse, whereas women tended towards anxiety and mood disorders. This finding was interpreted by Tolin and Foa as being probably related to varying social expectations (2006:979). Although the authors explain that their interpretation is speculative, it sounds fairly reasonable in the light of what we know about gender differences in response to stress: while men try to suppress their anxiety and to fight rather than to remain passive, women show more passive reactions to threatening events and environments because both genders have gone through processes of socialisation imposing exactly these behaviour patterns upon them. It is the deeply internalised ideologies of femininity and masculinity, rather than biopsychological differences, which seem to explain these different outcomes.

In a study examining gender differences in post-traumatic vulnerability in the face of terror attacks in Israel, women were found to be six times more likely to develop PTSD than men. The elevated vulnerability of women was interpreted as being attributable to gender differences in terms of safety, coping strategies and self-efficacy. Israeli women were observed to manifest an emotion-focused coping strategy as opposed to the problem-focused strategies of men. While men tend to overcome stress by being active outside the home, talking about problems and looking for solutions, women tend to stay at home, to worry about their friends and families and to share their anxiety with others. The male strategy appears to strengthen self-efficacy, optimism and feelings of personal safety, whereas the female strategy appears to increase worry and other negative feelings, making it more difficult for women to overcome traumatic stress (Solomon et al. 2005: 6–7). Another way of expressing the difference might be that women are suffering from gender-typical behaviours: spending a lot of time in the private sphere and caring for the problems of others is the age-old and almost universal behaviour pattern of women that has been shaped by the social division of labour between the sexes.

There are also some arguments that the increased PTSD prevalence among women is due to a report bias, in that men tend to under-report and women tend to over-report symptoms. This may be true to some extent because of social expectations about women being vulnerable and men being tough and resilient (Ditlevsen and Elklit 2010:8).

Some traumatic events like life-threatening illnesses, accidents or assault are very personal. They happen to a single individual or to a small group. Giving birth is also a very personal major life event, and it may be experienced as very stressful or even as traumatic by some women. There are different study reports indicating perinatal trauma and PTSD during the early period after birth. Up to 10 % of women have severe traumatic stress responses to birth (Ayers 2004), and 24–34 % of post-partum women may have one or more traumatic stress symptoms (Takegata et al. 2014). The prevalence rates of reported PTSD range from 1.5 % to 9 % (Ayers and Pickering 2001; Beck 2004; Ayers et al. 2007; Garthus-Niegel et al. 2012; Takegata et al. 2014). These are findings of studies in developed countries, and data from underdeveloped populations are necessary for obtaining a fuller picture of this highly gendered issue.

There are significant differences between birth and other events that cause PTSD. Birth is predictable, in many cases entered into voluntarily, experienced by the majority of women, and socially approved. What is more, a healthy newborn is a reward that can make up for the pain and anxiety associated with labour. On the other hand, birth may threaten and sometimes damage bodily integrity in a way which is different from other traumatic events, and it requires a great deal of readjustment. Since infant care is an intensive and full-time activity, mothers will also be steadily reminded of the event of birth and may have a hard time recovering (Ayers et al. 2009).

Delivery-related stressors and previous depression have been found to predict post-partum post-traumatic stress (PTS). Risk factors contributing to PTS and PTSD have been grouped as (1) prenatal factors (e.g. previous traumatic deliveries, history of infertility and complicated pregnancies, delivery of an ill or stillborn baby, depression, childhood sexual abuse, etc), (2) nature and circumstances of delivery (e.g. long, hard, extremely painful labour, forceps delivery, emergency caesarian section, lack of control) and (3) subjective factors during delivery (e.g. feelings of powerlessness, lack of social support, fear of harming the infant, fear of harming oneself, fear that one may die or the infant may die) (van Son et al. 2005). A longitudinal study showed that women's subjective birth experiences had the highest association with PTSD symptoms (Garthus-Niegel et al. 2012). More research is required to confirm risk factors and to explain the role of particular variables such as history of sexual abuse, lack of control in birth and blame after birth (Ayers 2004). A qualitative study examined thoughts and emotions during birth, postnatal cognitive processing and memories of birth. As compared to women without symptoms, women with postnatal PTSD reported more panic, anger, thoughts of death, mental defeat and dissociation during birth, fewer strategies that focus on the present, more painful memories, intrusive memories and rumination, with the implication that women with signs of mental defeat or dissociation should be offered postnatal support in order to prevent PTSD (Ayers 2007).

Women with negative expectations about birth tend to have negative experiences during it. The negative expectations are associated with anxiety (Ayers and Pickering 2005). It has been shown that women who fear the process of birth and women with symptoms of anxiety and depression tend to have subjectively negative birth experiences, and these experiences predict post-partum post-traumatic symptoms (Garthus-Niegel et al. 2012).

Research on postnatal distress has identified that the degree of social support (especially partner support), life events, circumstances of mothering and infant temperament are important factors for the development of depression in the first year (Small et al. 1994). Mothers in whom post-partum distress symptoms persist tend to describe their infants as 'slow to warm up'. Such infants are characterised by a low level of adaptation, low activity, moderately negative responses to new stimuli and moderate irregularity of biological functions (Di Blasio and Ionio 2005). It is hard to decide whether babies are perceived and described as 'difficult' because the mothers are in distress or whether their distress is actually an outcome of the difficult temperament of the infant.

Postnatal PTSD does not only influence the woman's mental health, but probably has adverse effects upon the infant, the existing children and the family unit. On the other hand, the comorbidity of PTSD with other psychiatric disorders may result in misdiagnosis and ineffective treatment (Ayers 2004). In a qualitative study, women with postnatal PTSD reported fear of childbirth as well as changes in physical well-being, mood, behaviour and social interaction. Their relationships with their partners were negatively affected including disagreements, sexual dysfunction and blame for events of birth. Most of them admitted to having initially rejected their infants, and in the long term, they seemed to develop avoidant or anxious attachments (Ayers et al. 2006).

All this points to the necessity of much better and person-centred care for mothers. The medical care and social support mothers receive during pregnancy and labour and the months following these may vary in association with socio-economic variables such as level of education, income and occupation, as well as with the status of the woman in her cultural group. In other words, the highly mystified 'joy of mothering' is a gender issue, and women receive unequal shares of it, depending on their social locations. This joy is likely to be limited not only by social location, but also by uncontrollable natural and social events. Detailed research on theoretically vulnerable women (e.g. mothers in forced marriages, adolescent mothers, women living in poverty and/or social isolation, migrant and refugee mothers, women giving birth without assistance, women experiencing pregnancy and birth during catastrophic periods such as wars or disasters, women with histories of rape and torture) may supply more information about the problem and lay the foundations of adequate policies for supporting women.

Even though labour-related trauma might appear to be a sex-specific problem, there are some studies showing that men can also experience stress and depression related to the birth of a child or to miscarriage. Ayers et al. (2007) have shown that 5 % of men and women had severe symptoms of PTSD which were not associated with the parent-baby bond or the couple's relationship.

Bereavement is considered to be one of the most stressful life events which people face. The loss of a loved one, especially of a partner, can be experienced as a traumatic event and have long-term effects on an individual's mental health. A review of studies on psychopathology related to widowhood revealed that especially during the first year, the rates of mood and anxiety disorders are elevated in widowed people. Major depression (22 %) and PTSD (12 %) are widespread, and there are increased risks of panic and generalised anxiety disorders. However, the authors state that based on the study data, it is impossible to understand whether there are differences in vulnerability between genders (Onrust and Cuijpers 2006). Depression is particularly common in widowed men. In studying this issue Umberson et al. (1992) have taken into consideration the gender differences in marital relations as well as in psychological distress. The authors stress that men often suffer from a lack of psychosocial support in widowhood, because often it is wives who organise and maintain couples' social networks. Women usually have confidants outside the family, while men tend to prefer to confide in their wives only. The loss of a wife often means isolation and lack of support. Widowed men do not only have to deal with the stress of social isolation, but they also have difficulties in managing the household. Women on the other hand have greater psychosocial support and are more effective in running their everyday lives, but very often they suffer from financial strains. The authors conclude that men's apparent vulnerability to depression in widowhood is actually an outcome of the different circumstances and meanings of widowhood for both genders. Another study focusing on sex differences in depression due to widowhood explored whether environmental strains such as a lack of social support or concerns about finances and housekeeping explain these differences. The findings revealed that widowhood is associated with higher levels of depressive symptoms and that this association is stronger for men than for women. The effect of widowhood is mediated by different types of environmental strain for men and women. The authors concluded that women adapt to widowhood more successfully than men (van Grootheest et al. 1999).

For parents, the death of a child is an extremely traumatic event, causing more intense and long-lasting grief than perhaps any other loss. A reasonable question might be whether there are any gender differences in the response to the death of a child. Comparisons between fathers' and mothers' responses to this event yield inconsistent results (Büchi et al. 2007). In many samples, fathers seem to suffer as deeply as do mothers, but there is a need for more cross-cultural data on this point, because motherhood does not have the same meaning everywhere. In a context where motherhood is almost the only way for a woman to be fully accepted by the family and the community, the loss of a child may be perceived as directly threatening the mother's existence.

Gender and Mass Traumas

Responses to individually experienced traumas may be different from the responses to traumas affecting a group or a community. In order to see whether there are gender-related differences in the prevalence of probable lifetime PTSD after a major traumatic event affecting a large community, a study was conducted involving a sample living in the New York metropolitan area, 6–9 months after the terrorist attacks on September 11, 2011. To understand the factors that explain gender differences in PTSD risk, the following were assessed: the number of previous life stressors, the type of previous life stressors (sexual assault, non-sexual assault, non-assaultive trauma), pre-existing mental health problems, social support (perceived support, group participation, marital status), the number of recent life stressors, the type of recent life stressors (work, family, parenting) and peri-event panic. Of these, peri-event panic appeared to have the strongest relation with PTSD vulnerability. Women were not found to have a greater likelihood to develop symptoms of PTSD related to the attacks, but they had higher rates of re-experiencing and hyperarousal symptoms. The researchers concluded that this gender disparity in symptoms was largely due to higher rates of peri-event panic among women. Previous experiences of sexual assault, peri-event panic, pre-existing mental health problems, race/ethnicity and marital status (divorced, widowed or separated) explained the higher prevalence of lifetime PTSD among women. The authors commented that panic may be related to cognitive appraisal of the consequences of the event or to biological sex differences in panic susceptibility, and they concluded that women may be more vulnerable to personal assault, but their vulnerability to other types of trauma may be closer to men's (Stuber et al. 2006).

It has been pointed out that studies examining the impact of terrorism on nationally representative samples in developed countries are relatively few in number, except for the studies conducted in the USA after the terrorist attack on the World Trade Center. In a study concerned with Israeli people exposed to terrorist attacks (Bleich et al. 2003:616–617), women were found to present significantly more PTSD symptoms than men (16.2 % and 2.4 %, respectively). Women also had a higher frequency of TSR symptoms and feelings of depression than men. Interestingly, both PTSD and TSR symptoms were also associated with lower income, and women born in Israel had lower degrees of TSR than those born outside Israel. The associations of PTSD and TSR with income and birthplace suggest that in this sample the higher rate of traumatisation for females does not reflect a simple sex difference, but rather different social locations within one gender. Another study by the same authors (Solomon et al. 2005) examining gender differences in post-traumatic problems in response to terrorist attacks during the Al-Aksa Intifada

(September 2000–April 2002) revealed that women had more post-traumatic and depressive symptoms than men and were six times more likely than men to develop PTSD.

The findings of a study on the terrorist attacks on the World Trade Center revealed that even though people all over the country were traumatised immediately after the event, which could be witnessed through the media, these stress responses were mild and transient, showing that there is a relation between physical proximity to an event and the degree of distress. The trauma-related responses in the initial weeks after the event were once again stronger in female than in male participants (Matt and Vazquez 2008).

The Nazi Holocaust is one of the most significant large-scale traumatic events of the twentieth century, and its psychological impact has been studied from the late 1940s onwards. Because of a law passed by the West German government in 1956 that granted restitution to victims, the emphasis of initial case studies was on finding evidence of impairment. Hence, the dominant theme was severe debilitation in survivors. From the 1970s on however, a less pessimistic picture of post-war adjustment emerged (Lurie-Beck et al. 2008). Obviously, many of the survivors have managed to adapt to life, and one should not forget the philosophical, scientific and artistic contributions of persons who have turned their suffering into valuable lessons for and about humanity. On the other hand, the criticism is also levelled that the Holocaust is generally discussed from a gender-blind perspective, disregarding or perhaps choosing to forget about women's specific experiences in this horrific process (Ringelheim 1997).

Armed Conflicts, Wars and Trauma

The problems experienced by military veterans, especially veterans of the Vietnam War, and the studies focused thereupon have enabled scientists to identify traumatic events and their effects. Fifteen years after the end of their service, about 500,000 soldiers still had post-traumatic stress disorder (Nolen-Hoeksema 2011:119). Initially, the cases studied were predominantly men. Meanwhile there is also some literature on war trauma in women, because one cannot ignore the exposure of civilians to trauma during wars. Kirmayer et al. report that about 50 % of the casualties were civilians in the World War II, rising to 80 % in the 1980s and 90 % in the 1990s, the largest number being women and children (2010:162). Another interesting source of information about war trauma in women is constituted by studies on the increasing numbers of females in the US army (an army which continues to engage in active warfare in different parts of the world).

Not only is the number of women in the USA army increasing, but the roles and functions they take are also becoming more similar to men's. Whereas about 7,000 women were deployed to Vietnam and served as nurses or in clerical positions in the army, 200,000 women were deployed in the more recent conflicts in Afghanistan and Iraq. Women in the US army are officially still barred from direct ground combat positions, but many of the women deployed to Iraq or Afghanistan served alongside men, gaining considerable combat experience. Research on deployment and combat stress in the USA army members shows that men report exposure to a larger number of combat-related stressors, while women report greater stress relating specifically to hygiene and gynaecological issues, and both report similar levels of perceived threat. The likelihood of PTSD and other trauma-related disorders is almost the same among men and women (Vogt et al. 2011; Vogt and Street 2013). This may be interpreted as reflecting the significance of professional training in overcoming gender stereotypes and bringing about similar responses in both genders.

On the other hand, there is a gender difference relating to sexual assault in military life (Street et al. 2013). Since the risk of exposure to sexual violence within the military was observed to be high, the US veteran health administration adopted the term 'military sexual trauma' (MST). MST refers to severe forms of sexual assault that tend to have lasting deleterious consequences. Veterans all over the country were screened for MST, and positive screens were associated with higher rates of mental health comorbidities including PTSD and dissociative, eating and personality disorders and higher suicide risk. A significant gender difference was observed, with approximately 22 % of the screened veteran women as opposed to 1 % of men reporting MST (Kimerling et al. 2007). This difference can be interpreted as showing that MST is predominantly a woman's problem, but since the total number of male veterans is still much higher (than the total number of female veterans), even a prevalence rate of 1 % calls for intensive measures to identify and rehabilitate male victims. The authors of the study comment that prolonged exposure to MST is very similar to family violence, as both are associated with dissociative symptoms, personality disorders and self-harm.

War trauma is not peculiar to people who actively participate in the army. As already stated, modern war technologies have victimised masses of civilians along with soldiers. What is more, civilians generally have to put up with great adversities and stress during times of war. Worries about what may happen, grief for the lost ones and scarcity of material resources create a lot of distress. In 2004, 42 % of Afghan citizens had PTSD, and 72 % had other anxiety symptoms. Because they were controlled, oppressed and abused by the Taliban warriors, there was an increased likelihood of women developing psychopathology; 90 % reported some symptoms and 42 % were diagnosed to have PTSD (Nolen-Hoeksema 2011:120). A study in Bosnia revealed that women who had been exposed to long-term war trauma had serious post-traumatic and other psychological symptoms, 10 years after the war. About 28 % of the study participants met the criteria for PTSD diagnosis, and 7.5 % had partial PTSD. The researchers also observed that everyday post-war stressors (e.g. personal health concerns, changes in occupational and social spheres, loss of loved ones) contributed to the intensity of post-traumatic symptoms and other disorders (Klaric et al. 2007). A study on war-affected samples from Bosnia-Herzegovina, Macedonia, Croatia, Kosovo and Serbia revealed generally high prevalence rates of anxiety and mood disorders as well as substance abuse, even several years after the Yugoslavian War. The results were interpreted as being consistent with other studies pointing to the long-term mental health consequences of wars (Priebe et al. 2010).

Mass torture and sexual violence against civilians also accompany most wars. Sometimes men and children are attacked too, but it is generally women who are traumatised on a large scale. Women are taken hostage, raped, forced into prostitution, left pregnant or sterilised in order to demoralise and humiliate their nations or ethnicities. Rapists may belong to the enemy as well as to 'friendly' forces, and even members of UN peacekeeping forces have been reported to commit rape and sexual abuse (Chinkin 1994). New conceptualisations of war rape in international laws define rape as a war strategy and a weapon (Farwell 2004). A few of the well-known examples from the twentieth century include the 'comfort camps' established by the Japanese during World War II where about 200,000 women of different ethnicities were imprisoned, raped and tortured by the Japanese soldiers; the 200,000–400,000 Bengali women who were raped by Pakistani soldiers during the 1971 War of Liberation; Vietnamese women raped by US soldiers during the Vietnam War; Kuwaiti women raped by Iraqi soldiers during the invasion in 1990; the massive rape, torture and murder of Moslem women by Serbs in Bosnia-Herzegovina during the civil war of former Yugoslavia; and state-sponsored violence during conflicts in Rwanda, Guatemala and Burma (Chinkin 1994; Sancho 1997; Farwell 2004). During the final preparation of the present paper, hundreds of Iraqi women have been raped, killed or forced to become sex slaves by the terrorist ISIS warriors.

In Turkish culture, men are often praised for being actual or potential soldiers of the nation. The violence they endure in battles is glorified not only in the name of the nation, but also in the name of religion. Similar notions may exist in many of the world's cultures, since wherever we look, it is men who decide to start wars and who engage in active fighting. However, women's suffering in war is shameful, degrading and traumatic, and people often prefer not to talk about it or do not acknowledge survivors for what they have had to put up with. Actually, in many such instances, surviving women cannot return to their parents or husbands, or if they do, they remain silent for the rest of their lives. Not only are the psychological and social impacts of war rape profound, but they carry grave health and reproductive consequences as well.

While it is a widely used practice to weaken the enemy by degrading female bodies in times of war, there is also a tendency towards increased violence among civilians during wars. Crime statistics for 110 countries from 1900 onwards have revealed that there are substantial increases in homicide rates in countries after wars. This has been explained as follows: war '1. weakens the population's inhibitions against aggression, 2. leads to imitation of aggression, 3. makes aggressive responses more acceptable and, 4. numbs our senses to the horror of cruelty and destruction, making us less sympathetic toward the victims' (Aronson et al. 2002:445). Putting together all this evidence, one might say that during wars, women suffer much more than usual from various types of violence (combat violence, domestic violence and sexual violence). This is another trauma and gender issue that requires being studied in depth and detail.

Wars and armed political conflicts often lead to waves of illegal migration, either because people want to escape the violence or because they are being persecuted. In many countries, governments try to discourage refugees and asylum seekers and apply harsh policies of deterrence which may add to the existing traumatic symptoms of these people. Even if they are accepted as refugees, their everyday life is generally filled with adversities such as unemployment, housing problems, difficulties in adapting to the new language and culture, discrimination and missing and worrying about those they have left behind. Epidemiological studies about refugees in different parts of the world indicate many mental health problems (Kirmayer et al. 2010). A review of 20 psychiatric surveys on refugee people settled in the Western countries has shown that the average rate of PTSD is around 9 % (Fazel et al. 2005).

Victims of torture are another group of trauma survivors, a frequent occurrence during wars and armed conflicts and inevitably among refugees. Organised violence may result in repetitive and extended traumatic stress followed by high rates of PTSD. If the victims are internally displaced or seeking asylum, then they are found to be suffering from a variety of additional and potentially continuous everyday adversities. The prevalence rates of PTSD are around 40 % in asylum seekers (Hensel-Dittmann et al. 2011). Compared to men, women are at greater risk of being the victim of organised violence. Unless politically active, they are also poorly prepared for the risk of torture. Women are also at increased risk for gender-based violence, in particular rape. As with all torture methods, the goal of torture rape is generally to destroy individual identity and specifically to disturb sexual functioning. The international legal community has only very recently accepted rape as a form of torture, during the ethnic cleansing incidents in Bosnia and Rwanda. The war criminals there were the first to be prosecuted for war rape and sexual slavery (Quiroga and Jaranson 2005).

Disasters, Trauma and Gender

Disasters are mass traumatic events which need to be studied extensively with respect to gendered vulnerability. The gender-neutral stance of most disaster theory and research has been claimed to mask the gendered organisation of social life (Enarson and Morrow 1998:171). In many research reports about disasters, gender is used as a quantitative demographic category only, but there is also a growing body of literature in which gender is a central analytic concept. This literature is concerned with the social inequalities, power relations and women's subordinate position prior to disasters that influence how women and girls will be affected within a disaster-stricken community (Enarson et al. 2007). This approach also enables one to understand that the higher rates of post-traumatic symptoms and distress among women are due to social and cultural rather than biopsychological differences. This is not to say that men have no gender-specific risks in the face of disasters. However, especially when faced with natural disasters, women and girls suffer more. There are more female casualties in many cases and higher rates of trauma-related psychological problems in women.

Generally women also have more serious economic problems in the aftermath of disasters (Enarson 2000: 9–23).

A good example for gender differences in disasters are earthquakes as a category of natural events that happen suddenly and bring about great casualties as well as property damage, if they hit densely populated and poorly prepared areas. The prevalence of PTSD reported in earthquake victims varies between 13 and 95 %, depending on the degree of severity and impact. Some victims may not develop the full range of PTSD symptoms, but only some of them, and are thus diagnosed as having subthreshold or partial PTSD (PTSS). Both categories of disorders are observed more frequently in females than males (Lai et al. 2004).

Norris et al. (2002) reviewed empirical literature on disasters between 1981 and 2001 and analysed the results of 160 samples covering 60,000 victims. Being female was among the factors that they found to increase most consistently the likelihood of adverse outcomes for adults (psychological problems, health concerns, problems in living, non-specific distress, loss of resources). The other factors increasing adverse outcomes were severity of exposure, middle age, minority status, secondary stressors, prior psychiatric problems and weak or deteriorating psychosocial resources. With regard to gender, the authors found that 'not every study looked for gender effects, and not every study that looked for them found them' (Norris et al. 2002: 229). Still, 49 articles described a statistically significant gender difference in post-disaster stress, distress or disorder. Ninety-four percent of these studies reported that female survivors were more strongly affected. The differences concerned not only adults but also female children and adolescents. After many disasters, women were almost twice as likely than men and boys to develop PTSD. The gender effects were greater within samples that had additional risk factors for impairment. In some studies, culture was shown to interact with gender in predicting outcomes. The risk to women appeared to emerge at the stage of subjective interpretation, because they tended to estimate the duration and/or severity of their exposure to the disaster in a more pessimistic way than did men.

Analysing disasters and demographic data in 141 countries over the period 1981–2002, Neumayer and Plümper (2007) found that (1) natural disasters and their subsequent impact on average kill more women than men and female casualties are also younger on average; (2) major calamities led to more severe impacts on female life expectancy than do smaller disasters and (3) the higher women's socio-economic status, the weaker the effect on the gender gap in life expectancy. Hence, 'it is the socially constructed gender-specific vulnerability of females built into everyday socio-economic patterns that lead to the relatively higher female disaster mortality rates compared to men' (2007:1).

Although many disasters affect larger populations or communities, the individual responses to them vary depending on the personal and collective meanings attached to the event. Some population groups (women, children, elderly people, handicapped people, the poor and ethnic minorities) are considered to be at greater risk in the face of disasters. This does not imply that young to middle-aged healthy men who are not minority members and who have sufficient command over material resources will be the only survivors. It is obvious however that they have greater chances of survival and recovery.

Gender in mortality rates varies according to type and location of disasters. Greater numbers of male casualties are reported in some weather-related disasters such as tornadoes and thunderstorms. Gender norms and the masculine ideology may encourage more risky behaviour on the part of men during the disaster, and men may tend to seek less advice and support afterwards. They may also be more active in rescue and later in reconstruction, which are risky types of work. Their increased alcohol consumption and violent behaviours can also be considered risk factors (Nelson et al. 2002). Enarson and Morrow state that while much of women's disaster experience is ignored and distorted, men's gender-specific experiences are also concealed by gender-neutral research, and there is a 'female victim/male rescuer paradigm' that masks women's active roles before, during and after disasters (1998: 171).

Poverty is another important factor of vulnerability, and there is a good deal of literature about disasters in the poor South. A review of literature on poverty and disasters carried out in the 1980s and 1990s illustrated that the poor in the USA are also more vulnerable to natural disasters. This increased vulnerability is due to factors such as qualities of residence, building construction and social exclusion (Fothergill and Peek 2004).

> The review shows that socio-economic status is a significant predictor in the pre- and post-disaster stages as well as for the physical and psychological impacts. The poor are more likely to perceive hazards as risky; less likely to prepare for hazards or buy insurance; less likely to respond to warnings; more likely to die, suffer injuries, and have proportionately higher material losses; have more psychological trauma and face more obstacles during the phases of response, recovery and reconstruction. These differences are significant, and they illustrate a systematic pattern of stratification within the US. (Fothergill and Peek 2004:103)

Emotional vulnerability is related to class status, and lower-income disaster victims suffer more psychological impacts than do higher-income victims. Poverty is deepened by the loss of resources in disaster: unemployment and economic crisis in the aftermath strike the poor much more strongly, and few of them have access to adequate health- and psychosocial care facilities (Fothergill and Peek 2004). These findings about the poor in the USA apply to a much greater extent to the poor in the underdeveloped countries, and 70 % of the world's poor are women anyway.

Besides gender and poverty age, race and ethnicity are also important socio-demographic variables that are related to disaster vulnerability. In many cases however, data is reported without an analysis of the intersections between these variables and gender. Research subjects are divided into categories such as 'black', 'white', 'male', 'female', 'lower class' and 'middle class'. It is therefore hard to see what happens to a black female belonging to the upper class or to an elderly man belonging to a religious minority (Fothergill 1998:12–13). Feminist studies on disasters have shed some light upon women's specific problems, but there is a huge need for studies that are sensitive to the needs and circumstances of groups with varying social locations.

As well as economic problems, there are also cultural and organisational reasons for women's vulnerability. Women who are at the same time household heads and who bear responsibilities for the domestic group are especially vulnerable. Discrimination against women and female children can be aggravated in the crisis phase when the community is trying to share limited resources. Women often lose their security and may be forced to prostitution. The health and subsistence problems of their children represent ongoing stressors for most women (Wiest et al. 1994). The caretaking role of women becomes also more complicated after disasters, because they often have to take care of disabled persons or may be disabled themselves (Enarson et al. 2007). If food is scarce, as it usually is during the crisis period, women may eat last and least in order to make sure that their husbands and children are sufficiently served (Sultana 2010).

In many societies, women have no or very poor access to information and decision-making. This prevents them from being well prepared for disasters and directing communities' decisions with regard to disaster work. Conventional behaviour and dress codes sometimes prevent women from leaving their shattered houses, running away or climbing or swimming to safety if necessary. Their responsibilities for their children or the sick and elderly also limit their capacity to rescue themselves. The 2004 Asian earthquake and tsunami killed about 400,000 people in 12 countries, and in certain regions up to 80 % of the deaths were women and children. On the morning of the tsunami, many of them were on the beaches, fishing or working at morning markets, and most of them could not rescue themselves due to their traditional long garments that restricted their movements, as well as their not having been allowed to learn to swim. Still others were at home and drowned while trying to save their children. In communities where the sex ratio of the population is altered drastically, surviving women and girls have additional hardships, because they may be coerced into marriages, encouraged to have additional children, assaulted or raped (Amaratunga and O'Sullivan 2006). There are other examples of large earthquakes, cyclones and floods in Russia, Japan, Guatemala, Egypt and Bangladesh where many more females than males died, again because they could not leave their homes due to caretaking responsibilities or for fear of blame and punishment in case anything happened to the family property (Fothergill 1998).

Regarding the psychological impact of disasters, many studies report that women and female children complain of more emotional problems, stress, depression and PTSD, often aggravated by the difficulties of caregiving, while men tend to use more alcohol. But the results are mixed, and some studies report greater distress in men (Fothergill 1998). A review of studies about disasters in different countries over 40 years (1963–2003) (Galea et al. 2005) revealed that women were consistently reported to have a higher prevalence of PTSD. Research on gender differences in risk perception reveals that women perceive disaster risks as more serious than men. They report experiencing more fear about earthquakes and other natural or man-made hazards. They are also more likely to take warnings seriously and to evacuate. Despite their increased awareness, they are assigned very few roles in decision-making and preparation (Fothergill 1998).

After a disaster, women often have difficulty finding or building shelters, finding employment and restructuring life. Very often the frequencies of sexual assault and rape increase in communities (Thornton and Voigt 2007). Even if the family unity is saved, the extreme hardships following disasters very often lead to domestic unrest and violence (Fothergill 1998; Fothergill and Peek 2004; Enarson et al. 2007; Kümbetoglu and User 2010). Violence in the community and sexual assault may result in unwanted pregnancies, miscarriages and the spread of sexually transmitted diseases, especially HIV/AIDS (Sultana 2010). Disasters also cause many hygiene, health and reproductive problems for women. Clean underwear may not be available, especially after floods and earthquakes. Polluted waters may lead to infections. Women's poor nutritional status and poor access to health care combined with disaster stress often leave them very weak. Giving birth during or right after a disaster means that labour will take place under the most adverse circumstances, and the infant and the mother will be deprived of adequate medical care. A pregnancy may also be highly complicated under disaster circumstances. Very similar risks have also been mentioned for times of wars and other armed conflicts.

Under the circumstances outlined above, it is inevitable that women will be affected most badly by disasters and that they will experience high degrees of traumatic stress. Their problems are not due to constitutional vulnerabilities, but to social, economic and cultural factors. In any disaster-stricken region, women belonging to the upper socio-economic strata, living in safe dwellings and commanding over adequate resources, will suffer far less than their less well-off peers.

Gender and Perceiving Benefits in Adversity

The belief in positive changes following adverse experiences and suffering is quite old. There are various religious and philosophical notions about the self being tested by hardship, learning from this, and attaining a higher level of development. In the twentieth century a number of authors pointed to the possibility of psychological development resulting from life crises. From the 1990s on, a growing body of literature emerged that emphasised the positive outcomes of highly stressful events. Referring to these positive outcomes, Tedeschi and Calhoun coined the term 'post-traumatic growth' (PTG). Even though numerous other concepts such as 'stress-related growth', 'transformational coping', 'perceived benefits', 'blessings', 'positive adjustment' or 'thriving' refer to a process of psychological maturation after suffering (Siegel and Schrimshaw 2000:1453; Linley and Joseph 2004:11), the most widely used concept appears to be 'post-traumatic growth' (PTG).

PTG is defined as a positive change in ones belief or functioning as a result of the struggle with highly challenging life crises. Tedeschi and Calhoun (2004:5) describe trauma as a psychologically seismic event that leads to the collapse of and necessitates the reconstruction of the individual's cognitive processes. The new schemas of the individual incorporate the trauma and possible future events. The individual experiences these cognitive changes as growth. The authors have identified five domains of growth: (1) greater appreciation of life and change of priorities, (2) more intimate and meaningful relationships, (3) a sense of increased personal strength,

(4) identification of new possibilities in life and (5) change and growth in the domains of spiritual and existential matters. Personality characteristics such as extroversion, openness to experience and optimism may be facilitative for PTG. The authors have constructed a measurement instrument (the post-traumatic growth inventory) to assess growth in these five domains (Tedeschi and Calhoun 1996). This instrument was translated, validated and used in many other contexts too (e.g. Karanci and Acarturk 2005; Jaarsma et al. 2006; Nishi et al. 2010; Karanci et al. 2012; Taku et al. 2007; Kimhi et al. 2010). The cross-cultural studies on PTGI indicate that post-traumatic growth is not an American construct only. This phenomenon can be observed in other cultures, but the factors may be somewhat different than those identified by Tedeschi and Calhoun.

The positive changes due to PTG are often reflected in personal relationships, self-perception and philosophy of life (Sawyer et al. 2012). In other words, PTG means that one has not only recovered from the stressful episode, but also surpasses the level of functioning one had before the occurrence of the traumatic event (Hefferon et al. 2009:243). A person's perception of his or her ability to deal with hardship can be positively altered after having survived a trauma or adversity. This altered perception of the self can also empower the person in the face of future problems and suffering.

Initially the researchers using this concept were concerned with growth after events which were considered as typical in the trauma literature. Hence, people who had experienced combat, natural disasters or sexual violence were studied in order to determine the degree of growth. Later, Calhoun and Tedeschi explained that they were using the words 'trauma', 'crisis', 'highly stressful events' and other similar terms as roughly synonymous expressions describing sets of circumstances that represent significant challenges to the adaptive resources of individuals and their ways of interpreting the world (2004:1). Recently and associated with the change in the definitions of trauma and PTSD, other highly stressful events such as diagnosis and treatment of cancer, heart attack, work problems or migration have also begun to be considered as facilitating PTG. Research on PTG has rapidly grown including patients with melanoma; bone marrow transplantation; spinal cord injury and brain injury; adult childhood cancer survivors; breast, prostate, and testicular cancer patients; patient-partner dyads; and children's medical problems as well as survivors of house fires, sexual assault and combat. Refugees, people who had been taken hostage, Holocaust survivors and former German child soldiers of World War II were also examined for PTG (Zwahlen et al. 2010; Sawyer et al. 2012; Forstmeier et al. 2009; Chun and Lee 2008; Tedeschi and Calhoun 1996; Tedeschi and Calhoun 2004; Widows et al. 2005; Lurie-Beck et al. 2008; Hefferon et al. 2009; Garland et al. 2007; Jaarsma et al. 2006).

Despite the large numbers of reports on PTG, one should not assume that growth is an inevitable result of trauma. What is more, growth may often coexist with continuing personal distress. According to Tedeschi and Calhoun, there are important differences between PTG and the phenomena resilience, hardiness and sense of coherence. PTG has to do with positive changes, whereas the latter are related with coping, and people with a high capacity for these mechanisms will probably not report a high degree of growth, because their coping will prevent them from being too badly challenged by trauma or adversity (Tedeschi and Calhoun 2004). There are also studies that have aimed at identifying which coping strategies are positively related with PTG (for a brief review see Chun and Lee 2008:878). Among factors found to be contributing to PTG are experience of meaningful engagement, social acknowledgement as a survivor (e.g. appreciation of and positive reactions to one's traumatic experience) and experience of meaningful family relations including emotional intimacy and gaining trust, emotional expression and openness to experience (Jaarsma et al. 2006; Chun and Lee 2008; Forstmeier et al. 2009).

PTG should not be expected to take place after all kinds of traumatic events. In a study with Bosnian people after the war in former Yugoslavia, considerably lower degrees of PTG were observed. This finding was interpreted with reference to the degree of traumatisation. The Bosnian people had experienced multiple traumas, and the system surrounding them had also collapsed. The authors suggested an inverted-U relationship between severity of exposure and growth, in which medium stress is linked with the highest average growth (Powell et al. 2003).

Women tend to score higher on the post-traumatic growth inventory, and the greatest differences exist in their ability to perceive spiritual and relationship changes (Tedeschi and Calhoun 1996: 468), probably because women rely more on social and spiritual support when they are faced with stressful events. There are also gender differences in the perception of new possibilities and personal strength, but these differences are smaller. It seems that women have a greater capacity for positive learning from adversity. In a review of 39 studies, in which not only PTGI but also other measurement instruments had been used, the evidence with regard to gender differences in psychological growth after adversity was found to be mixed (Linley and Joseph 2004:16). However, differences as well as similarities of outcome should be considered with caution, as long as the sample characteristics, measurement instruments and types of adversity studied vary.

A review of 57 qualitative studies published over a period of 32 years revealed that besides the five elements of PTG identified by Tedeschi and Calhoun, a sixth element emerges in relation to people who have suffered from life-threatening diseases. This is described as a new awareness and a heightened perception of the importance of the body as well as a new and positive identification with it, leading the person to take increasing responsibility for his or her health, to omit health-compromising habits and to engage in health-promoting behaviour (Hefferon et al. 2009). Even though a gender analysis is not attempted in this review, 16 of the studies reviewed are about women with breast cancer, 1 about lymphoedema in women, 1 about arthritis, osteoporosis and fibromyalgia in women and 3 about women with HIV/AIDS. One may say that a considerable body of evidence has been accumulated and a review from the gender perspective might be very useful, especially considering the fact that women tend to have a heightened sensitivity about their bodies because of cultural pressures emphasising physical beauty, fitness and youthfulness in the female gender.

PTG in cancer patients was found to be related to gender, with women reporting significantly more PTG than men (Jaarsma et al. 2006). A study with breast cancer patients showed that PTG moderates the relationships between post-traumatic stress symptoms and depression as well as impaired quality of life. In this study, Morrill et al. (2008) interviewed survivors of breast cancer and assessed PTG as well as PTDS, depressive symptoms and quality of life, finding that PTG moderates between post-traumatic symptoms and both depressive symptoms and quality of life. At the same time, they found that women with better educational and financial status enjoyed greater well-being. This evidence implies that social differences within one sex may determine the degree of negative as well as positive effects of a traumatic event. Neither breast cancer nor any other life crisis will affect women of different social status in uniform ways, because there is no essential and uniform female existence, but rather various existences shaped by social, cultural and material means and circumstances. Although all women may be expected to experience breast cancer as a life-threatening as well as disfiguring disease, their individual differences in intellectual endowment, world view, perception of the female role or material means of improving their health and their looks will probably affect their responses to the disease.

Another gender-specific context within which PTG has been studied is childbirth. In one study, about 50 % of a sample of 219 women were assessed as having experienced PTG in four of the five domains measured by Tedeschi and Calhoun's PTG Inventory. The greatest change was in the appreciation of life, and the smallest was in the domain of spirituality. Growth was not associated with PTSD symptoms, and this was interpreted to imply that women experience growth after birth, even if labour has not been perceived as traumatic (Sawyer and Ayers 2009). However, in a prospective study aimed at examining the correlates of post-traumatic growth after birth, the strongest predictors of growth were found to be operative delivery and post-traumatic stress symptoms, and average levels of growth were lower than generally reported in other studies (Sawyer et al. 2012). Parents who have been traumatised by losing a child have also been studied. Two to 6 years after the death of a premature infant, parents were found to be suffering still. The mothers experienced higher grief and scored higher on PTG (Büchi et al. 2007).

A qualitative study on African-American, Puerto Rican and non-Hispanic white women living with HIV/AIDS in New York, USA (Siegel and Schrimshaw 2000), revealed that almost all of them experienced some growth related to the distress of their illness. The forms of growth varied in relation to the women's ethnic backgrounds, class situations and intravenous drug use histories. The authors criticised previous research on PTG for being confined to educated, middle-class, mostly male samples (often students) and supplying very little information about women and ethnic minorities. Their study showed that for disadvantaged groups, PTG may have different meanings. The study participants declared that they experienced problems including stigma, disability and distress. Nevertheless, most of them believed that the illness had also contributed something positive to their lives. Since the adversities they experienced continued due to the chronicity of their illness, their situation was different to that of people who have experienced and recovered from a trauma. Hence, they were evidence that growth may take place in the continued presence of adversity. The forms of growth were various (e.g. women with a history of drug abuse reported positive changes in health behaviours;

African-American and Puerto Rican women emphasised spiritual change; educated, middle-class women were concerned with career changes). Some of the women described very modest changes as growth, but for their circumstances, these changes also meant a lot. These findings show that context is important for the form as well as the degree of growth. What is more, they also point to the usefulness of qualitative techniques in such research, because fixed scale items do not allow the researcher to understand what participants with different backgrounds mean by benefiting from adversity.

Massive traumas have also been found to lead to growth in personal and group functioning in the afflicted communities. In the case of terrorism, the development of new skills and strengths, altruism, sharing emotions, changes in cognitive schemas and positive emotions were identified as dimensions of growth after trauma, and governments were urged to focus not only on minimising the negative effects, but also on promoting positive outcomes and growth (Vazquez et al. 2008). A study on multi-traumatised psychiatric outpatients with a refugee background in Norway revealed that all reported some degree of growth. Sixty percent of these patients were unemployed, 80 % reported post-traumatic symptoms and 93 % reported depressive symptoms. The authors comment that PTG takes time. In their sample they have observed people with a relatively recent refugee experience to have an illusory construct of benefiting from adversity which functions as a coping mechanism. However, people who have had this experience for a long time also have a genuine and constructive growth experience. The authors conclude that clinicians working with traumatised persons should pay greater attention to positive changes after trauma and to monitoring the quality of life among their patients (Teodorescu et al. 2012).

Lurie-Beck et al. (2008) found consistent positive relationships between PTSD symptoms and post-traumatic growth in a sample of 23 Holocaust survivors. The authors suggest that if larger samples of Holocaust survivors can be reached (which is becoming increasingly difficult for demographic reasons) and studied, the results might inform clinicians dealing with more recent examples of mass trauma such as former Yugoslavia, Cambodia, Rwanda, Darfur, Iraq, Afghanistan, Israel and Palestine. A study on survivors of Hurricane Katrina in the USA reported that survivors with relatively good mental and physical health and stronger coping self-efficacy experienced less PTG than survivors with relatively low coping self-efficacy and stronger symptoms of PTSD. This is also interpreted as evidence that people who cope effectively with trauma and prevent themselves from intensive symptoms of PTSD or other stress-related mental problems experience little growth (Cieslak et al. 2009).

In a study about PTSD and PTG in an Israeli sample 1 year after the war in 2009, women reported a higher level of traumatic stress symptoms and lower rates of PTG than men. Since the studies on gender differences in PTG appear to have mixed results, the authors theorise that the association between gender and PTG depends on the type of trauma. On the other hand, a study on former German child soldiers in World War II (Forstmeier et al. 2009) revealed that social acknowledgement as a survivor and the belief in a meaningful world enhance PTG. These two feelings are incompatible with events considered as shameful by the victims (e.g. rape, torture) or events that have resulted in death or serious injury of loved ones (e.g. accidents or disasters)

Concluding Remarks

Even though there is a vast amount of research considering trauma, PTSD and PTG, comparing the results is difficult: there are great differences in the types of trauma, the cultural contexts of the traumatic events and sample characteristics. On the other hand, clinical assessments and community surveys based on self-report supply data of a very different nature which is hard to compare. Many of the community surveys in the literature are based on phone or web interviews. Phone and web surveys seem to be well established, and there is no reason to doubt that they are being carried out in accordance with the technical and ethical rules pertaining to sampling, training of the interviewers and obtaining informed consent. However, this does not mean that these techniques are beyond criticism. To begin with, they can only be employed in communities where phone or web access is universal. What is more, the average individual in a target community must display a level of intellectual development and literacy that will enable him or her to appreciate the significance of scientific inquiry and of understanding and honestly responding to every question. Even in cases where the presence of such a community can be assumed, it is impossible to ascertain whether the researcher has actually contacted the targeted respondents. Additionally, communication via telephone or the Internet is very limited and does not enable the researcher to establish sufficient rapport or to notice non-verbal cues. All this means that the dependability of such survey results is questionable and that many communities in the world can still not be reached via these techniques. The latter point limits the comparability of research results obtained in different settings. Phone or web interviews are convenient in order to reach large samples from a distance and to collect data quickly, but the qualitative superiority of data generated via face-to-face contact with respondents and backed up by real observations in the field is not negligible.

No matter how the interviews are administered, researchers have to rely on self-ratings and self-reported symptoms in community surveys. Whether these symptoms have any clinical significance and how gender, culture or class biases in reporting will be ruled out remain open questions. Women's greater vulnerability to trauma may be related to willingness to report symptoms, whereas men may tend to under-report because of considerations that identifying oneself as a suffering victim may jeopardise one's masculinity. This concern has been reported in the literature (Tolin and Foa 2006; Vogt et al. 2011). Trying to compare community samples with clinical samples is therefore problematic.

The available evidence indicates that men and women experience different risks, vulnerabilities and reactions in the face of traumatic events. These differences are very poorly analysed with respect to gender as a sociocultural status. Some studies give at least partial information about how sociodemographic variables affect the impact of trauma, which may enable future researchers to be more sensitive to differences not only between men and women, but also between different groups within one sex. Rather than identifying women as the 'usual victims', researchers should concentrate on understanding the interactions between trauma and the socio-demographic variables of gender, age, ethnicity, marital status, education, income and occupation. Such an approach may enable scientists as well as decision-makers to see how social inequalities create vulnerabilities, and policy measures may be taken in order to improve people's and communities' circumstances before the occurrence of any traumatic event. For a comprehensive understanding of the relationship between trauma and gender, multisite epidemiological research in different cultures might also be very useful. The focus of any research on trauma and gender should be not only on vulnerability and victimisation, but also on agency and growth. However, the possibilities of agency and growth should not blind researchers or decision-makers to the distress and suffering of people.

It should also be kept in mind that instruments of quantitative measurement operationalise concepts, narrowing down the boundaries within which phenomena will be observed. Hence, more qualitative research is required to understand what people experience and how they interpret their experiences. Data obtained with gender- and culture-sensitive techniques may be useful in improving diagnosis and treatment, as well as in preparing different population groups for imminent traumatic events such as deployment or natural disasters.

References

Amaratunga CA, O'Sullivan TL (2006) In the path of disasters: psychosocial issues for preparedness, response, and recovery. Prehosp Disaster Med 21(03):149–153

Aronson E, Wilson TD, Akert RM (2002) Social psychology, 4th edn. Pearson Education, Prentice Hall, Upper Saddle River, NJ

Astbury, J (1999) Gender and mental health. Harvard Center for Population and Development Studies

Ayers S (2004) Delivery as a traumatic event: prevalence, risk factors, and treatment for postnatal post-traumatic stress disorder. Clin Obstet Gynecol 47(3):552–567

Ayers S, Pickering, AD (2005) Women's expectations and experience of birth. Psychology and Health 20(1):79–92

Ayers S (2007) Thoughts and emotions during traumatic birth: a qualitative study. Birth 34(3):253–263

Ayers S, Pickering AD (2001) Do women get post-traumatic stress disorder as a result of childbirth? A prospective study of incidence. Birth 28(2):111–118

Ayers S, Eagle A, Waring H (2006) The effects of childbirth-related post-traumatic stress disorder on women and their relationships: a qualitative study. Psychol Health Med 11(4):389–398

Ayers S, Wright DB, Wells N (2007) Symptoms of post-traumatic stress disorder in couples after birth: association with the couple's relationship and parent–baby bond. J Reprod Infant Psychol 25(1):40–50

Ayers S, Harris R, Sawyer A, Parfitt Y, Ford E (2009) Post-traumatic stress disorder after childbirth: analysis of symptom presentation and sampling. J Affect Disord 119(1):200–204

Beck CT (2004) Post-traumatic stress disorder due to childbirth: the aftermath. Nurs Res 53(4):216–224

Bleich A, Gelkopf M, Solomon Z (2003) Exposure to terrorism, stress-related mental health symptoms, and coping behaviors among a nationally representative sample in Israel. JAMA 290(5):612–620

Brewin CR, Andrews B, Valentine JD (2000) Meta-analysis of risk factors for post-traumatic stress disorder in trauma-exposed adults. J Consult Clin Psychol 68(5):748

Büchi S, Mörgeli H, Schnyder U, Jenewein J, Hepp U, Jina E, Neuhaus R, Fauchere J-C, Bbucher HU, Sensky T (2007) Grief and post-traumatic growth in parents 2–6 years after the death of their extremely premature baby. Psychother Psychosom 76(2):106–114

Chinkin C (1994) Rape and sexual abuse of women in international law. Eur J Int Law 5:326

Chun S, Lee Y (2008) The experience of post-traumatic growth for people with spinal cord injury. Qual Health Res 18(7):877–890

Cieslak R, Benight C, Schmidt N, Luszczynska A, Curtin E, Clark RA, Kissinger P (2009) Predicting post-traumatic growth among Hurricane Katrina survivors living with HIV: the role of self-efficacy, social support, and PTSD symptoms. Anxiety Stress Coping 22(4):449–463

Connell, RW (1987) Gender and power: society, the person and sexual politics. Stanford University Press

Courtenay WH (2000) Constructions of masculinity and their influence on men's well-being: a theory of gender and health. Soc Sci Med 50(10):1385–1401

Creamer M, Burgess P, McFarlane AC (2001) Post-traumatic stress disorder: findings from the Australian National Survey of Mental Health and Well-being. Psychol Med 31(07):1237–1247

Davison GC, Neale JM (1998) Abnormal psychology. Wiley, New York

Deaux K, Major B (2000) A social-psychological model of gender. In: Kimmel MS (ed) The gendered society reader. Oxford University Press, New York, pp 81–90

Di Blasio P, Ionio C (2005) Post-partum stress symptoms and child temperament: a follow-up study. J Prenat Perinat Psychol Health 19(3):185–198

Ditlevsen DN, Elklit A (2010) The combined effect of gender and age on post traumatic stress disorder: do men and women show differences in the lifespan distribution of the disorder. Ann Gen Psychiatry 9(32):32. doi: 10.1186/1744-859X-9-32

Ditlevsen DN, Elklit A (2012) Gender, trauma type, and PTSD prevalence: a re-analysis of 18 nordic convenience samples. Ann Gen Psychiatry 11:26. doi: 10.1186/1744-859X-11-26

Enarson, EP (2000). Gender and natural disasters. ILO, Geneva.

Enarson E, Morrow BH (1998) Why gender? Why women? An introduction to women and disaster. In: The gendered terrain of disaster: through women's eyes. Praeget, New York, pp 1–8

Enarson E, Morrow BH (1998) Women will rebuild Miami: a case study of feminist response to disaster. In: Enarson E, Morrow BH (eds) The gendered terrain of disaster: through women's eyes. Praeger Publishers, Westport, pp 171–184

Enarson E, Fothergill A, Peek L (2007) Gender and disaster: foundations and directions. In: Dynes, RR, Quarantelli, EL, Rodriguez, H (eds) Handbook of disaster research. Springer, New York, pp 130–146

Farwell N (2004) War rape: new conceptualizations and responses. Affilia 19(4):389–403

Fazel M, Wheeler J, Danesh J (2005) Prevalence of serious mental disorder in 7000 refugees resettled in western countries: a systematic review. Lancet 365:1309–1314

Forstmeier S, Kuwert P, Spitzer C, Freyberger HJ, Maercker A (2009) Post-traumatic growth, social acknowledgment as survivors, and sense of coherence in former German child soldiers of World War II. Am J Geriatr Psychiatry 17(12):1030–1039

Fothergill A (1998) The neglect of gender in disaster work: an overview of the literature. In: Enarson E, Morrow BH (eds) The gendered terrain of disaster: through women's eyes. Praeger Publishers, Westport, pp 12–13

Fothergill A, Peek LA (2004) Poverty and disasters in the United States: a review of recent sociological findings. Nat Hazards 32(1):89–110

Galea S, Nandi A, Vlahov D (2005) The epidemiology of post-traumatic stress disorder after disasters. Epidemiol Rev 27(1):78–91

Garland SN, Carlson LE, Cook S, Lansdell L, Speca M (2007) A non-randomized comparison of mindfulness-based stress reduction and healing arts programs for facilitating post-traumatic growth and spirituality in cancer outpatients. Supportive Care in Cancer 15(8):949–961

Garthus-Niegel S, von Soest T, Vollrath ME, Eberhard-Gran M (2012) The impact of subjective birth experiences on post-traumatic stress symptoms: a longitudinal study. Arch Women's Ment Health 16(1):1–10

Gold SD, Marx BP, Soler-Baillo JM, Sloan DM (2005) Is life stress more traumatic than traumatic stress? J Anxiety Disord 19(6):687–698

Hefferon K, Grealy M, Mutrie N (2009) Posttraumatic growth and life threatening physical illness: a systematic review of the qualitative literature. Br J Health Psychol 14(2):343–378

Hensel-Dittmann D, Schauer M, Ruf M, Catani C, Odenwald M, Elbert T, Neuner F (2011) Treatment of traumatized victims of war and torture: a randomized controlled comparison of narrative exposure therapy and stress inoculation training. Psychother Psychosom 80(6):345–352

Jaarsma TA, Pool G, Sanderman R, Ranchor AV (2006) Psychometric properties of the Dutch version of the posttraumatic growth inventory among cancer patients. Psycho-Oncology 15(10):911–920

Karanci NA, Acarturk C (2005) Post-traumatic growth among Marmara earthquake survivors involved in disaster preparedness as volunteers. Traumatol Int J 11(4):307–323

Karanci AN, Işıklı S, Aker AT, Gül Eİ, Erkan BB, Özkol H, Güzel HY (2012) Personality, posttraumatic stress and trauma type: factors contributing to posttraumatic growth and its domains in a Turkish community sample. Eur J Psychotraumatol 3, pp 1–14. doi:10.3402/ejpt.v3i0.17303

Kimerling R, Gima K, Smith MW, Street A, Frayne S (2007) The Veterans Health Administration and military sexual trauma. Am J Public Health 97(12):2160–2166

Kimhi S, Eshel Y, Zysberg L, Hantman S (2010) Postwar winners and losers in the long run: determinants of war related stress symptoms and post-traumatic growth. Community Ment Health J 46(1):10–19

Kimmel MS (2000) Introduction. In: Kimmel MS, Aronson A (eds) The gendered society reader. Oxford University Press, New York, pp 1–6

Kirmayer LJ, Kienzler H, Afana AH, Pedersen D (2010) Trauma and disasters in social and cultural context. In: Morgan C, Bhugra D (eds) Principles of social psychiatry, 2nd edn. Wiley-Blackwell, New York, pp 155–177

Klarić M, Klarić B, Stevanović A, Grković J, Jonovska S (2007) Psychological consequences of war trauma and postwar social stressors in women in Bosnia and Herzegovina. Croat Med J 48(2):167–176

Kumbetoglu B, User I (2010) Gender aspects of the disaster recovery process. In: Dasgupta S, Siriner I, Partha SD (eds) Women's encounter with disaster. Frontpage, London

Lai TJ, Chang CM, Connor KM, Lee LC, Davidson JR (2004) Full and partial PTSD among earthquake survivors in rural Taiwan. J Psychiatr Res 38(3):313–322

Lee C (1998) Women's health. Psychological and social perspectives. Sage, London

Linley PA, Joseph S (2004) Positive change following trauma and adversity: a review. J Trauma Stress 17(1):11–21

Lurie-Beck JK, Liossis P, Gow K (2008) Relationships between psychopathological and demographic variables and posttraumatic growth among holocaust survivors. Traumatol Int J 14(3):28–39

Matsuoka Y, Nishi D, Nakajima S, Kim Y, Homma M, Otomo Y (2008) Incidence and prediction of psychiatric morbidity after a motor vehicle accident in Japan: the Tachikawa Cohort of Motor Vehicle Accident Study. Crit Care Med 36(1):74–80

Matt GE, Vázquez C (2008) Anxiety, depressed mood, self-esteem, and traumatic stress symptoms among distant witnesses of the 9/11 terrorist attacks: transitory responses and psychological resilience. Span J Psychol 11(02):503–515

Mejía XE (2005) Gender matters: working with adult male survivors of trauma. J Couns Dev 83(1):29–40

Morrill EF, Brewer NT, O'Neill SC, Lillie SE, Dees EC, Carey LA, Rimer BK (2008) The interaction of post-traumatic growth and post-traumatic stress symptoms in predicting depressive symptoms and quality of life. Psycho-Oncology 17(9):948–953

Nelson V, Meadows K, Cannon T, Morton J, Martin A (2002) Uncertain predictions, invisible impacts, and the need to mainstream gender in climate change adaptations. Gend Dev 10(2):51–59

Neumayer E, Plümper T (2007) The gendered nature of natural disasters: the impact of catastrophic events on the gender gap in life expectancy, 1981–2002. Ann Assoc Am Geogr 97(3):551–566

Nishi D, Matsuoka Y, Kim Y (2010) Research post-traumatic growth, post-traumatic stress disorder and resilience of motor vehicle accident survivors. BioPsychoSoc Med 4:7

Nolen-Hoeksema S (2011) Abnormal psychology. McGraw-Hill, New York

Norris FH, Perilla JL, Ibañez GE, Murphy AD (2001) Sex differences in symptoms of post-traumatic stress: does culture play a role? J Trauma Stress 14(1):7–28

Norris FH, Friedman MJ, Watson PJ, Byrne CM, Diaz E, Kaniasty K (2002) 60,000 disaster victims speak: part I. An empirical review of the empirical literature, 1981–2001. Psychiatry Interpersonal Biol Process 65(3):207–239

Onrust SA, Cuijpers P (2006) Mood and anxiety disorders in widowhood: a systematic review. Aging Ment Health 10(4):327–334

Powell S, Rosner R, Butollo W, Tedeschi RG, Calhoun LG (2003) Post-traumatic growth after war: a study with former refugees and displaced people in Sarajevo. J Clin Psychol 59(1):71–83

Priebe S, Bogic M, Ajdukovic D, Franciskovic T, Galeazzi GM, Kucukalic A, Lecic-Tosevski D, Morina N, Popovski M, Wang D, Schützwohl M (2010) Mental disorders following war in the Balkans: a study in 5 countries. Arch Gen Psychiatry 67(5):518–528

Quiroga J, Jaranson JM (2005) Politically-motivated torture and its survivors. Torture 15:2–3

Ringelheim J (1997) Genocide and gender: a split memory. In: Lentin R (ed) Gender & catastrophe. Zed Books Ltd., London, pp 18–33

Russell D (1995) Women, madness & medicine. Polity Press, Cambridge

Sancho N (1997) The 'comfort women' system during World War II: Asian women as targets of mass rape and sexual slavery by Japan. In: Lentin R (ed) Gender & catastrophe. Zed Books Ltd., London, pp 144–153

Sawyer A, Ayers S (2009) Post-traumatic growth in women after childbirth. Psychol Health 24(4):457–471

Sawyer A, Ayers S, Young D, Bradley R, Smith H (2012) Post-traumatic growth after childbirth: a prospective study. Psychol Health 27(3):362–377

Schambler A (2008) Women and health. In: Schambler G (ed) Sociology as applied to medicine. Saunders, Edinburgh, pp 133–158

Siegel K, Schrimshaw EW (2000) Perceiving benefits in adversity: stress-related growth in women living with HIV/AIDS. Soc Sci Med 51(10):1543–1554

Small R, Astbury J, Brown S, Lumley J (1994) Depression after childbirth. Does social context matter? Med J Aust 161(8):473–477

Solomon Z, Gelkopf M, Bleich A (2005) Is terror gender-blind? Gender differences in reaction to terror events. Soc Psychiatry Psychiatr Epidemiol 40(12):947–954

Street AE, Gradus JL, Giasson HL, Vogt D, Resick PA (2013) Gender differences among veterans deployed in support of the wars in Afghanistan and Iraq. J Gen Intern Med 28(2):555–556

Stuber J, Resnick H, Galea S (2006) Gender disparities in post-traumatic stress disorder after mass trauma. Gend Med 3(1):54–67

Sultana F (2010) Living in hazardous waterscapes: gendered vulnerabilities and experiences of floods and disasters. Environ Hazards 9(1):43–53

Takegata M, Kitamura T, Haruna M, Sakanashi K, Tanaka T (2014) Childbirth as a trauma: psychometric properties of the impact event scale in Japanese mothers of neonates. Psychol Behav Sci 3(2):46–50

Taku K, Calhoun LG, Tedeschi RG, Gil-Rivas V, Kilmer RP, Cann A (2007) Examining post-traumatic growth among Japanese university students. Anxiety Stress Coping 20(4):353–367

Tedeschi RG, Calhoun LG (1996) The posttraumatic growth inventory: measuring the positive legacy of trauma. J Trauma Stress 9(3):455–471

Tedeschi RG, Calhoun LG (2004) Posttraumatic growth: conceptual foundations and empirical evidence. Psychol Inq 15(1):1–18

Teodorescu DS, Siqveland J, Heir T, Hauff E, Wentzel-Larsen T, Lien L (2012) Post-traumatic growth, depressive symptoms, post-traumatic stress symptoms, post-migration stressors and quality of life in multi-traumatized psychiatric outpatients with a refugee background in Norway. Health Qual Life Outcomes 10:84

Thornton WE, Voight L (2007) Disaster rape: vulnerability of women to sexual assaults during Hurricane Katrina. J Public Manag Soc Policy 13(2):23–49

Tolin DF, Foa EB (2006) Sex differences in trauma and post-traumatic stress disorder: a quantitative review of 25 years of research. Psychol Bull 132(6):959

Umberson D, Wortman CB, Kessler RC (1992) Widowhood and depression: explaining long-term gender differences in vulnerability. J Health Soc Behav 33(1):10–24

van Grootheest DS, Beekman AT, Van Groenou MB, Deeg DJ (1999) Sex differences in depression after widowhood. Do men suffer more? Soc Psychiatry Psychiatr Epidemiol 34(7):391–398

van Son M, Verkerk G, van der Hart O, Komproe I, Pop V (2005) Prenatal depression, mode of delivery and perinatal dissociation as predictors of post-partum post-traumatic stress: an empirical study. Clin Psychol Psychother 12(4):297–312

Vázquez C, Pérez-Sales P, Hervás G (2008) Positive effects of terrorism and post-traumatic growth: an individual and community perspective. In: Linlay PA, Joseph S (eds) Trauma, recovery, and growth: positive psychological perspectives on post-traumatic stress. Wiley, Hoboken, pp 63–91

Vogt D, Vaughn R, Glickman ME, Schultz M, Drainoni ML, Elwy R, Eisen S (2011) Gender differences in combat-related stressors and their association with post-deployment mental health in a nationally representative sample of US OEF/OIF veterans. J Abnorm Psychol 120(4):797

Vogt D, Street AE (2013) Women in Combat. In: Moore BA, Bernett EJ (eds) Military psycohologists' desk reference. Oxford University Press, pp 148–152

Widows MR, Jacobsen PB, Booth-Jones M, Fields KK (2005) Predictors of post-traumatic growth following bone marrow transplantation for cancer. Health Psychol 24(3):266

Wiest RE, Mocellin JS, Motsisi DT (1994) The needs of women in disasters and emergencies. Disaster Research Institute, University of Manitoba

Zwahlen D, Hagenbuch N, Carley MI, Jenewein J, Buchi S (2010) Post-traumatic growth in cancer patients and partners-effects of role, gender and the dyad on couples' post-traumatic growth experience. Psycho-Oncology 19(1):12

Exposure to Trauma and Forced Migration: Mental Health and Acculturation Patterns Among Asylum Seekers in Israel

Ido Lurie and Ora Nakash

Forced Migration to Israel

Political tension, civil unrest and persecution based on religious affiliation are some of the reasons that force people to leave their countries of origin and flee to safer places where asylum is offered. Section 94(1) of the Immigration and Asylum Act of the United Nations Agency for Refugees defines an asylum seeker as a displaced person who '…is not under 18 and has made a claim for asylum which has been recorded by the Secretary of State but which has not been determined' (United Nations High Commissioner for Refugees 2001). The number of asylum seekers is growing rapidly, and the United Nations High Commissioner for Refugees (2011) estimated that there are approximately 895,000 asylum seekers worldwide.

In keeping with global immigration trends, during the last few decades, the State of Israel has become a target for economic migrants, refugees, asylum seekers and victims of human trafficking. Particularly, Israel has been facing an influx of African asylum seekers in recent years. There are currently approximately 55,000 asylum seekers in Israel, the majority having come from Eritrea and Sudan (Moshe 2013). African asylum seekers began crossing the Egypt-Israel border in 2006. Most, if not all, arrive in Israel via the Sinai desert in Egypt (Lijnders 2012). From 2007 to 2013, the number of asylum seekers that arrived in Israel through the Sinai desert increased dramatically and reached a peak of over 2,000 people each month during 2010

I. Lurie (✉)
Adult Mental Health Clinic, Shalvata Mental Health Center, Hod Hasharon, Israel

Sackler School of Medicine, Tel Aviv University, Tel Aviv, Israel
e-mail: ido.lurie@gmail.com

O. Nakash
School of Psychology, Interdisciplinary Center (IDC), Herzliya, Israel

© Springer International Publishing Switzerland 2015
M. Schouler-Ocak (ed.), *Trauma and Migration:
Cultural Factors in the Diagnosis and Treatment of Traumatised Immigrants*,
DOI 10.1007/978-3-319-17335-1_10

(Human Rights Watch 2014; Lijnders 2012). This trend decreased following the completion of the Egyptian-Israeli border fence and an increase in restrictive policies that substantially reduced the number of new arrivals since 2013.

There are numerous reasons for the influx of asylum seekers entering Israel. Eritreans claim asylum based on their escape from an extremely repressive situation, including a life-long compulsory military service in their native country, grave violations of human rights, religious and political persecution, disappearances of citizens and the use of torture by the government (Connell 2012; Tronvoll 2009). Men and women from the Darfur region in Sudan flee persecution and mass murder of civilian populations perpetrated by the government and armed militia groups. Israel also hosts a smaller community of asylum seekers who have escaped years of governmental persecution, civil war, insecurity and lack of social infrastructure in South Sudan (Furst-Nichols and Jacobsen 2011; Reynolds 2013). Other reasons for this influx can be traced to the growing restrictions on migration to Europe and the decline of living conditions for African refugees in Libya and Egypt with the political unrest, the state of insecurity and chaos in North Africa.

The journey of African asylum seekers to Israel has led them through the Northern Sinai, a region that despite being under Egyptian rule has been characterised by a political vacuum, growing lawlessness and impunity since the Arab Spring in 2010 (Furst-Nichols and Jacobsen 2011; Reynolds 2013). While some people who flee from East Africa are able to pay smugglers to guide them in relative safety to refugee camps, a significant number cross the border without help and often fall prey to human traffickers who roam the Sinai desert and the border region (van Reisen et al. 2012). Traffickers also operate within Ethiopian and Sudanese refugee camps (van Reisen et al. 2013). A sizable network of smugglers operates across Eritrea, Sudan, Egypt and Israel to smuggle sub-Saharan asylum seekers to their destination in Israel.

African asylum seekers in Israel live mainly concentrated in southern Tel Aviv, in one of the city's poorest neighbourhoods (Israel Parliament Information Centre 2010). The government of Israel has adopted restrictive policies while labelling the Sudanese and Eritrean as 'infiltrators'; meanwhile, the legal status of asylum seekers lacks clear definition (Centre for Civil and Political Rights 2013). Initially, Israel's collective group protection policy granted Eritrean and Sudanese asylum seekers the right to remain in Israel until their home countries are deemed safe for their return. This was based on the principle of non-refoulement, under which it is forbidden to deport a person whose life or freedom could be endangered by such a deportation. This applies to the majority of the asylum seekers who come from Eritrea to Israel, and the same reasoning was also originally applied by the Israeli authorities toward the Sudanese. Later on, these authorities claimed that the Sudanese, in comparison to Eritreans, cannot be deported because Israel does not have diplomatic relations with Sudan. This situation prevents them from applying for official refugee status and results in a provisional status which must be frequently renewed. Until 2013, the Israeli authorities all but blocked access to asylum procedures for Eritrean and Sudanese people. To date, an exceptionally small number of asylum seekers have received refugee status in Israel (Mundlak 2008). For a full description of the living conditions of asylum seekers, please see the Human Rights Watch report 'Make their lives miserable' (HRW 2014).

In 2012, the Israeli Knesset (parliament) passed an 'anti-infiltration law', which allowed up to 3 years' detainment of 'infiltrators' who are non-deportable. In September 2013, the High Court of Justice went on to declare that the long-term custody of migrants in detainment (called 'Saharonim') was unconstitutional (Israel Supreme Court 2013). By the end of 2013, following amendments of the legislation, the authorities shortened the detainment period of new-coming 'infiltrators' to 1 year only but also established the 'Holot Residence Centre' in Israel's Negev desert, where asylum seekers could be detained for an unlimited period of time (based on the argument that it is an open facility rather than a prison). By June 2014, there were 2,369 people detained in 'Holot'. Although it was defined as an open facility by the authorities, the centre was located in a remote location, and residents were required to check in three times a day and to remain in the centre at night. During 2014, the government's policy was also criticised by the State of Israel's Comptroller's Annual Report (2014). In September 2014, the Supreme Court ruling cancelled the legal amendment allowing asylum seekers to be jailed for 1 year without trial and under which the 'Holot Residence Centre' operated and ordered the state to close the facility (Israel Supreme Court 2014). This reiterated a previous Supreme Court ruling that it is unlawful to detain an individual in pursuance of a deportation order if no effective procedure is pending. This ruling is still under debate in the Knesset.

As a result, African asylum seekers in Israel often remain in an economically and psychologically unstable situation for a prolonged period of time and are excluded from fully participating in Israel's social, political and health systems, meaning that many cannot legally work and have limited access to the national healthcare system (Furst-Nichols and Jacobsen 2011; Mundlak 2008; Reynolds 2013); Physicians for Human Rights (2013).

Forced Migration and Mental Health

Migration and Mental Health in Adults

Though mostly focused on refugees, previous research reported that forced migration serves as a risk factor for poor mental health (Ellis et al. 2008; Kirmayer et al. 2011; Leaman and Gee 2012; van Willigen et al. 2006). Factors related to premigration experiences such as political and religious persecution, rape, torture, famine, war and ethnic conflicts, poverty (Masocha and Simpson 2012; Porter and Haslam 2005; Thomas and Thomas 2004), the loss of family and friends, traumatic experiences during the migration and post-migration experiences including discrimination and restrictive policies (Nakash et al. 2012, 2013; Porter and Haslam 2005) are all likely to play a role in the increased risk of mental ill-health which is reported among refugees and asylum seekers.

In particular, studies have documented an elevated risk of anxiety, depression and post-traumatic stress disorder (PTSD) among asylum seekers and refugees (Burnett and Peel 2001; Fazel et al. 2005; Laban et al. 2004; Tempany 2009). For example, 19 % of the newly arrived adult African asylum seekers in Australia were reported to have mental health problems (Tiong et al. 2006). Prolonged waiting periods for refugee status led to more severe mental distress (Sultan and O'Sullivan 2001) and higher risk of psychopathology (Laban et al. 2004). Similarly, approximately 30 % of asylum seekers who received treatment at the mental health clinic in the Physicians for Human Rights (PHR) Open Clinic for asylum seekers in Israel were diagnosed with PTSD (Lurie 2009). Reesp (2003) suggested that asylum seekers are at high risk for developing psychopathology owing to their limited social support and the uncertainty that accompanies their legal status.

In a meta-analysis examining pre- and postdisplacement factors associated with mental ill-health among refugees and internally displaced persons, Porter and Haslam (2005) identified several factors including age (children and adolescents reported less psychopathology than adults), gender (women have a higher prevalence of depression and PTSD than men) and employment status post-migration (unemployment was associated with worse mental health). In addition, during migration, family structure is often disrupted, and early separation from significant others is common (Chan et al. 2009). Furthermore, a study that examined medical records of refugees from Africa and Asia who participated in the Bellevue Hospital/ New York University Program for Survivors of Torture in New York showed that past exposure to multiple traumatic events among participants of the programme was common and was associated with mental ill-health (Chu et al. 2013).

Another post-migration stressor that has received growing attention is detention. In order to deal with the influx of irregular migrants, many countries have adopted a strategy of restrictionism including the establishment of detention centres where asylum seekers are held for undetermined periods of time while their application for refugee status is evaluated (Robjant et al. 2009). Although limited, some research has suggested that a prolonged stay in these centres can contribute to mental ill-health, especially among individuals who experienced traumata before and during migration (Masocha and Simpson 2012). For example, in a 2-year longitudinal study among refugees from Iran and Afghanistan living in Australia, Steel et al. (2011) found that detained refugees had higher baseline and follow-up scores on PTSD scales compared to non-detained refugees. Similarly, Keller et al. (2003) interviewed asylum seekers from Africa, Europe and Asia who lived in the USA and documented that longer periods of detention were associated with more severe symptoms of PTSD at follow-up and suggested that the detention of asylum seekers exacerbates psychological symptoms.

Additionally, asylum seekers, like other migrants, often need to adapt to a new cultural environment that can place them at odds with their heritage culture (Berry 1990), with significant implications for mental health (Heptinstall et al. 2004; Pumariega et al. 2005).

Migrant Adolescents and Mental Health

Although some studies indicate the relative lesser vulnerability of adolescent immigrants (e.g. Porter and Haslam 2005), youth migrancy comprises a particularly vulnerable group that is likely to have many risk factors for psychological distress including trauma, loss and social exclusion as a result of prejudice (Beiser et al. 1995). Most of the evidence for psychological distress among migrant youths comes from the post-migration experience in industrialised countries and suggests that behavioural problems, depression and PTSD are common (Beiser et al. 1995; Berman 2001; Bronstein and Montgomery 2011; Kinzie et al. 1986; Lustig et al. 2004; Rousseau 1995).

As with adults, factors related to premigration experiences (e.g. political turmoil and poverty in the country of origin), the process of migration (e.g. the loss of family and friends, traumatic experiences during the migration) and post-migration experiences (e.g. discrimination and restrictive policies) are all likely to play a role in increasing the risk of mental health problems among child and adolescent migrants (Chan et al. 2009; Ellis et al. 2008; Leavey et al. 2004; Pumariega et al. 2005; Stevens and Vollebergh 2008). For example, prevalence rates of psychiatric morbidity as high as 50 % have been found in refugee children from former Yugoslavia and Southeast Asia living in the USA (Sack et al. 1995; Weine et al. 1995) compared to native-born children. Similarly, a meta-analysis comparing the mental health status of refugees from a number of different countries living in six Western host countries found that between 19 % and 54 % of the children and adolescents scored above the clinical cut-off for PTSD, significantly higher than the rates recorded among the youth in the general population in the respective countries (Bronstein and Montgomery 2011).

Although very limited (in number), some research found that migration was also associated with increased engagement in risk behaviours (Romero et al. 2007). For example, Romero et al. (2007) documented that reports of smoking, drinking, drug use and violence were significantly associated with bicultural stress among Latino compared with non-Latino white middle school students in the USA. Viner et al. (2006) further suggested that patterns of risk and protective factors may vary among cultural and ethnic groups and called for research investigating risk and protective factors for risk behaviours among adolescents belonging to minority ethnic groups. In a school-based study of a representative sample in London, Viner et al. (2006) found that the highest rates of co-occurring risk behaviours were observed among adolescent boys of mixed ethnic heritage.

Migrant adolescents are often neglected within the healthcare and educational systems because of their lack of legal status, socio-economic marginalisation, language and cultural barriers and the fact that their parents or guardians are often overwhelmed and unable to care for their needs (UNICEF 2010; Schwartz et al. 2010). In addition, low socio-economic status might play a role in predicting emotional distress among migrant youths. For example, Darwish et al. (2003) found that the low socio-economic status of migrant Turkish parents explained a higher prevalence of behavioural problems of their children compared to Dutch native adolescents.

In the case of migrant and refugee adolescents, findings also support a strong association between perceived discrimination and negative mental health outcomes including depression and PTSD (Ellis et al. 2008, 2010; Te Lindert et al. 2008; Berry et al. 2006; Fisher et al. 2000; Kessler et al. 1999). Migrant youths may also be targets of discrimination for additional reasons such as religious beliefs, immigrant status, ethnicity and/or poverty (Ellis et al. 2010). Berry et al. (2006) further suggested that young people who experience discrimination are more likely to reject the receiving culture.

Gender has also been implicated as a significant factor in predicting mental health status among migrant adolescents as socialisation demands on daughters compared to sons might vary particularly among traditional cultures and thus lead to a differential impact of immigration on emotional distress (Dion and Dion 2001; Vollebergh et al. 2005). For example, Ellis et al. (2010) found that for Somali adolescent girls in the USA, greater cultural identification with the heritage culture was associated with improved mental health, while for Somali adolescent boys, greater identification with the American receiving culture was associated with improved mental health.

In addition, family structure is often disrupted during migration, and early separation from significant caregivers is common (Chan et al. 2009). These migrants are at an even greater risk of developing mental health problems as the turmoil of adolescence is exacerbated by risks associated with immigration and the acculturation processes that affect them during the developmental phase of identity formation (Bronstein and Montgomery 2011; Rumbaut 1994; Stevens and Vollebergh 2008). These young migrants often need to adapt to a new cultural environment that might place them at odds with their heritage culture (Berry 1990), with significant implications for mental health (Heptinstall et al. 2004; Pumariega et al. 2005).

Notably, among adolescents, the relationship between acculturation patterns, gender and mental health problems is further compounded by individual variables such as self-esteem, with research showing a positive association between self-esteem and ethnic identity (Phinney 1989) and a negative association between self-esteem and mental health problems (Oppedal et al. 2004; Smokowski et al. 2010).

Acculturation and Mental Health

The process of learning about and adapting to a new culture is termed 'acculturation' (Berry 1990). Two independent dimensions have been hypothesised to underlie the process of acculturation: heritage-culture retention and receiving-culture acquisition (Berry 1997). According to this bidimensional approach, four acculturation patterns can possibly emerge as a result of the intersection of the two dimensions: *assimilation*, whereby there is limited interest and involvement in maintaining the heritage culture alongside a high level of involvement with the receiving culture; *separation*, in which there is high involvement in maintaining the heritage culture and low involvement with the receiving culture; *marginalisation*, in which there is low involvement in both cultures; and *integration*, or *biculturalism*, in which there is high involvement in both heritage and receiving cultures (Berry et al. 2006).

The process of acculturation is acknowledged to be stressful and can be associated with social and psychological problems (Berry 1997). The extent, pace and type of cultural changes necessary can all impact the psychological well-being of the immigrating individual. Lack of support, pressure to adapt too quickly or inability to follow the desired acculturative strategy can lead to emotional problems. Berry argued that the most positive acculturation pattern in societal and psychological terms is integration, wherein new arrivals develop relationships with the receiving culture while maintaining their own cultural heritage and identity. Much research over the past three decades has provided support for the benefits of an integrated acculturative pattern and has shown that it is associated with improved mental health outcomes compared to other acculturation patterns (Berry 2006; Chen et al. 2008; Sullivan et al. 2007).

Although limited (*in number*), some studies have shown that acculturating to the receiving society proves to be more challenging among those who have been forced to leave their home country, partly because of their temporary status which inhibits their motivation to adapt to the ways of the receiving society. Furthermore, specific integration policies may be necessary to ensure that the development of intercultural relationships is possible; it is thus important that institutions act to facilitate interaction while at the same time ensuring that services can be adapted to meet newcomers' needs. This is particularly important in the case of forced migrants as they can have a preference for acculturative strategies (e.g. mixing with the receiving culture), yet they might have little choice regarding its implementation. The context of reception, which includes experiences of discrimination, has been hypothesised to play a seminal role in the acculturative process (Segal and Mayadas 2005) with implications for mental health distress and engagement in risk behaviours (Oppedal et al. 2004; Williams and Mohammed 2009). In the case of forced migration, acculturative strategies may be imposed if members of the receiving culture are reluctant to engage with new arrivals or if policies are not in place to support integration and institutions do not adapt to meet their needs. In a study among refugees living in England, Pillimore (2011) suggested that in the current restrictive policy environment, many refugees lack choice about acculturation strategy, struggle to integrate and remain vulnerable to psychosocial stress.

Studies Related to Forced Migration in Israel

Exposure to Trauma During the Journey to Israel Among Asylum Seekers

To document the exposure of African asylum seekers to traumatic events on their journey to Israel, a survey was conducted at the PHR Open Clinic between the Autumn of 2010 and the Spring of 2012 (Nakash et al. 2014a). We investigated the reported prevalence of exposure to traumatic experiences during migration among a consecutive sample of adult asylum seekers ($n=895$ Eritrean, of whom $n=447$ women and $n=448$ men, and $n=149$ Sudanese, of whom $n=18$ women and $n=131$ men) who sought health services in the Open Clinic. Participants were between 18 and 40 years old.

Upon accessing services at the Open Clinic, participants were interviewed in their native language by a nurse fluent in Tigrinya and Arabic about their experiences during migration. Structured interviews focused on respondents' experiences in the Sinai desert and included socio-demographic information as well as detailed information about exposure to violence and other traumatic events while in the Sinai desert.

Our findings showed that significantly more male than female Eritrean asylum seekers reported witnessing violence ($n = 185$, 41.3 %; $n = 131$, 29.3 %, respectively; $\chi^2(2) = 14.92 \, p < .001$). Over half of the Eritrean men ($n = 251$, 56.0 %) and a little over a third of the women ($n = 156$, 34.9 %) reported that they were victims of violence. Exposure to shootings and beatings were the most prevalently reported violent experiences. Significantly more Eritrean men than women reported being shot at ($n = 157$, 35 %; $n = 106$, 23.7 %, respectively; $\chi^2(2) = 15.21 \, p < .001$) and beaten ($n = 157$, 35 %; $n = 57$, 12.8 %, respectively; $\chi^2(2) = 65.32 \, p < .001$). Significantly more Eritrean women than men reported being sexually assaulted ($n = 24$, 5.4 %; $n = 2$, 0.4 %, respectively; $\chi^2(2) = 19.34 \, p < .001$). More than half of the Eritrean men and women reported being deprived of water ($n = 229$, 51.1 %; $n = 243$, 54.4 %, respectively; $\chi^2(2) = 1.16$ n.s.) and/or food ($n = 252$, 56.2 %; $n = 271$, 60.6 %, respectively; $\chi^2(2) = 1.92$ n.s.) during their time in the Sinai desert. Approximately half of the male (51.9 %, $n = 68$) and little less than half of the female (44.4 %, $n = 8$) Sudanese asylum seekers reported being victims of violence while in the Sinai desert. Shooting was the most prevalent experience of violence reported by Sudanese men and women ($n = 62$, 47.3 %, and $n = 8$, 44.4 %, respectively; $\chi^2(2) = 0.32$ n.s.). They were shot at, or they witnessed shootings. They were exposed to violence Incl. being shot. Approximately half of the Sudanese men and women reported being deprived of water ($n = 71$, 54.2 %, and $n = 9$, 50 %, respectively; $\chi^2(2) = 1.12$ n.s.) and/or food ($n = 75$, 57.3 %, and $n = 9$, 50 %, respectively; $\chi^2(2) = 0.33$ n.s.) during transit. Sexual assault was not reported by the Sudanese, but the very small number of reports among the Eritreans is considered an under-reported rate (see below).

It should be noted that the data in this study were collected only from a specific sample, namely, those who sought medical treatment at the Open Clinic and who may therefore represent a particularly vulnerable or resourceful group. In addition, data were self-reported approximately 1 year after arrival to Israel and may therefore be subject to reporting and recall biases. Many torture survivors, especially rape victims, may have been reluctant to reveal what they had undergone in Sinai (Schubert and Punamäki 2011), thus our data may represent an under-reporting of these experiences. Most importantly, our study included only those who survived the journey. A recent report based on the testimonies of Eritrean asylum seekers who were tortured during and after captivity suggests that during the last 5 years, an estimated 4,000 asylum seekers did not survive the torture camps and journey, losing their lives in the desert (van Reisen et al. 2012).

Studies of Acculturation Among Asylum Seekers in Israel

Research to date has provided evidence to support the idea that acculturation patterns have a significant impact on the mental health symptoms of migrants. However, little attention has been paid to the relationship between acculturation and mental health in the context of forced migration in general and among asylum seekers in particular. We examined the role of acculturation in predicting mental health symptoms among two groups in Israel: adult asylum seekers from Eritrea and Sudan and migrant adolescents.

Acculturation Among Adult Asylum Seekers

This study was conducted among a convenience sample of asylum seekers from Eritrea and Sudan who sought health services in the PHR Open Clinic between April 2012 and June 2013 (Nakash et al. 2014b). The participants were 91 Eritreans and 27 Sudanese from age 19 to 48 years. We used a Hopkins Symptoms Checklist (HSCL25; Parloff et al. 1954) of 25 Likert-type questions covering both anxiety and depression symptoms and the Harvard Trauma Questionnaire (HTQ-Part 1; Mollica et al. 1992) to assess the prevalence of exposure to traumatic events. In addition, a Bicultural Involvement and Adjustment Scale (Szapocznik et al. 1980) was used to assess the acculturation pattern and adoption of receiving-culture practices and retention of heritage-culture practices.

The majority of participants were Eritrean men with up to 12 years of formal education and who were unemployed. Most of the participants had been detained for up to 3 months upon their arrival to Israel. There were no significant differences in socio-demographic characteristics among the acculturation groups, except for age (assimilated participants were older compared with participants in other acculturation groups), duration of detention (assimilated participants reported longer detention periods compared with other acculturation groups) and formal education (a larger percentage of participants in the integrated acculturation group reported more than 12 years of formal education compared with participants in other acculturation groups).

Our findings showed significant differences between acculturation groups in terms of depression scores, with assimilated participants reported higher sum scores for depressive symptoms ($M = 33.6$ SD $= 10.5$) compared to marginalised participants ($M = 24.2$ SD $= 10.8$). We conducted hierarchical linear regression analysis using anxiety scores as the outcome measure and socio-demographic variables (i.e. gender, age, employment, family status and country of origin; first block), detention length, total traumatic events (second block) and acculturation (third block) as predictor variables; these were significant, predicting 18 % of the variance. Employment, country of birth and total exposure to traumatic events were associated with higher anxiety scores, such that being unemployed (*partial r* $=-.21$, $p < .05$), arriving from Eritrea (*partial r* $=-.20$, $p < .05$) and exposure to traumatic events (*partial r* $= .24$, $p < .05$) predicted higher anxiety.

A second hierarchical linear regression analysis using depression scores as the outcome variable and the same predictor variables was also significant, predicting 26 % of the variance. Employment and exposure to traumatic events were significantly associated with depression, such that unemployment (partial r $=-.22$, $p < .05$) and exposure to traumatic events (partial r $= .33$, $p < .01$) predicted higher depression scores. In addition, acculturation patterns were related to depression scores even after accounting for demographic factors, detention and exposure to trauma, with assimilated acculturation patterns being related to higher depression scores (partial r $= .33$, $p < .01$) compared to integrated acculturation patterns.

Acculturation Among Adolescents

We conducted another study in which we examined the role of acculturation, perceived discrimination and self-esteem in predicting mental health symptoms and risk behaviours among non-Jewish 1.5 and second-generation migrant adolescents from families that migrated for political and economic reasons (Nakash et al. 2012). By examining the unique contribution of acculturation, contextual variables (i.e. experiences of discrimination in the receiving country) and individual variables (i.e. self-esteem) to mental health distress and risk behaviours, we sought to assess the effect of the acculturative process on the mental health outcomes of migrant youths. Of the 125 participants in this study of adolescent migrants aged 12–19, 65 were born outside of Israel (1.5 generation), and 60 were born in Israel to migrant parents (second generation). Of the 1.5 generation participants, 9.3 % ($n = 6$) were born in Asia, 33.8 % ($n = 22$) were born in the former Soviet Union and Eastern Europe, 10.7 % ($n = 7$) were born in South America, 29.3 % ($n = 19$) were born in Africa, and 16.9 % ($n = 11$) were born the Middle East. The second-generation migrant participants were born to parents from Asia (33.3 %, $n = 20$), the former Soviet Union and Eastern Europe (10 %, $n = 6$), South America (13.3 %, $n = 8$), Africa (28.3 %, $n = 17$) and the Middle East (15 %, $n = 9$). An age, gender and socio-economic matched sample of $n = 146$ native-born Jewish Israeli adolescents also participated in the study and served as the comparison group.

All participants completed several measures that included a demographic questionnaire, the Brief Symptom Inventory (Derogatis and Melisaratos 1983) which is a brief self-report mental health symptom measure, and the Middle School Youth Risk Behaviour Survey (Centres for Disease Control and Prevention 2011) which assesses engagement in risk behaviours during the past 2 years. In addition, migrant adolescents also completed the following predictor measures: the Acculturation Index (Ward and Rana-Deuba 1999) which is used to determine one's acculturation pattern, the Everyday Discrimination Scale (Williams et al. 1997) which assesses perception of discrimination and the Single-Item Self-Esteem Scale (Robins et al. 2001) which assesses self-esteem.

An approximately equal number of adolescent boys and girls participated in each group. Migrants who belonged to 1.5 generation were slightly older than participants in the other groups. While the majority of migrant participants in both generations reported having an above-average socio-economic status, the majority of native-Israeli participants reported having average or below-average socio-economic status. The majority of migrant participants were Christian, while the entire sample of native-born Jewish Israelis was Jewish. A higher percentage of migrants who belonged to the 1.5 generation reported living with both parents and siblings in one house compared to second-generation migrants.

Using a bipartite split, the Acculturation Index rendered a score for each participant that was placed on a 2×2 quadrant to determine each participant's acculturation pattern, resulting in four acculturation patterns ($n = 25$ separated, $n = 27$ assimilated, $n = 44$ integrated/bicultural, $n = 23$ marginalised).

Univariate ANOVA was used to examine the difference between the four acculturation groups in the BSI General Severity Index. Migrants who were characterised by integrated acculturation patterns reported significantly lower scores on the BSI General Severity Index than assimilated migrants (F (3,116)=3.90; $p<.01$; partial η 2=.09). The Kruskal-Wallis test showed no significant differences between the different acculturation patterns in terms of risk behaviours ($\chi^2(3)=2.26$; n.s.).

Hierarchical linear regression analysis using the BSI General Severity Index (BSI-GSI) as outcome measure and age, gender, SES (first block), perceived discrimination, self-esteem (second block) and acculturation (third block) as predictor variables was significant, predicting 29 % of the variance. Our findings showed that gender was related to BSI-GSI higher scores, in that females had higher BSI-GSI compared with males. Neither age nor socio-economic status was related to severity scores. Perceived discrimination was also related to BSI-GSI, with higher reports of perceived discrimination being related to higher BSI-GSI score. Self-esteem was most strongly associated with BSI-GSI (partial $r=-.33$, $p<.01$). The assimilated acculturation pattern was also positively associated with BSI-GSI, with assimilated participants showing higher BSI-GSI scores. Other acculturation patterns (separated, marginalised) were not related to BSI-GSI.

A second hierarchical linear regression analysis using the same predictor variables (in addition to generation) and risk behaviour scale as outcome variable was also significant, predicting 29 % of the variance in risk behaviours. Gender, age and socio-economic status were not related to risk behaviours. Generation was significantly associated with risk behaviours, with 1.5 generation migrants reporting higher engagement in risk behaviours compared to second-generation migrants. Self-esteem was not related to risk behaviours. Perceived discrimination was the independent variable most strongly associated with risk behaviours (partial $r=.34$, $p<.01$). Acculturation pattern was not related to risk behaviours after accounting for demographic factors, self-esteem and perceived discrimination.

Discussion

A high percentage of Sudanese and Eritrean men and women reported witnessing violence and/or being victims of violence during their journey through the Sinai desert. These findings provide additional evidence on the role of exposure to traumatic events in the mental health status of displaced individuals (Porter and Haslam 2005), expanding upon previous research that has documented the high prevalence of exposure to traumas among displaced individuals, including harassment, witnessing violence to others, torture of family members and living in hiding (Hooberman et al. 2007; Nakash et al. 2014a). In terms of clinical work and future studies, these findings highlight the need to gather information regarding all phases of forced migration, from home country through the journey to the hosting country.

Our findings further manifest the important effect of the acculturation pattern on mental health symptoms in the integration experiences of asylum seekers and of the experience of discrimination and levels of self-esteem on mental health symptoms and risk behaviours in the immigration process of adolescents. Being forced to flee their countries of origin and integrate into 'strange foreign lands, where they can be isolated, ostracised and impoverished' (Williams and Berry 1991, p. 632), may result in acculturation risks that will have lingering mental health consequences. For both adults and adolescents migrants, rejection of the heritage culture and adoption of the Israeli culture as a possible mechanism for improving the likelihood of upward social mobility or local acceptance may carry heavy mental health consequences. Assimilated adult asylum seekers reported higher depressive symptoms when compared to integrated asylum seekers. Acculturation predicted depressive symptoms among asylum seekers beyond the effect of history of detention and reports of experiences of traumatic events. We did not find similar associations between acculturation and anxiety symptoms. The contrasting outcomes concerning anxiety and depression suggest that our findings are not merely the result of culturally based response bias.

Notably, assimilated asylum seekers reported the highest levels of depressive symptoms compared to those who had other acculturation patterns, whereas no significant differences emerged between integrated compared with marginalised and separated individuals. It is possible that our results also manifest the unique characteristics of non-Jewish migrants in Israel. Harper and Zubida (2010) suggested that even when forced migrants want to settle in Israel and become part of the Israeli society, they remain, for the most part, 'invisible' to the Israeli public, who perceive them as a cultural monolith and not as individuals with unique personalities and personal histories.

In the case of adolescents, migrant youths reported worse mental health symptoms and higher engagement in risk behaviours than native-born Jewish Israelis of the same age group. These results are consistent with previous research that documented increased mental health risks for migrant youth (Beiser et al. 1995; Berman 2001; Bronstein and Montgomery 2011; Kinzie et al. 1986; Lustig et al. 2004; Rousseau 1995) and expand this literature to show that this increased risk is also present among 1.5 and second-generation migrants who would be expected to be at a decreased risk due to acculturation and social capital (Rumbaut and Portes 2001). Our findings further showed that acculturation plays an important role in predicting the mental health status of migrant youths. Consistent with previous research, integrated migrant adolescents revealed fewer mental health symptoms when compared to their peers with an assimilated acculturation pattern. Similar to the case with adult asylum seekers, assimilated youths reported the most severe mental health symptoms compared to other acculturation patterns.

Rumbaut (1997) called attention to the paradox of assimilation and the mental health risks it poses among those wishing to integrate into the new culture at the expense of their original culture. Assimilation can be a highly stressful process for migrants (Wang and Freeland 2004), especially at the beginning stage of relocation, when the newcomer is overwhelmed with daily hassles (Abouguendia and Noels 2001), poverty (Porter and Haslam 2005) and discrimination (Nakash et al. 2012).

Restrictive policies in many industrial countries (Moshe 2013; Phillimore 2011; Tempany 2009) pose great hardship on the integration of asylum seekers into the new cultures. Based on qualitative analyses of interviews with refugees living in England, Phillimore (2011) examined the experiences that influenced refugee arrival and resettlement in the new country. Her findings showed how, in current restrictive policy environments, many refugees lack choice regarding acculturation strategies and are forced into marginalisation. They are thereby vulnerable to psychosocial stress and struggle to integrate. Miller and Rasmussen (2010) and Rasmussen et al. (2010) further suggested that stressful social and material conditions (daily stressors) partially mediate the relationship between war exposure and mental ill-health. In a study among Darfuri Refugees in Eastern Chad, Rasmussen and colleagues (2010) found that although war-related traumatic events were the initial causes of refugees' distress, the day to day challenges and concerns in the camps mediated the relationship between exposure to traumatic events and emotional distress.

Asylum seekers may thus constitute a particularly vulnerable group among forced migrants due to their temporary status, this eliminating the possibility of integrating into the local social and political spheres. As described previously, asylum seekers in Israel face restrictions regarding employment and social and civil involvement. These conditions might force asylum seekers to live in encapsulated ghetto communities and relative marginalisation.

Furthermore, identity conflicts reported among the migrant population, including the internalisation of prevalent Israeli negative stereotypes toward their heritage culture and/or the ethnic group, are transmitted and exacerbated among their children. For example, many migrants indicated that their children have adopted prevalent Israeli negative stereotypes toward their own heritage culture or ethnic group. The internalised negative attitudes and the disparity between the children's acculturation and mastery of Hebrew and Israeli culture and their parents' Israeli linguistic and cultural deficits, alongside restrictive policies, may intensify this culture clash.

In addition, our findings highlight the importance of measuring variables related to the context of immigration such as perception of discrimination in the receiving culture as well as individual factors such as self-esteem when investigating outcomes of the acculturation process. For example, in the case of migrant youths, lower self-esteem and higher perception of discrimination were most strongly associated with more severe mental health symptoms and higher risk behaviours, respectively. These findings corroborate the recent call to investigate the impact of the context of reception (Segal and Mayadas 2005) on the mental health outcomes of migrant youth and stress the critical role experiences of discrimination may have on the well-being of migrants in general.

To conclude, our findings on acculturation draw attention to the paradox of assimilation and the mental health risks it poses for adult asylum seekers and adolescent immigrants wishing to integrate into the new culture at the expense of their original culture. Future longitudinal studies may shed light on the dynamic nature of the adaptive function of acculturation patterns and show whether the assimilated acculturative pattern continues to be most maladaptive for these populations if and when they naturalise. Further qualitative studies, which will allow more in-depth investigation into the acculturative experience particularly of the marginalised group, might illuminate the possible protective function it serves among African asylum seekers and migrant youth in Israel. Mental health professionals should be culturally aware of this vulnerability in therapeutic interventions with forced migrants. Policy makers may consider the benefits of restrictive policies that have characterised many industrial countries in recent years.

References

Abouguendia M, Noels KA (2001) General and acculturation-related daily hassles and psychological adjustment in first-and second-generation South Asian immigrants to Canada. Int J Psychol 36:163–173

Beiser M, Dion R, Gotowiec A, Hyman I, Vu N (1995) Immigrant and refugee children in Canada. Can J Psychiatry 40:67–72

Berman H (2001) Children and war: current understandings and future directions. Public Health Nurs 18:243–252

Berry JW (1990) Psychology of acculturation. In: Berman JJ (ed) Cross-cultural perspectives: Nebraska symposium on motivation. University of Nebraska Press, Lincoln, pp 201–234

Berry JW (1997) Immigration, acculturation, and adaptation. Appl Psychol 46:5–34

Berry JW (2006) Stress perspectives on acculturation. In: Sam DL, Berry JW (eds) The Cambridge handbook of acculturation psychology. Cambridge University Press, New York, pp 43–57

Berry JW, Phinney JS, Sam DL, Vedder P (2006) Immigrant youth: acculturation, identity, and adaptation. Appl Psychol 55:303–332

Bronstein I, Montgomery P (2011) Psychological distress in refugee children: a systematic review. Clin Child Fam Psychol Rev 14:44–56

Burnett A, Peel M (2001) Asylum seekers and refugees in Britain: health needs of asylum seekers and refugees. Br Med J 322:544–547

Center for Civil and Political Rights, Human Rights Committee (2013) Concluding observations on the fourth periodic report of Israel. p 8. http://www.ccprcentre.org/country/israel/. Accessed 14 Dec 2014

Centers for Disease Control and Prevention (2011) Middle school youth risk behavior survey. http://www.cdc.gov/healthyyouth/yrbs/. Accessed 14 Dec 2014

Chan G, Barnes-Holmes D, Barnes-Holmes Y, Stewart I (2009) Implicit attitudes to work and leisure among North American and Irish individuals: a preliminary study. Int J Psychol Psychol Ther 9:317–334

Chen SX, Benet Martinez V, Harris BM (2008) Bicultural identity, bilingualism, and psychological adjustment in multicultural societies: immigration based and globalization based acculturation. J Pers 76:803–838

Chu T, Keller AS, Rasmussen A (2013) Effects of post-migration factors on PTSD outcomes among immigrant survivors of political violence. J Immigr Minor Health 15:890–897

Connell D (2012) Escaping eritrea – why they flee and what they face. Middle East Rep 264:2–9

Darwish Murad S, Joung I, Lenthe FJ, Bengi Arslan L, Crijnen AAM (2003) Predictors of self reported problem behaviours in Turkish immigrant and Dutch adolescents in the Netherlands. J Child Psychol Psychiatry 44:412–423

Derogatis LR, Melisaratos N (1983) The brief symptom inventory: an introductory report. Psychol Med 13:595–605

Dion KK, Dion KL (2001) Gender and cultural adaptation in immigrant families. J Soc Issues 57:511–521

Ellis BH, MacDonald HZ, Lincoln AK, Cabral HJ (2008) Mental health of Somali adolescent refugees: the role of trauma, stress, and perceived discrimination. J Consult Clin Psychol 76:184–193

Ellis BH, MacDonald HZ, Klunk Gillis J, Lincoln A, Strunin L, Cabral HJ (2010) Discrimination and mental health among Somali refugee adolescents: the role of acculturation and gender. Am J Orthopsychiatry 80:564–575

Fazel M, Wheeler J, Danesh J (2005) Prevalence of serious mental disorder in 7000 refugees resettled in western countries: a systematic review. Lancet 365:1309–1314

Fisher CB, Wallace SA, Fenton RE (2000) Discrimination distress during adolescence. J Youth Adolesc 29:679–695

Furst-Nichols R, Jacobsen K (2011) African refugees in Israel. Forced Migr Rev 37:55–56

Harper R, Zubida H (2010) Making room at the table: incorporation of foreign workers in Israel. Policy Soc 29:371–383

Heptinstall E, Sethna V, Taylor E (2004) PTSD and depression in refugee children. Eur Child Adolesc Psychiatry 13:373–380

Hooberman JB, Rosenfeld B, Lhewa D, Rasmussen A, Keller A (2007) Classifying the torture experiences of refugees living in the United States. J Interpers Violence 22:108–123

Human Rights Watch (2014) I wanted to lie down and die: trafficking and torture of Eritreans in Sudan and Egypt. http://www.hrw.org/sites/default/files/reports/egypt0214_ForUpload_1_0. pdf. Accessed 1 Mar 2014

Human Rights Watch report (Make their lives miserable, HRW, 2014). http://www.hrw.org/ node/128687. Accessed 14 Dec 2014

Israel Supreme Court (2013) High Court of Justice (HCJ) 7146/12 Adam and others v. The Knesset and others, Verdict dated 16 September 2013 [Hebrew]. http://www.refworld.org/ docid/524e7ab54.html. Accessed 14 Dec 2014

Israel Supreme Court (2014) High Court of Justice (HCJ) 7385/13 Eytan et al. vs. the Knesset et al., verdict dated September 22, 2014 [Hebrew]. http://elyon2.court.gov.il/files/13/850/073/ M19/13073850.M19.htm. Accessed 14 Dec 2014

Israel Parliament, Information Center (2010) Data on crimes committed by illegal immigrants and asylum seekers and crimes against illegal immigrants and asylum seekers. p 3. http://www. knesset.gov.il/mmm/data/pdf/m02625.pdf [Hebrew]. Accessed 14 Dec 2014

Keller AS, Rosenfeld B, Trinh-Shevrin C, Meserve C, Sachs E, Leviss JA, Kim G (2003) Mental health of detained asylum seekers. Lancet 362:1721–1723

Kessler RC, Mickelson KD, Williams DR (1999) The prevalence, distribution, and mental health correlates of perceived discrimination in the United States. J Health Soc Behav 40:208–230

Kinzie JD, Sack WH, Angell RH, Manson S, Rath B (1986) The psychiatric effects of massive trauma on Cambodian children: I. The children. J Am Acad Child Adolesc Psychiatr 25:370–376

Kirmayer LJ, Narasiah L, Munoz M, Rashid M, Ryder AG, Guzder J, Pottie K (2011) Common mental health problems in immigrants and refugees: general approach in primary care. Can Med J 183:E959–E967

Laban CJ, Gernaat HB, Komproe IH, Schreuders BA, De Jong JT (2004) Impact of a long asylum procedure on the prevalence of psychiatric disorders in Iraqi asylum seekers in The Netherlands. J Nerv Ment Dis 192:843–851

Leaman SC, Gee CB (2012) Religious coping and risk factors for psychological distress among African torture survivors. Psychol Trauma 4:457–465

Leavey G, Hollins K, King M, Barnes J, Papadopoulos C, Grayson K (2004) Psychological disorder amongst refugee and migrant schoolchildren in London. Soc Psychiatry Psychiatr Epidemiol 39:191–195

Lijnders L (2012) Caught in the borderlands: torture experienced, expressed, and remembered by Eritrean asylum seekers in Israel. Oxf Monit Forced Migr 2:64–76

Lurie I (2009) Psychiatric care in restricted conditions for work migrants, refugees and asylum seekers: experience of the open clinic for work migrants and refugees Israel. Isr J Psychiatry Relat Sci 46:172–181

Lustig SL, Kia-Keating M, Knight WG, Geltman P, Ellis H, Kinzie JD, Keane T, Saxe GN (2004) Review of child and adolescent refugee mental health. J Am Acad Child Adolesc Psychiatry 43:24–36

Masocha S, Simpson MK (2012) Developing mental health social work for asylum seekers: a proposed model for practice. J Soc Work 12:423–443

Miller KE, Rasmussen A (2010) War exposure, daily stressors, and mental health in conflict and post-conflict settings: bridging the divide between trauma-focused and psychosocial frameworks. Soc Sci Med 70:7–16

Mollica R, Caspi-Yavin Y, Bollini P, Truong T, Tor S, Lavelle J (1992) Validating a cross-cultural instrument for measuring torture, trauma, and posttraumatic stress disorder in Indochinese refugees. J Nerv Ment Dis 180:111–116

Moshe N (2013) Health services to foreign workers and undocumented migrants in Israel. http://www.knesset.gov.il/mmm/data/pdf/m03198.pdf. Accessed 6 Sept 2013.

Mundlak G (2008) Irregular migration in Israel – a legal perspective. http://cadmus.eui.eu/bitstream/handle/1814/10104/CARIM_AS%26N_2008_59.pdf?sequence=3. Accessed 1 Jul 2011

Nakash O, Nagar M, Shoshani A, Zubida H, Harper RA (2012) The effect of acculturation and discrimination on mental health symptoms and risk behaviors among adolescent migrants in Israel. Cultur Divers Ethn Minor Psychol 18:228–238

Nakash O, Wiesent-Brandsma C, Reist S, Nagar M (2013) The contribution of gender-role orientation to psychological distress among male African asylum-seekers in Israel. J Immigr Refug Stud 11:78–90

Nakash O, Langer B, Nagar M, Shoham S, Lurie I, Davidovitch N (2014a) Exposure to traumatic experiences among asylum seekers from Eritrea and Sudan during migration to Israel. J Immigr Minor Health [Epub ahead of print]

Nakash O, Nagar M, Shoshani A, Lurie I (2014b) The association between acculturation patterns and mental health symptoms among Eritrean and Sudanese Asylum seekers in Israel. Cultur Divers Ethnic Minor Psychol [Epub ahead of print]

Oppedal B, Røysamb E, Sam DL (2004) The effect of acculturation and social support on change in mental health among young immigrants. Int J Behav Dev 28:481–494

Parloff MB, Kelman HC, Frank JD (1954) Comfort, effectiveness, and self-awareness as criteria of improvement in psychotherapy. Am J Psychiatry 111:343–352

Phillimore J (2011) Refugees, acculturation strategies, stress and integration. J Soc Policy 40:575–593

Phinney JS (1989) Stages of ethnic identity development in minority group adolescents. J Early Adolesc 9:34–49

Physicians for Human Rights (2013) http://www.phr.org.il/default.asp?PageID=26&action=more. Accessed 6 Sep 2013

Porter M, Haslam N (2005) Predisplacement and postdisplacement factors associated with mental health of refugees and internally displaced persons. JAMA 294:602–612

Pumariega AJ, Rothe E, Pumariega JAB (2005) Mental health of immigrants and refugees. Community Ment Health J 41:581–597

Rasmussen A, Nguyen L, Wilkinson J, Vundla S, Raghavan S, Miller KE, Keller AS (2010) Rates and impact of trauma and current stressors among Darfuri refugees in Eastern Chad. Am J Orthopsychiatry 80:227–236

Reesp S (2003) Refuge or retrauma? The impact of asylum seeker status on the wellbeing of East Timorese women asylum seekers residing in the Australian community. Australas Psychiatry 11:96–101

Reynolds S (2013) Hope on hold: African asylum seekers in Israel. http://refugeesinternational.org/policy/field-report/hope-hold-african-asylum-seekers-israel. Accessed 4 Mar 2014

Robins RW, Hendin HM, Trzesniewski KH (2001) Measuring global self-esteem: construct validation of a single-item measure and the Rosenberg Self-Esteem Scale. Pers Soc Psychol Bull 27:151–161

Robjant K, Hassan R, Katona C (2009) Mental health implications of detaining asylum seekers: systematic review. Br J Psychiatry 194:306–312

Romero AJ, Martinez D, Carvajal SC (2007) Bicultural stress and adolescent risk behaviors in a community sample of Latinos and non-Latino European Americans. Ethn Health 12:443–463

Rousseau C (1995) The mental health of refugee children. Transcult Psychiatry 32:299–331

Rumbaut R (1994) The crucible within: ethnic identity, self-esteem, and segmented assimilation among children of immigrants. Int Migr Rev 28:748–794

Rumbaut R (1997) Assimilation and its discontents: between rhetoric and reality. Int Migr Rev 31:923–960

Rumbaut R, Portes A (2001) Ethnicities: children of immigrant absorption. University of California Press, Berkeley

Sack WH, Clarke GN, Seeley J (1995) Posttraumatic stress disorder across two generations of Cambodian refugees. J Am Acad Child Adolesc Psychiatry 34:1160–1166

Schubert CC, Punamäki R-L (2011) Mental health among torture survivors: cultural background, refugee status and gender. Nord J Psychiatry 65:175–182

Schwartz SJ, Unger JB, Zamboanga BL, Szapocznik J (2010) Rethinking the concept of acculturation: Implications for theory and research. Am Psychol 65:237–251. http://dx.doi.org/10.1037/a0019330

Segal UA, Mayadas NS (2005) Assessment of issues facing immigrant and refugee families. Child Welf 84:563–583

Smokowski PR, Rose RA, Bacallao M (2010) Influence of risk factors and cultural assets on Latino adolescents' trajectories of self-esteem and internalizing symptoms. Child Psychiatry Human Dev 41:133–155

State Comptroller's Annual Report 2014, Section 64C. Foreigners not subject to expulsion [Hebrew]

Steel Z, Momartin S, Silove D, Coello M, Aroche J, Tay KW (2011) Two year psychosocial and mental health outcomes for refugees subjected to restrictive or supportive immigration policies. Soc Sci Med 72:1149–1156

Stevens GWJM, Vollebergh WAM (2008) Mental health in migrant children. J Child Psychol Psychiatry 49:276–294

Sullivan S, Schwartz SJ, Prado G (2007) A bidimensional model of acculturation for examining differences in family functioning and behavior problems in Hispanic immigrant adolescents. J Early Adolesc 27:405–430

Sultan A, O'Sullivan K (2001) Psychological disturbances in asylum seekers held in long term detention: a participant-observer account. Med J Aust 175:593–595

Szapocznik J, Kurtines WM, Fernandez T (1980) Bicultural involvement and adjustment in Hispanic-American youths. Int J Intercult Relat 4:353–365

Tang SS, Fox SH (2001) Traumatic experiences and the mental health of Senegalese refugees. J Nerv Ment Dis 189:507–512

Te Lindert A, Korzilius H, Van de Vijver FJR, Kroon S, Arends-Tóth J (2008) Perceived discrimination and acculturation among Iranian refugees in the Netherlands. Int J Intercult Relat 32:578–588

Tempany M (2009) What research tells us about the mental health and psychosocial wellbeing of Sudanese refugees: a literature review. Transcult Psychiatry 46:300–315

Thomas SL, Thomas SD (2004) Displacement and health. Br Med Bull 69:115–127

Tiong A, Patel MS, Gardiner J, Ryan R, Linton KS, Walker KA et al (2006) Health issues in newly arrived African refugees attending general practice clinics in Melbourne. Med J Aust 185:602–606

Tronvoll K (2009) The lasting struggle for freedom in Eritrea: human rights and political development, 1991 – 2009. http://www.jus.uio.no/smr/forskning/publikasjoner/boker/2009/docs/Eritrea-the-lasting-struggle-for-freedom_2009.pdf. Accessed 1 Mar 2014

UNICEF (2010) Children, adolescents and migration: filling the evidence gap. http://www.child-migration.net/files/UNICEF_Data_on_migrant_children_and_adolescents_Poster_Update_June_2010_.pdf. Accessed 10 Sept 2011

United Nations High Commissioner for Refugees (2001) The 1951 convention relating to the status of refugees and its 1967 protocol. http://www.unhcr.org.hk/files/useful_resources/Important_documents/Benefits_of_accession_to_the_Convention.pdf. Accessed 1 Jul 2011

United Nations High Commissioner for Refugees. Global trends 2011. http://www.unhcr.org. Accessed 22 Aug 2013 van Reisen M, Estefanos M, Rijken C (2012) Human trafficking in the Sinai: refugees between life and death. http://www.eepa.be/wcm/dmdocuments/publications/Report_Human_Trafficking_ in_the_Sinai_Final_Web.pdf. Accessed 17 Sept 2014

van Reisen M, Estefanos M, Rijken C (2013) The human trafficking cycle: Sinai and beyond [Draft]. Wolf Legal Publishers, Oisterwijk

van Willigen LH, Hovens JE, van der Ploeg HM (2006) Physical and mental health of Afghan, Iranian and Somali asylum seekers and refugees living in the Netherlands. Soc Psychiatry Psychiatr Epidemiol 41:18–26

Viner RM, Haines MM, Head JA, Bhui KB, Taylor S, Stansfeld SA, Booy R (2006) Variations in associations of health risk behaviors among ethnic minority early adolescents. The Journal of Adolescent Health 38:55.e15–55.e23

Vollebergh WAM, Ten Have M, Dekovic M, Oosterwegel A, Pels T, Veenstra R, De Winter A, Ormel H, Verhulst F (2005) Mental health in immigrant children in the Netherlands. Soc Psychiatry Psychiatr Epidemiol 40:489–496

Wang L, Freeland D (2004) Coping with immigration: new challenges for the mental health profession. In: The psychology of prejudice and discrimination. Praeger, Westport: Conn pp 162–191

Ward C, Rana-Deuba A (1999) Acculturation and adaptation revisited. J Cross Cult Psychol 30:422–442

Weine SM, Becker DF, McGlashan TH, Laub D, Lazrove S, Vojvoda D, Hyman L (1995) Psychiatric consequences of "ethnic cleansing": clinical assessments and trauma testimonies of newly resettled Bosnian refugees. Am J Psychiatry 152:536–542

Williams CL, Berry JW (1991) Primary prevention of acculturative stress among refugees: application of psychological theory and practice. Am Psychol 46:632

Williams DR, Mohammed SA (2009) Discrimination and racial disparities in health: evidence and needed research. J Behav Med 32:20–47

Williams DR, Yu Y, Jackson JS, Anderson NB (1997) Racial differences in physical and mental health: socio-economic status, stress and discrimination. J Health Psychol 2:335–351

Part III

Trauma and Migration: Treatment Issues

Cultural Competence in Trauma

11

Adil Qureshi, Irene Falgàs Bagué, Khalid Ghali, and Francisco Collazos

Introduction

The term "Cultural competence", or some variation thereof, has unfortunately been abused to the point that the construct really has no clear definition and, indeed, can signify rather contrasting notions (Kirmayer 2012; Kleinman and Benson 2006; Qureshi and Eiroa-Orosa 2012; Williams 2006). Given that the point of this chapter is to apply the concept to trauma work with immigrants with the goal of improving service provision, the chapter will simply focus on this very point and in the process explicate a model of cultural competence that it is hoped will be useful, in accord with research and with overall approaches to effective clinical work with diverse patients.

The model used here has as its starting point the finding, as noted by Gregg and Saha (2006), that mental health disparities arise from two distinct but partially related sources: cultural and racial difference. The former refers to those differences in the presentation of distress, in communication style, in values, and, so forth, in what could be termed the "4 exes": experience, expression, explanation, and

A. Qureshi, PhD (✉)
Servei de Psiquiatria, Hospital Universitari Vall d'Hebron, Barcelona, Spain

Institute for the International Education of Students, Barcelona, Spain
e-mail: asfqureshi@gmail.com

I. Falgàs Bagué • K. Ghali
Servei de Psiquiatria, Hospital Universitari Vall d'Hebron, Barcelona, Spain

Vall d'Hebron Institut de Recerca, Barcelona, Spain

F. Collazos
Servei de Psiquiatria, Hospital Universitari Vall d'Hebron, Barcelona, Spain

Department of Psychiatry and Legal Medicine, Universitat Autònoma de Barcelona, Barcelona, Spain

© Springer International Publishing Switzerland 2015
M. Schouler-Ocak (ed.), *Trauma and Migration:*
Cultural Factors in the Diagnosis and Treatment of Traumatised Immigrants,
DOI 10.1007/978-3-319-17335-1_11

expectations. Thus differences in service provision revolve around clinicians having difficulties making sense of their culturally different patients, of understanding them, and of communicating with them. The latter, however, does not have to do with such differences, but rather with the impact of racial and ethnic prejudice and of racism, in which patients are accorded a lower quality of care due to racism. There is, by now, sufficient research that demonstrates that involuntary hospitalizations, use of restraints, and so forth are more common in "people of colour" than in the native born (Hustoft et al. 2013; Iversen et al. 2011; Tarsitani et al. 2013) (Fig. 11.1).

Culturalist

The cultural perspective holds that health disparities are a result of culture and cultural differences. Culture and cultural difference impact the experience, the expression, and the explanation of trauma and its effect, as well as in the expectations about the course and outcome of the trauma and about the treatment process. All of these will be explained below. As is perhaps obvious, all people are cultural, to the extent that culture is not simply the domain of the "exotic other" but of all people. To that end the very conceptual foundation of cultural competence is predicated on the notion that clinicians are as impacted by their own culture, in terms of experience, expression, explanation, and expectations as are their patients.

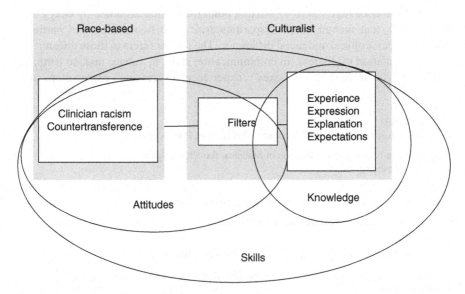

Fig. 11.1 Model of cultural competence (Reproduced by permission from *Cultural Variations in Psychopathology* by Sven Barnow & Nazli Balkir, ISBN 978-0-88937-434-8, p. 254)

Race Based

In many respects, the race-based "side" of the equation is the most complicated and perhaps even controversial. Whereas the culturalist is easier to digest in as much as the focus is on different ways of being in the world, the race based is far more uncomfortable as it has to do with differential access to resources on the basis of an arbitrary feature that is usually physical, although not necessarily so. The race-based domain resituates the "issue" in psychiatric work in the psychiatrist, and not in the patient; the issue at hand is not the behaviour of the patient but of the filters through which the mental health professional experiences the patient. What the reports on health disparities left very clear is that certain patients receive a lower quality of care simply because they are perceived to be members of a particular "race"(Atdjian and Vega 2005; Institute of Medicine 2002; Mallinger and Lamberti 2010). Much has been written as to whether "race" exists or not, and there is sufficient research that clearly shows that it is of no interest biologically, nor does belonging to a given race mean anything about an individual's behaviour (Betancourt and Lopez 1993; Helms et al. 2005). Race is meaningful in psychiatry as a social construct (Smedley and Smedley 2005). What this means is that being identified as a member of a given race can result in a certain sort of treatment.

The patient who is perceived as being racially different may well be treated differently, not on the basis of any characteristic specific to the patient, but rather due to prejudices that the therapist will project onto the patient (Fernando 2010). Race is a particularly complicating factor because even as it is visible, its impact often remains invisible. Researchers have routinely demonstrated that there is often a difference between what they term explicit and implicit race-related behaviour (Banaji et al. 1997; Penner et al. 2010). The former is that which is under the individual's conscious control; the latter is not. Thus, although we may consider ourselves to be "colour-blind" and ignore race in our encounters with patients, there is a strong body of research which suggests that even those individuals who consider themselves to be antiracist themselves show an own-race preference (Dovidio et al. 2002; Quillian 2008).

The upshot of this is that most of us are under the influence of what could be termed unconscious racism, and as it is unconscious, we are blind to it, and nevertheless it impacts our interactions with patients. Clearly, then, it is incumbent on the clinician to develop awareness of this process in order to minimize the interference of prejudices in the therapeutic encounter.

Experience

Recent developments in the neurosciences have contributed to the notion of the "cultural brain" which notes that neural development is conditioned by the experiences that occur in a given cultural context (Chiao et al. 2010). This contributes to the overall understanding that experience is never "pure" but is always conditioned and/or mediated by culture, previous experience, context, and so forth. What this means, then, is that humans do not simply have experiences and then subsequently interpret them through their cultural filters, but rather the event itself is experienced culturally, so to speak. This does not presuppose determinism, that being from a particular culture will automatically result in certain sorts of experiences, but rather culture will set forth the parameters in within which experience occurs. What it really reminds of us is that experience can be highly variable, even if it would appear to be otherwise. The trauma experience is not pure either, nor is it simply a question of the initial pure trauma experience which is then conditioned by the cultural context and interpretation. Rather, what is and is not a "trauma," as we shall see below, is very much culturally contingent, as is how the trauma is experienced.

Expression

Just as culture conditions and sets forth the parameters for experience, so too is it the case with expression. Most every aspect of human expression is culturally mediated, from style of communication to nonverbal communication to more complex aspects of interaction. This means that everything from eye contact (or its lack) to gestures to tone of voice can vary cross-culturally. In addition to the "how" of communication, culture influences the form and content. Thus, there is considerable variability in "how much" emotion is expressed, how directly one expresses oneself, and how much formality is used. In many European countries and in North America in particular, the notion that one should "say what one means" is relatively normative. The message is given "as is". This is not always the case, particularly in more interdependent and collectivist cultures, in which human relationships often take precedence, and therefore the priority is maintaining those relationships, even if it means being flexible with the truth. As we will see below, this is particularly the case with trauma although not universally so. The central issue here is that in psychiatry the idea is that a specific cluster of symptoms are indicative of a specific diagnostic category. This generally holds in the Euro-American cultural context and may indeed hold universally, but at times it does not. At times there is what could be called a symptom miss-match, meaning that the disorder finds a different sort of expression.

Expression, then, is germane to the psychiatrist working with an immigrant or culturally different patient in two ways. One has to do with the interaction, always understood to be a two-way street. Each person will have her or his own normative communication style and their way of expressing themselves verbally, nonverbally, and stylistically. This process is generally rather automatic; neither are we conscious of how we communicate, nor are we conscious that we are interpreting the expression of the other and in the process making decisions about the other person. Thus as clinicians we may observe that the patient has "flat affect" or indeed is "emotionally labile". Both of these evaluations are indeed predicated on what we implicitly consider normative for emotional expression. The other way in which expression is relevant is that the very expression of symptoms can vary considerably (Katz et al. 1988; Minsky et al. 2003). Perhaps the most "common" of these has to do with verbal or psychological versus somatic expression. As Western biomedicine developed in the context of mind-body dualism, mind and body are separated, and this separation means that the mind is treated by psychiatrists and the body by other medical specialists. Indeed, the very existence of "mental" health and its related healing traditions (psy) is predicated on this dualism. Indeed, in other parts of the world, there are not "mind healers" as differentiated from "body healers" (although the difference might be between body and soul). What this means, then, is that in the West we expect a differentiation of mental and somatic expression, with the latter being reserved for physical problems and the former for psychological or psychiatric problems. The very notion of "psychosomatic" is predicated on the notion that psyche and soma should be separated, and when they are not, this is symptomatic of a psychiatric problem.

The place of embodied expression in trauma is particularly relevant in this respect, and as we shall see below, this complex interplay of body and mind in trauma can be very highly influenced by culture.

Explanation

Just as culture circumscribes expression of distress, that is, the symptomatology, it also circumscribes what Arthur Kleinman calls the explanatory paradigm (1976). This refers to how the person makes sense of their distress. As mental health professionals, we tend to accept the biomedical approach, even if it is tempered by this or that school of psychology. We tend to opt for a natural and internal sort of explanation, meaning that the cause is natural, be it biological, psychological, or social (as opposed to supernatural, magical, etc.), and that the origin of the problem lies "within" the individual (Bhui and Bhugra 2002). This will also mean that the "cure" lies "within" the individual, be it through their "internal" focus in psychotherapy or through altering their neurochemistry.

The explanation, for example, that we provide for the impact of trauma follows these lines.

> The human response to psychological trauma is one of the most important public health problems in the world. Traumatic events such as family and social violence, rapes and assaults, disasters, wars, accidents and predatory violence confront people with such horror and threat that it may temporarily or permanently alter their capacity to cope, their biological threat perception, and their concepts of themselves. (Van der Kolk 2000)

What we see here is that the traumatic event is understood to have a psychological and perhaps biological impact and is framed as such. It is important to note that the question is not so much "which explanation is correct" but rather to recognize the different sorts of explanations that may emerge and that there may be considerable variability in the explanations.

On the other hand, there are multiple "ontological domains" (Hinton and Kirmayer 2013) such as economic and environmental context, judicial/political situation, spirituality and religion, and ethnopsychology, ethnophysiology, and cultural idioms of distress that may be involved in a given person's explanation, particularly when they are not from a culture heavily influenced by Western biomedicine.

Expectations

The fourth "ex" is related to the multiple expectations surrounding both the course and outcome of the distress as well as any treatment-related issues such as the nature of the doctor-patient relationship and the nature of the treatment itself. As with the other exes, culture is central.

Expectations about the impact of the distress, how long it will last, indeed, what it means, can vary considerably according to how the distress is experienced, made sense of, and explained. This determines, in part, what needs to be done in the face of the distress. Thus, for example, one might expect that not thinking about a problem will be the optimal way of managing it, if it is understood that the problem has its origins in factors beyond one's control such as the will of God, as there is then nothing that the individual can do about it, and God will remove the negative experience when he or she so sees fit. Such a perspective could also impact the expectations about what is needed to effectively deal with the problem. If it is a result of God's will, then perhaps what makes most sense is to appease God or engage in some activity that will facilitate God removing the distress. To that end, engaging in individually centred talk therapy that assumes an internal locus of control and that involves engaging with the distressing experience would make little sense (Kirmayer 2007).

Cultural norms also dictate expectations about the nature of human interaction. Cultures differ considerably in how hierarchical they are, in how credibility is ascertained, in how formal or informal interactions are, in how much self-disclosure is normative, and so forth. Most modes of mental health treatment require that the individual reflects honestly on their psychoemotional experiences and shares these with the mental health professional. It is also expected that people speak clearly, directly, and to the point. All of these are simply "Western norms" and are by no means universal and, for many, could be considered to be rather strange and even uncomfortable (Qureshi and Collazos 2011). Further, the mental health professional may be expected to provide expert advice; any sort of exploratory talk therapy may be seen as rather strange. Many times we have heard comments such "enough with this talk, Doctor, please tell me what I must do" or something to that effect. Many Western psychotherapy modalities seek a collaborative type of relationship in which power differentials are minimized. This makes perfect sense in the context of a Western, Educated, Industrialized, Rich, and Democratic (WEIRD) culture (Henrich et al. 2010), but it does not with patients who have rather different cultural backgrounds.

Knowledge

As one of the key components of cultural competence, the knowledge domain has generated some controversy and indeed considerable criticism surrounding the notion that clinicians need to have knowledge about a given culture (Kleinman and

Benson 2006). This notion is problematic for a variety of reasons, to the extent that some commentators reject the very notion of cultural competence for the cultural reductionism that such a notion implies (ibid.). Cultural knowledge is problematic for a few reasons. For many clinicians it is simply unreasonable to expect that they will have the time and energy to inform themselves about the cultures of the many different patients they see. But more importantly, cultural knowledge is a deceptive notion. In addition to the very important observation that culture is "distal" from the actual therapeutic interaction (Sue and Zane 1987), "knowing" a culture is a decidedly complicated notion. Cultures are complex, heterogeneous, and indeed contradictory and every changing. Thus to make any clinically relevant comment such as "Spaniards are emotive" or "Swedes hide their pain" is dangerous because although this may apply to some or indeed many people in a given culture, it does not apply to all. The very idea that "Swedes" or "Spaniards" are psychologically meaningful categories is inherently problematic. It assumes that all members of a given culture will share certain psychologically relevant characteristics. Not even addressing the complex issue of what defines a culture and distinguishes it from another ("Spain"? or should it be broken down to autonomous regions? Or specific linguistic groups? Or?), the idea of cultural knowledge runs a very serious risk of subjecting patients to stereotypes that simply may not be applicable and can lead to inadequate treatment.

But this is not to say that knowledge is not an important part of cultural competence. Knowledge that the four exes impact mental health and its treatment is essential. What should be clear is that all we can know is that the four exes are important for all humans; however, how this is the case is something that is not clearly known.

One of the central tenets of transcultural psychiatry is that, one way or the other, all explanations are cultural explanations, which means that all understanding of "trauma" is cultural, indeed, "trauma" itself, is a cultural construct. This is not to say that trauma does not exist, nor is it to descend into irrationalism, but rather to recognize that Western biomedicine is not, as Richard Rorty would say, "the mirror of nature", but rather an explanatory model that serves us very well (1981). Thus, to put it more concretely, it is important to know that trauma in general and PTSD more specifically are understood in psychiatry according to the specific epistemological basis of Western biomedicine, and as such trauma and its consequences may show up very differently in different cultural contexts. Again, it is important to note that we can only say "may" precisely because of the considerable human diversity that exists even within the same culture.

Attitudes

The attitude domain is perhaps the most complex of the three, precisely because it is the most intangible and is the antithesis of a more standard, "objective" concrete domain such as that of knowledge. This is because both the skills and knowledge domains of cultural competence require a willingness on the clinician's part to approach patients and their cultures openly, to put their preconceived notions on hold, and to allow themselves to be challenged. Although this is clearly a positive characteristic of any clinician, it is particularly challenging in as much as it requires the clinician to acknowledge not only that he or she may not know, but also that he or she may indeed be disposed to prejudices. In this respect, clinician countertransference is of particular importance. The so-called racial countertransference has to do with how we unconsciously deal with uncomfortable racial material. In large part because most clinicians are socialized in a context that rejects racism, racist and racialist thoughts and feelings are dealt with by relegating them to the unconscious where they show up indirectly and implicitly (Altman 2002; Comas-Díaz and Jacobsen 1991; Gorkin 1996). Researchers and theorists have identified a number of ways in which clinicians can do this, which include both "positive" and "negative" explicit responses. The former are ones in which we lose sight of the patient himself or herself and see the patient as a sort of specimen of the culture in question. We can end up exoticizing the patient, adopting a patronizing attitude in which we feel compelled to "save" the patient, convince ourselves that although there may be racism occurring in the world at large, we are different from others, and provide our patients with a different sort of experience. We can tell ourselves that we are colour-blind and do not see the person's race, just them. Conversely, we can end up seeing the patient as a "problem", and we can see their religion (if it is different from ours) as perhaps explanatory for their problematic ways of dealing with their problems. We can see them as somehow "primitive" and backwards with their quaint "cultural explanations" of their distress.

Thus an essential attitude is one of openness in every sense of the word, both to the patient but also to how one approaches the patient. This further requires that the psychiatrist be willing to adopt that very uncomfortable position of "not knowing" and of approaching the patient interaction with as open a mind as possible.

In the context of trauma, this means in effect suspending what we think we know about trauma, its symptoms, its impact, and its treatment. Further, it demands that we are willing to question our interpretive filters and our attitudes towards the patient.

Skills

The skills domain focuses on the application of knowledge and all aspects related to the interaction with the patient or the "doing" side of things. In the graphic above, it encompasses both the race-based and the culturalist approaches and involves having the competence to effectively manage cultural differences in interaction as well as to attend to and deal with prejudices and with cultural filters. In addition, and perhaps most importantly, it consists of communication and relationship development skills. There is a considerable research base that shows that the therapeutic relationship is the substrate upon which therapeutic effectiveness is built (Clemence et al. 2005; Lim et al. 2006; Suchman 2006) and that communication forms an important part of the development of the relationship. Further, just as culture is present in explanations and expression, so it is in understanding and empathy (Rasoal et al. 2011). Thus taken together, this means that the culturally competent clinician is skilled at engaging with her or his culturally different patient, with the ability to adapt to the relational and communicative style of the patient. But it is not only "culture" here, but also race, in as much as prejudices, stereotypes, and transference may well be involved. This means that clinicians are skilled at identifying how racial prejudices and transference may interfere with good communication and the development of the therapeutic relationship.

In the context of trauma, this also means that the clinician has the capacity to detect what sort of relational dynamic will be optimal for the particular patient in question, given his or her cultural context, and will be one that facilitates trust. In particular this means that the clinician is sufficiently open to "where the patient is at" to not impose the received relational model but rather to adapt to the specifics of the patient. It may mean, for example, adopting a more formal tone, in which honorifics (Mrs.; Mr.; Ms.; Miss) and surnames are used. It most certainly also involves adapting to the cultural communication style of the patient. It is beyond the scope of this chapter to address this in detail, and indeed, there is no shortage of excellent material available that delineates different aspects of intercultural communication.

Trauma as a Sociocultural Construct

In this section we will attempt to deconstruct or reconstruct this concept from an interdisciplinary perspective. One of the difficulties of the concept is that it is used in various different forms in different contexts that specifying the work is rather complicated (Erikson 1994). The word derives from the Greek *traumat* and refers to an injury to the tissues. From the eighteen century, the term began to show up in some medical texts in France, in which it was understood as tissue damage due to an external agent (Corominas 1980). Progressively the term became more general. It came to signify damage to nervous system tissue with a series of associated symptoms. In the nineteenth century, the term was increasingly associated with strange behaviours and dissociated and involuntary memory. Around then the associated term traumatic memory appeared which referred to the way in which the body recorded highly intense and emotionally difficult experiences. In this way we see how the concept passed from making reference from external to internal damage, from body tissues to the nervous system.

During this epoch Freud became interested in the concept and began to use it in his theory. Initially he considered that the traumatic events were real and damaged the psyche, but he would subsequently come to view the memory of damage as a function of the repression of inappropriate desires. What this meant was that trauma had to be interpreted in conjunction with the individual's biography and as an internal process (Ortega 2008).

The large-scale violence of the twentieth century, from major wars to genocides, has led to the concept of cultural trauma and the concept taking on sociological, philosophical, and historical dimensions. In these contexts, trauma is understood as damage that is interpreted and defined collectively, in which material and moral damages are determined.

A central component of understanding trauma from a "culturally competent" perspective has to do with the degree to which the construct is understood as a natural phenomenon versus social construct, on the one hand, and, on the other, the degree to which the construct itself in Western biomedicine has in its historical development, taken on its own particular coherence and logic, such that it then appears to be real and objective.

The solution, however, need not be one which creates its own problems, that of cultural relativism which itself would render any cross-cultural discussion of trauma untenable (or indeed, we would end up with trauma being a Western construct which would then not be applicable to peoples from other cultures). Thus the challenge is to find a mid-range response, a "universalist" or "derived emic" approach in which the construct of trauma is accepted as existing across cultures yet is understood to vary in its experience, expression, explanation (meaning), and expectations as to its course and optimal treatment. To that end, trauma can be understood as moral dissonance between what socially acceptable or legitimate and the actual suffering, which has cognitive, ideological, and emotional consequences. Trauma is damage to a sacred value within a sociocultural context, which requires reparation and emotional, institutional, and symbolic reconstruction (Alexander et al. 2004).

Trauma can also be understood as an alteration of the established social order and as the violation of the normative symbolic value system of culturally constructed values. Trauma derives, then, from actions and events that damage social order. What this means, is that trauma does not simply follow from the event itself, but is rather entirely caught up in the nexus of the cultural context of experience, expression, and explanation. Thus the occurance and impact of trauma varies cross-culturally; indeed, the development of PTSD would appear to be related, in part, to an interaction between life experiences and cultural context (Jobson and O'Kearney 2008).

Trauma can be associated with social changes or severe events such as natural disasters or genocides. At the same time, the specific sources of trauma can vary considerably with both culture and social structures, related to both the system of representation and social dynamics. What can be called a traumatic event may be lived rather differently depending on the overarching cultural characteristics (especially along the individualism/independent self-collectivism/interdependent self-dimension), religiosity, and the overall social context (e.g. prolonged war). Events will be interpreted in accordance with a logic that is defined by the local sociocultural context (Sztompka 1993).

The definition provided here suggests that trauma is in part a function of goals not being met, with serious interruptions or challenges to life projects. To that end, research shows that impediments with goal-directed behaviour are more present in the development of PTSD in "Western" individualist cultures than "Eastern" collectivist ones, precisely because it would seem that cultures with less expectations of control over their environment and world such as those with fatalistic religiosity are less susceptible to the sort of trauma as understood in the West (DeVries 1996). Indeed, contravention of social norms constitutes one important aspect of trauma, and clearly, social norms are not universal.

Culture is the basis on which social relationships as well as relationships with nature are established and defined. This being the case, it does not make sense that a traumatic event be interpreted the same way the world over. Interpretations, as we have seen, are predicated on a particular sociocultural and personal context. To that end, there are cultural differences with regard to catastrophes. White (1959), for example, distinguished between nomadic and sedentary societies and their reactions to fleeing. Sedentary societies, as one might imagine, are more susceptible to experiencing feeling threatened in flight than nomadic societies. Other studies have demonstrated that collectivist societies, above all Asian ones, are more accepting of catastrophes and negative events (Markus et al. 1996), and Africans response to epidemics with greater passivity (Delumeua 1993). This suggests that the sociocultural structure plays a central role in determining the behavioural, emotional, and interpretive responses in the face of a natural disaster.

Trauma in Context

Naj is a 24-year-old man born in a small village in the high mountains in the Eastern part of Kunar province in Afghanistan. He comes from a Pashto family of goat herders making a subsistence living. He never went to school, and the furthest he had ever travelled was, by foot, to a livestock market. When Naj was 11 years old, the USA invaded his country in the aftermath of the Twin Tower attacks in September 2001. Although at the outset the war took place primarily in the south and in the major cities, the noise of snipers, attack sirens, and B-52 bombers became commonplace. He lived his adolescence between the danger of attack and the silent calm of the goats peacefully grazing on the steep mountainous slopes. Given the difficult geography of the region, Kunar would become one of the most violently contested provinces, with some 3,500 people having died by the end of 2013. Naj was married when he was 19 years old to a cousin consistent with Pashtun customs. They have one daughter who was 10 months old when the Taliban kidnapped him in the mountains.

Naj explains that the purpose of kidnapping them was to demand that he carry out a suicide attack in the name of the Taliban cause. As a consequence of Naj's refusal to do so, he was in effect made a slave and forced to carry the heaviest items or be tied up or otherwise prevented from escaping. He was also tortured and sexually abused on various occasions. This continued for a year until one day, Naj saw some people he knew and he ran and escaped to the family village. The family, fearing reprisals, sold all of their goats (their source of survival) and the jewels of the mother's dowry with which they paid a human smuggler to take him to Europe.

The voyage was long and arduous lasting some nine months and included long journeys by foot through the mountains in small groups, with little food or shelter along the way. He had to jump off of a boat without knowing how to swim with the hope that the Greek Coast Guard would rescue him. Some of the others died during the voyage. Along the way he passed through Iran, Turkey, and Greece and finally was detained by the police in Hungary. From there he crossed the rest of Europe arriving at a train station in Barcelona with nothing but the clothes on his back and a birth certificate. He did not know where he was, only having been told that Spain was where he had the best chance of being granted papers. After wandering around for a few days, he made contact with a local refugee agency, which referred him to a local health care service which in turn identified that he required mental health services.

At the first visit at the transcultural psychiatry centre, Naj explained that he had severe headaches, stomachaches, leg pain, insomnia, nightmares, and confusion. He expressed a constant fear of being found by the Taliban. He continually relived the experiences of being pursued night and day. He avoided areas where he would be in contact with other Muslims, which meant that he could not attend Mosque services, despite being rather pious, in order to avoid possible contact with the Taliban. He had few opportunities to be in touch with his family, although he was clearly concerned about them, but any contact with "the place where the Taliban were" terrified him. Naj is in a very precarious social situation and is rather isolated as he does not speak anything but Pashto, and there are few Pashto speakers in Barcelona. He is currently awaiting a decision on his asylum petition and is totally dependent on social services. Any stressor, even relatively minor ones, result in decompensation, with ideas of death, hopelessness, and desperation appearing, that lead to repetitive behaviour (continuously asking if he will be deported, asking for help, showing his fear that he will be tortured) and self-harm.

Certainly, this is a complex case involving both depressive and anxious symptoms as well as previous traumatic experience that makes the symptoms compatible with the diagnosis of post-traumatic stress disorder. The constant hyperarousal, the avoidance of experiences that can remind him of the trauma, the indifference towards traumatic situations, nightmares, anxiety, fear and confusion are all observed components in people who suffer from this controversial disorder.

The culturally competent approach and analysis of this case and of many others perhaps not as clear but of similar characteristics are comprised of different levels:

The first level of approach to the case is a practical one but of considerable importance. Diagnosis and treatment both require good communication. The clinician needs to understand the patient allowing him or her to express himself or herself in the most comfortable manner and to transmit his or her words with clarity. Communication problems are clearly a tremendous obstacle to the treatment process and can be very trying for all involved. To that end, it is essential to have available a professional who can facilitate linguistic communication (medical interpreter or intercultural mediator) between the vehicular language of the patient and the clinician. This issue could be said to comprise part of institutional or organizational cultural competence in that it is a resource that does not depend on the clinician's competence beyond the recognition of the importance of this level. Relatedly, good intercultural communication is not uniquely dependent on language skills but also an open attitude that involves the capacity to communicate using good listening skills along with empathy. In this particular case, the entire process has been complicated by the lack of a professional Pashto interpreter. Fortunately, a very well-intentioned Pashto speaker has been accompanying the patient along the way, but unclear communication has muddied the process considerably.

The second level is to keep in mind when dealing with a case of post-traumatic pathology in culturally different individual that his or her social situation can have an important role in his or her experience and possibly explanation of his or her distress. For example, being an asylum seeker as is the case of Naj, or indeed living on the street or in any precarious socioeconomic and legal situation, can serve to augment to distress.

The first question to address the following model of the four "exes" is the perception of the traumatic experience in itself. We have to be aware that Naj's personality, for example, developed in the context of war and conflict of potentially constant traumatic events. His story may appear to consist of one terrible event upon another, to the extent that, for some, it may be difficult to believe or hear. Naj's treatment team found it difficult to believe his story due to a combination of his personality, the lack of shared language, and the very apparently incredible story he told (although, upon further exploration, the story is rather more common than the treatment team had thought). Indeed, a culturally competent diagnosis will include the possibility that what may appear to be traumatic for some may, for others, be adaptive to the violent context that has been the hallmark of his life. As has been described in other cases (Kirmayer 2007), the trauma story may, at times, sound contradictory to a person from a different culture. Indeed, Rousseau et al. (2002) has pointed out that refugee hearings have made errors in their determination of asylum claims due to distrust not only of the recounting of the events themselves but also of a moral-cultural nature (e.g. questioning how a person could abandon their children and flee alone or how a person might escape from the bondage of slavery) which further complicate an "open" listening to the case. In this respect, it is important to recall that what we consider "common sense" about traumatic experiences is rather specific to our own cultural context and thus best held in abeyance such that we can listen openly to the patient's narrative of stressful events that he or she found traumatic. Only in this way will we be close to the reality of the patient.

Secondly, we have to consider the expression of psychological distress of this person. It can be useful to consider the somatic expression of distress and to be aware of mind-body dualism in order to perceive the clinical symptom as a whole (after having dismissed possible organic pathology associated to migratory journey and to the physical conditions suffered). In this case, a psychological symptomatology is very clearly present, as is the case with most patients with a diagnosis of PTSD such as hyperarousal, the avoidance of phenomena that can remind them of traumatic experiences, nightmares. On the other hand, a clear somatic component exists in the presentation of symptoms that indicates the complex relationship between body and mind in terms of trauma that we have described above.

The third "ex" to keep in mind is the explanation of the phenomenon. This question, though simple, is of the utmost importance at the time of exploring the person in order to be able to deal with the diagnosis and, above all, the provision of effective treatment. If the clinician does not comprehend the explanation provided by the patient, it will be very difficult to effectively develop a positive therapeutic alliance, essential for increasing the likelihood of treatment adherence and efficacy. One must then ask about the meaning of what is happening and the possible causes and external and internal contributions to its symptomatology. How does one explain what happens? How is it understood? In addition, it is important to decipher the point in the process in which the patient's behaviour became dysfunctional and abnormal and what might be the benefits and drawbacks of the psychological state in which he or she finds himself or herself in. Once again, awareness of these issues can contribute to a better understanding of the patient and as such contribute to the development of an effective treatment process.

Lastly, and in conjunction with the previous questions, we will consider the patients' expectations about their health status and improvement. At this point we will also explore the resources of the patient during their process of recovery. What does the patient expect from us? Who are the real participants of the treatment process? What emerges from this expression of distress? What is the patient's real complaint? How does he or she expect to be treated? Answering these questions will bring us closer to the actual capacities of both the therapist and the patient to bring about positive change. Knowing the actual expectations of the patient can at times put the therapist in an uncomfortable situation as these may impede the therapeutic work we are accustomed to doing. Being conscious of that will help to focus the treatment around the actual expectations with the greatest possibility of success.

Awareness of the complications and consequences of intercultural psychiatric work is also key. How does treatment alter the symptomatology, the behaviour, and, indeed, the process through which the patient is living? How will the patient manage having a psychiatric diagnosis? Will it have an iatrogenic function and increment a "sick role" behaviour? Will this have an impact on the individual's cultural adaption, on the one hand, and on the other, will it be stigmatizing? Will it affect how the person views himself or herself or, indeed, function to marginalize the individual from her or his community? Or, conversely, will it result in secondary benefits that will increase adaptation?

Conclusions

Trauma in mental health, particularly as manifested in post-traumatic stress disorder, can be a considerable challenge for mental health professionals when treating immigrant patients. Culture, in the guise of the "exes"—experience, expression, explanation, and expectations—means that the mental disorder as delineated by institutional nosological systems (DSM; ICD) may or may not concord with the actual presentation of the culturally different patient. The process is all the more complex given that the clinician may be impacted by her or his racial prejudices that have been shown to filter clinical interactions. From the perspective of the cultural competence model presented here, a priori it is impossible to determine if a culturally different patient will present with classical symptomatology or rather different ones. It remains incumbent on the clinician to be willing and able to problematize his or her own way of interacting with and seeing the patient.

References

Alexander JC, Eyerman R, Giesen B, Smelser NJ, Sztompka P (2004) Cultural trauma and collective identity. University of California Press, Berkeley, Retrieved from http://books.google.es/books/about/Cultural_Trauma_and_Collective_Identity.html?id=shkt8_4srhoC&pgis=1

Altman N (2002) Black and white thinking: a psychoanalyst reconsiders race. Psychoanal Dialogues 10(4):589–605

Atdjian S, Vega WA (2005) Disparities in mental health treatment in U.S. racial and ethnic minority groups: implications for psychiatrists. Psychiatr Serv 56(12):1600–1602. doi:10.1176/appi.ps.56.12.1600

Banaji MR, Blair IV, Glaser J (1997) Environments and unconscious processes. In: Wyer RS (ed) The automaticity of everyday life: advances in social cognition, vol 10. Lawrence Erlbaum Associates, Mahwah, pp 63–74

Betancourt H, Lopez SR (1993) The study of culture, ethnicity, and race in American psychology. Am Psychol 48(6):629–637 [Article]

Bhui K, Bhugra D (2002) Explanatory models for mental distress: implications for clinical practice. Br J Psychiatry 181:6–7

Chiao JY, Hariri AR, Harada T, Mano Y, Sadato N, Parrish TB, Iidaka T (2010) Theory and methods in cultural neuroscience. Soc Cogn Affect Neurosci 5(2–3):356–361. doi:10.1093/scan/nsq063

Clemence AJ, Hilsenroth MJ, Ackerman SJ, Strassle CG, Handler L (2005) Facets of the therapeutic alliance and perceived progress in psychotherapy: relationship between patient and therapist perspectives. Clin Psychol Psychother 12(6):443–454. doi:10.1002/cpp.467

Comas-Díaz L, Jacobsen FM (1991) Ethnocultural transference and countertransference in the therapeutic dyad. Am J Orthopsychiatry 61(3):392–402, Retrieved from http://doi.wiley.com/10.1037/h0079267

Corominas J (1980) Diccionario Crítico Etimológico Castellano e Hispánico (Editorial). Gredos, Madrid

Delumeua J (1993) La peur en Occident. Fayard, Paris

DeVries MW (1996) Trauma in cultural perspective. In: van der Kolk BA, McFarlane AC, Weisaeth L (eds) Traumatic stress. Guilford Press, New York

Dovidio JF, Gaertner SL, Kawakami K, Hodson G (2002) Why can't we just get along? Interpersonal biases and interracial distrust. Cult Divers Ethn Minor Psychol 8(2):88–102, Retrieved from http://www.ncbi.nlm.nih.gov/entrez/query.fcgi?cmd=Retrieve&db=PubMed&dopt=Citation&list_uids=11987594

Erikson KT (1994) A new specific of trouble: Exploration in community, disaster and trauma. W.W. Norton: New York

Fernando S (2010) Mental health, race and culture. Palgrave Macmillan: Basingstoke, Hampshire, p 248. Retrieved from http://www.amazon.co.uk/Mental-Health-Culture-Suman-Fernando/dp/0230212719

Gorkin M (1996) Countertransference in cross-cultural psychotherapy. In: Foster RMP, Moskowitz M, Javiev RA (eds) Reaching across boundaries of culture and class: widening the scope of psychotherapy. J. Aronson, Northvale, pp 159–176

Gregg J, Saha S (2006) Losing culture on the way to competence: the use and misuse of culture in medical education. Acad Med 81(6):542–547

Helms JE, Jernigan M, Mascher J (2005) The meaning of race in psychology and how to change it: a methodological perspective. Am Psychol 60(1):27–36. doi:10.1037/0003-066x.60.1.27

Henrich J, Heine SJ, Norenzayan A (2010) The weirdest people in the world? Behav Brain Sci 33(2–3):61–83. doi:10.1017/S0140525X0999152X; discussion 83–135

Hinton DE, Kirmayer LJ (2013) Local responses to trauma: symptom, affect, and healing. Transcult Psychiatry 50(5):607–621. doi:10.1177/1363461513506529

Hustoft K, Larsen TK, Auestad B, Joa I, Johannessen JO, Ruud T (2013) Predictors of involuntary hospitalizations to acute psychiatry. Int J Law Psychiatry 36(2):136–143. doi:10.1016/j.ijlp.2013.01.006

Institute of Medicine (2002) Unequal treatment: confronting racial and ethnic disparities in health-care. National Academies Press, Washington, DC

Iversen VC, Berg JE, Småvik R, Vaaler AE (2011) Clinical differences between immigrants voluntarily and involuntarily admitted to acute psychiatric units: a 3-year prospective study. J Psychiatr Ment Health Nurs 18(8):671–676, Retrieved from http://www.ncbi.nlm.nih.gov/pubmed/21896109

Jobson L, O'Kearney R (2008) Cultural differences in personal identity in post-traumatic stress disorder. Br J Clin Psychol/Br Psychol Soc 47(Pt 1):95–109. doi:10.1348/014466507X235953

Katz MM, Marsella A, Dube KC, Olatawura M, Takahashi R, Nakane Y, Wynne LC et al (1988) On the expression of psychosis in different cultures: schizophrenia in an Indian and Nigerian community. Cult Med Psychiatry 12:331–355

Kirmayer LJ (2007) Psychotherapy and the cultural concept of the person. Transcult Psychiatry 44(2):232–257

Kirmayer LJ (2012) Rethinking cultural competence. Transcult Psychiatry 49(2):149–164. doi:10.1177/1363461512444673

Kleinman A (1976) Concepts and a model for the comparison of medical systems as cultural systems. Soc Sci Med 12:85–93

Kleinman A, Benson P (2006) Anthropology in the clinic: the problem of cultural competency and how to fix it. PLoS Med 3(10):e294. doi:10.1371/journal.pmed.0030294

Lim SC, Goh SK, Lai YR, Tee WW, Koh A, Xu XH, Wu YS et al (2006) Relationship between common functional polymorphisms of the p22phox gene (-930A > G and +242C > T) and nephropathy as a result of Type 2 diabetes in a Chinese population. Diabet Med 23(9):1037–1041. doi:10.1111/j.1464-5491.2006.01916.x, DME1916 [pii]

Mallinger JB, Lamberti JS (2010) Psychiatrists' attitudes toward and awareness about racial disparities in mental health care. Psychiatr Serv (Washington, DC) 61(2):173–179. doi:10.1176/appi.ps.61.2.173

Markus HR, Kitayama S, Heiman R (1996) Culture and "basic" psychological principles. In: Higgins ET, Kruglanski A (eds) Social psychology: handbook of basic principles. Guilford Press, New York, pp 857–914

Minsky S, Vega W, Miskimen T, Gara M, Escobar J (2003) Diagnostic patterns in Latino, African American, and European American psychiatric patients. Arch Gen Psychiatry 60(6):637–644. doi:10.1001/archpsyc.60.6.637

Ortega FA (2008) Violencia social e historia: el nivel del acontecimiento. Univ Humanística 66:31–56, Retrieved from http://dialnet.unirioja.es/servlet/articulo?codigo=2931442

Penner LA, Dovidio JF, West TV, Gaertner SL, Albrecht TL, Dailey RK, Markova T (2010) Aversive racism and medical interactions with black patients: a field study. J Exp Soc Psychol 46(2):436–440. doi:10.1016/j.jesp.2009.11.004

Quillian L (2008) Does unconscious racism exist? Soc Psychol Q 71(1):6–11. doi:10.1177/019027250807100103

Qureshi A, Collazos F (2011) The intercultural and interracial therapeutic relationship: challenges and recommendations. Int Rev Psychiatry 23(1):10–19. doi:10.3109/09540261.2010.544643

Qureshi A, Eiroa-Orosa FJ (2012) Training for overcoming health disparities in mental health care: interpretive-relational cultural competence. In: Barnow S, Balkir N (eds) Cultural variations in psychopathology. From research to practice. Hogrefe Publishing, Göttingen, Retrieved from http://www.hogrefe.com/program/cultural-variation-in-psychopathology.html

Rasoal C, Eklund J, Hansen E (2011) Toward a conceptualization of ethnocultural empathy. J Soc Evol Cult Psychol 5(1):38, Retrieved from http://jte.sagepub.com/content/39/1/38.short

Rorty R (1981) Philosophy and the mirror of nature. Princeton University Press, Princeton

Rousseau C, Crépeau F, Foxen P, Houle F (2002) The complexity of determining refugeehood: A multidisciplinary analysis of the decision-making process of the Canadian Immigration and Refugee Board. Journal of Refugee Studies 15(1):43–70

Smedley A, Smedley BD (2005) Race as biology is fiction, racism as a social problem is real: anthropological and historical perspectives on the social construction of race. Am Psychol 60(1):16–26. doi:10.1037/0003-066x.60.1.16

Suchman AL (2006) A new theoretical foundation for relationship-centered care. J Gen Intern Med 21(S1):S40–S44. doi:10.1111/j.1525-1497.2006.00308.x

Sue S, Zane N (1987) The role of culture and cultural techniques in psychotherapy: a critique and reformulation. Am Psychol 42:37–45

Sztompka P (1993) The sociology of social change. Blackwell Publishing, Oxford

Tarsitani L, Pasquini M, Maraone A, Zerella MP, Berardelli I, Giordani R, Polselli GM et al (2013) Acute psychiatric treatment and the use of physical restraint in first-generation immigrants in Italy: a prospective concurrent study. Int J Soc Psychiatry 59(6):613–618, Retrieved from http://isp.sagepub.com/content/59/6/613.short

Van der Kolk B (2000) Posttraumatic stress disorder and the nature of trauma. Dialogues Clin Neurosci 2(1):7–22, Retrieved from http://www.pubmedcentral.nih.gov/articlerender.fcgi?arti d=3181584&tool=pmcentrez&rendertype=abstract

White L (1959) The evolution of culture. McGraw Hill, New York

Williams CC (2006) The epistemology of cultural competence. Families in Society: The Journal of Contemporary Social Services 87(2). pp 209–220

Intercultural Trauma-Centred Psychotherapy and the Application of the EMDR Method

Meryam Schouler-Ocak

Introduction

According to the micro-census of 2014, the number of people with a migration background in 2013 was at least 16.5 million (Federal Statistics Office 2014), thus representing 20.5 % of the total population of Germany. Behind a supposedly uniform 'population group' are in reality many heterogeneous groups – people from different countries, who migrated in different generations and with different levels of education, residence status and socio-economic backgrounds. Since the 1990s, barriers to and within the social and health systems have been observed, hindering an equal quality of care for people with a migration background. One such pattern which has been observed is that people with a migration background usually make less frequent use of health services[1] (Lindert et al. 2008). Various different aspects could be held responsible for this situation, such as a lack of information on the healthcare system, legal factors pertaining to residence status (Grüsser and Becker 1999), communication difficulties and 'cultural' misunderstandings (Wohlfart and Zaumseil 2006; Schouler-Ocak 2011) – all of which can prevent or delay people finding their way into the system.

In addition, information-related, cultural, communicative and religious barriers can all lead to problems of under-treatment, over-treatment and unsuitable treatment of people with a migration background, sometimes leading to

---

[1] Currently in Germany, the term 'people with a migration background' refers to all those who moved to the current territory of the Federal Republic of Germany after 1949, as well as all foreigners born in Germany and all those born in Germany as German nationals but with at least one parent who moved to Germany or was born in Germany as a foreigner (Federal Statistics Office 2011).

M. Schouler-Ocak
Department of Psychiatry and Psychotherapy of the Charité, St. Hedwig Hospital,
Berlin, Germany
e-mail: meryam.schouler-ocak@charite.de

© Springer International Publishing Switzerland 2015
M. Schouler-Ocak (ed.), *Trauma and Migration:*
Cultural Factors in the Diagnosis and Treatment of Traumatised Immigrants,
DOI 10.1007/978-3-319-17335-1_12

substantially increased costs for treatment and care (Brucks and Wahl 2003). Experiences of discrimination also have an influence on migrants' subjective health. According to an investigation by Igel et al. (2010), the health of those who have experienced discrimination is significantly worse. Stigma and shame can represent other causes of the under-treatment amongst at least some groups of people with a migration background and mental health disorders (Schomerus 2009; Machleidt 2011).

It is becoming increasingly clear that in addition to cultural aspects, psychosocial and migration-specific factors also have a significant influence on the prevalence, onset and course of mental disorders in people with a migration background (Selten et al. 2007; Cantor-Graae and Selten 2005; Bhugra and Mastrogianni 2004; Jablensky et al. 1992; Selten et al. 2012; Heinz et al. 2013). Some international studies even suggest that severe mental health problems occur more frequently amongst people with a migration background. For example, Cantor-Graae and Selten (2005) and Selten et al. (2007) reported that migration is an important risk factor in the aetiology of schizophrenic disorders, and Veling et al. (2008) observed in The Hague (Netherlands) that the rate of schizophrenia amongst people with a migration background was significantly higher in districts with only a small number of people with a migration background compared to districts with a high ethnic density.

Epidemiology

McFarlane and Yehuda (2000) emphasise that post-traumatic stress disorder (PTSD) does not develop as a direct result of an event, but rather arises from the pattern of acute distress which is triggered by the event (McFarlane and Yehuda 2000, p. 143). It is assumed that different risk factors influence the development of PTSD. Objective risk factors include type, intensity and duration of the traumatic event, the extent of physical injury, whether the trauma was caused by people, and constantly being reminded of the event (triggering). Subjective risk factors include the unexpected occurrence of the traumatic event, a low level of personal control over what happens, guilt, and a lack of external help. Furthermore, youth or old age, belonging to a marginalised social group, low socio-economic status, a lack of social support and a family history of traumatic experiences all count as individual risk factors (Brewin et al. 2000; Ozer et al. 2003; Ehlers et al. 1998; Breslau et al. 1991).

According to Ehlers (1999), the prevalence of PTSD depends on the frequency of traumatic events and the nature of the trauma:

- Approximately 50 % prevalence for survivors of rape
- Approximately 25 % prevalence for survivors of other violent crimes
- Approximately 20 % prevalence for survivors of war
- Approximately 15 % prevalence for survivors of traffic accidents

The lifetime prevalence across all cultures lies between 1 and 7 % (Flatten et al. 2001).

Trauma and Migration

Trauma and migration can be connected in two different ways. Some people are faced with traumatic events associated with war, flight, expulsion and very often with sexual violence in their home countries; such experiences are often the reason for emigration to another country. On the other hand, people who leave their homeland can also be faced with a series of stressful events in the wake of this emigration.

Gilgen et al. (2005) examined various migrant groups in Switzerland and showed that conditions and events after migration have a serious impact on psychological well-being. Fifty percent of the surveyed Turkish/Kurdish migrants admitted to having experienced periods of extreme despair and suicidal thoughts after migration (ibid.), whereas before migration, only 12 % of them reported difficulties of this kind. Since then, several studies have provided evidence that migrants are at higher risk of experiencing traumatic experiences and developing PTSD. Al-Safar et al. (2001) examined three immigrant groups (Arabs, Iranians and Turks) in Stockholm and compared them with Swedish citizens. Of all the subjects surveyed, 89 % had experienced at least one trauma. The prevalence of PTSD was found to vary depending on group membership. Sixty-nine percent of Iranian immigrants, 59 % of the Arabs, 53 % of Turks and 29 % of Swedes were suspected of having PTSD (ibid.). The results indicate not only that multiple traumatic events increase the probability of developing PTSD, but also that belonging to an ethnic minority represents a risk factor (Brewin et al. 2000; Ozer et al. 2003; Ehlers et al. 1998; Breslau et al. 1991; Fearon et al. 2006; Veling et al. 2008; Selten et al. 2012).

Numerous studies confirm that PTSD in primary healthcare is common, but rarely diagnosed (Tagay et al. 2008). Instead, other comorbid mental disorders are diagnosed (Gomez-Beneyto et al. 2006; Katzman et al. 2005). A frequently cited reason for the poor rate of recognition for PTSD is the fact that patients themselves can rarely recognise or express the relationship between a past traumatic event and their illness (Carey et al. 2003; Munro et al. 2004). GPs therefore find themselves in a key position. The appropriate diagnosis and treatment of PTSD can significantly improve the outcome (Carey et al. 2003). The rate of trauma amongst refugees has been reported as being over 20 % (Gierlichs 2003); Gäbel et al. (2006) even speak of over 40 %. In a systematic review, the rate of PTSD amongst refugees and asylum seekers is described as being ten times more frequent than amongst the rest of the population (Crumlish and O'Rourke 2010).

Diagnosis of Post-traumatic Stress Disorder

The criteria described in ICD-10 and DSM-IV do not cover the entire spectrum of trauma-related disorders – there are a greater number of clinical disorders that can arise in connection with traumatic influences (Wöller et al. 2001). According to Sack (2004), a plethora of symptoms that would otherwise be classified as comorbid disorders can be drawn together into a unified etiological model with the help of the diagnostic category. Additional examination by an experienced clinician therefore forms an integral part of the diagnostic process.

A whole series exists of tried and tested questionnaires and structured interviews – such as the Impact of Event Scale Revision (IES-R), Structured Clinical Interview for DSM-PTSD (SCID-PTSD) or questionnaire for dissociative disorders (FDS) – with which to diagnose the consequences of extreme situations on mental health (Hofmann et al. 2001; Schützwohl 1997). In practice, these psychometric instruments are not generally suitable for the diagnosis of people from other cultures. The few available translations are rarely validated in their respective cultures, having been developed specifically for Western culture with regard to issues such as disease, symptoms, the concept of disease or mentality; this makes them only partially transferable to other cultures.

This highlights the dilemma of diagnostic testing in the field of intercultural psychiatry and psychotherapy (Birck et al. 2001). In addition, such methods cannot be used in cases where insufficient language skills are possessed. Özkan (2002) has pointed out the problematic areas in trauma-centred work with ethnic minorities. Schouler-Ocak et al. (2008) have insisted on the importance of cultural factors in intercultural treatment processes.

Special Aspects in Intercultural Treatment Processes

A useful picture of the physical and mental state of people with a migration background can often be gained through intercultural communication (Schouler-Ocak 1999; Schouler-Ocak et al. 2015). Knowledge of aspects which are specific to the relevant culture, disease, migration and the individual biography is essential. The use of a professionally trained, qualified interpreter as a linguistic and cultural mediator enables a mutual understanding in diagnosis and therapy (Salman 2001; Tuna and Salman 1999; Kluge 2011; Schouler-Ocak et al. 2015). Without such an understanding, taking a medical history, diagnosis and treatment are very difficult to manage; in a psychiatric-psychotherapeutic treatment context, these become virtually impossible.

In a pilot study in 12 large facilities, when asked about comprehension difficulties with patients with a migration background, teams of health professionals cited language-related problems in 27 % of cases, culture-related difficulties in 38 % of cases and both culture- and language-related communication problems in 44 % of cases (Koch et al. 2008). One example of the effects of such difficulties is shown by the results of a study of patients with a Turkish migration background and native-German patients in a women's clinic in Berlin (Pette et al. 2004). Low competence in spoken German amongst the women with a Turkish migration background correlated with holding a poor level of information about the diagnosis and treatment, as well as a loss of information during an inpatient stay and the associated process of therapeutic education (ibid.). Communication problems in the therapeutic context also lead to fewer consultations with doctors, a poorer understanding of medical explanations, more frequent laboratory tests and increased utilisation of emergency departments (Yeo 2004).

In order to avoid misdiagnosis, inappropriate treatment and frustration, not only is good verbal communication necessary, but also the consideration of different explanatory models regarding the cause, course and cure of certain health problems (Kleinman

1980; Bhui and Bhugra 2002; Penka et al. 2008, 2012; Schouler-Ocak et al. 2015). The terms used for the description of the respective diseases can have a thoroughly different meaning in a specific cultural context. Explanatory models and expectations regarding the treatment are also subject to permanent variation connected to cultural changes, traditional elements, personal experiences and information from the social environment or the media (Heinz and Kluge 2011; Heinz et al. 2013).

In addition, patients and their relatives may have differing ideas and expectations during a period of illness with regard to the cause, symptoms, onset mechanisms, course of disease and potential treatment options (Kleinman 1980, 1988; Penka et al. 2008, 2012). Explanations can differ on the one hand between different cultural contexts and on the other hand due to class-, age- or gender-specific factors, for example (Vardar et al. 2012). These ideas and expectations are in a dynamic process and may also influence each other; experiences can therefore change too (Kleinman 1980; Heinz and Kluge 2011). In Appendix F of the DSM-VI-TR (Saß et al. 2003), there is a proposal for guidelines on taking a medical history and offering treatment in a culturally sensitive way. Its application allows the systematic consideration of the sociocultural background of patients with a migration background and should be used regularly in the work with them. The Cultural Formulation Interview (CFI) published in chapter on cultural formulation in DSM-5 can be used in research and clinical settings as potentially useful tool to enhance clinical understanding and decision-making and not as the sole basis for making a clinical diagnosis (APA 2013).

Working with Interpreters (Linguistic and Cultural Mediators)

Intercultural treatment in Germany can only succeed if appropriate treatment can be ensured even for those with little knowledge of the German language. Even amongst those with a working knowledge of German for everyday life, not all people with a migration background have sufficient knowledge of German in the fields of body, health, well-being and sexuality (Razum et al. 2008). For health professionals, this situation necessitates the ability to work alongside interpreters (linguistic and cultural mediators); it also demands the availability of such mediators. This may, for example, involve community interpreting services such as those that exist in Berlin, but in larger hospitals, it is also conceivable that interpreting services might be offered by bilingual professional staff (Wesselmann 2000; Bahadir 2009).

The use of linguistic and cultural mediators should therefore take place as a matter of course when communication problems are evident. Guidelines for the professional use of linguistic and cultural mediators should be internalised not only by the mediators themselves, but also by the therapists (Bhugra et al. 2014; Schouler-Ocak et al. 2015). Interpreter-assisted treatment then becomes a viable option (Morina et al. 2010). In this context, a terminological ambiguity is inherent in the term 'linguistic and cultural mediators', as opposed to the more common term 'interpreter' (Penka et al. 2012); the term assumes a level of understanding in intercultural contexts which goes beyond the verbal (Penka et al. 2012; Qureshi et al. 2008, Qureshi and Collazos 2011). The aim is to recognise these cultural differences which are inherent to language differences and to make them accessible to the treatment process. According to Penka et al. (2012), in such cases, linguistic and cultural mediators are referred to for the cultural knowledge that they bring to the treatment setting and can help to clarify cultural differences and the resulting misunderstandings that can occur. The therapist must then integrate this knowledge into the therapeutic process (ibid.; Qureshi et al. 2008; Qureshi and Collazos 2011), a task for which an openness towards other symbolisations is a prerequisite (Kluge and Kassim 2006).

In this setting, it is therefore inappropriate to consider the interpreter simply as a mechanical, linguistic intermediary (Hsieh 2008; Qureshi et al. 2008; Qureshi and Collazos 2011; Haenel 2001); indeed, like the therapist, he/she is also involved in the transference of the patient and can in turn also trigger countertransference feelings. It is extremely important to take this into account too; otherwise, decisive factors which can influence the course of therapy might remain unnoticed and both the opportunity represented by the interpreter and the danger of trauma to the interpreters may be overlooked (Pross 2009). The therapeutic process can also be disrupted or stagnated when asymmetries in the relational patterns between the parties – therapist, interpreter and patient – occur. In such a setting, there are usually three rather than two players protagonists in the therapeutic space. These protagonists communicate in at least two different languages, creating a complex framework of levels of understanding and interaction that sometimes make such a setting difficult to comprehend (Qureshi et al. 2008, Qureshi and Collazos 2011; Hsieh 2008; Kluge 2011). In Germany, a lack of clarity in terms of the allocation of costs is a major cause for the low use of professional linguistic and cultural mediators (Kluge et al. 2012).

Intercultural Trauma-Centred Psychotherapy

Not only cultural, but also linguistic, religious and ethnic misunderstandings may play a role in intercultural psychotherapy (Gün 2007). In particular, there is an indispensable need for 'joining' – the willingness of the therapist to empathise and enter into the lives of the patients and families with a migration background (Schlippe von and El Hachimi 2000; Erim and Senf 2002; Erim 2005). If the therapist and patient come from different cultural contexts, two types of bias may occur. On the one hand, the differences between the cultural contexts can be overemphasised – in extreme cases, a native therapist might even consider psychotherapy to be impossible. On the other hand, differences can be denied, and the influence of culturally defined social circumstances on the patients ignored. Both attitudes are viewed as problematic (Fisek and Schepker 1997; Bhugra and Mastrogianni 2004; Bhui and Bhugra 2002).

Intercultural trauma-centred psychotherapy refers to psychotherapeutic work with traumatised people with a migration background. It presupposes that the therapist has intercultural competence, this being understood as a component of social competence, since perception, judgement and action are always culturally conditioned (Grosch and Leenen 1998; Bhugra et al. 2014). According to Oesterreich and Hegemann (2010), openness, interest and respectful curiosity towards the unfamiliar represent the foundations of intercultural competence. Amongst other things, this includes working with linguistic and cultural mediators, observing and recognising the idioms of distress (locally typical patterns of symptoms), taking into account patients' understandings of illness and expectations about treatment, and working out culturally appropriate explanations and treatment services (Kirmayer et al. 2008; Eiser and Ellis 2007; Betancourt et al. 2003; Odawara 2005). Trauma-centred psychotherapy consists of four phases (Sachsse 2004; Hofmann 2014; Reddemann and Sachsse 1997; Schouler-Ocak et al. 2008):

1. Taking a medical history, diagnosis, relationship building and developing a treatment plan
2. Stabilising/preparation phase (building resources, developing strategies for dealing with intrusions)
3. Trauma exposure phase (carefully measured re-exposure to the traumatic experiences in a protected space),
4. Grief, closure, reintegration and reorientation phase (integration of the cognitive components of traumatic experiences into the patient's life story).

The first phase involves taking the medical history, reaching a diagnosis, building a relationship and developing a treatment plan. The stabilisation phase involves promoting awareness of the patient's own resources by building their capacity to regulate and control external and internal processes, both psychological and bodily, as well as relativising self-accusations and negative judgements of symptoms by positively reinterpreting them as useful protection and survival mechanisms at the time of the trauma (including an inner safe space, internal vault, internal helpers, resources exercises). In the trauma exposure phase, the processing of the traumatic event is undertaken using various methods such as behavioural therapy, screen technique and/or EMDR (Eye Movement Desensitisation and Reprocessing) (Silver et al. 2008; Shapiro 2001; Hofmann 2014). In this phase, the principle of retroactively accelerated (neurophysiological) information processing leads to the reintegration of sensations previously stored as fragments and thus to the reduction of anxiety. The fourth phase involves mourning, rage and taking leave of those aspects of life which have been lost or were never experienced. Lastly, the construction and development of new meanings and ways of and perspectives on life can begin.

EMDR

EMDR (Eye Movement Desensitisation and Reprocessing) is a branch of therapy, a complementary technique to conventional medicine, and one of the most studied methods to resolve trauma within therapy. EMDR method was developed in the early 1990s by Francine Shapiro. It is a visual-confrontational, relaxing and highly supportive method which, through introducing bilaterally alternating stimuli (induced eye movements, tapping the hands, clicking the fingers), allows the processing and integration of traumatic experiences to be set in motion once again and move towards completion (Silver et al. 2008; Schubbe 2009; Shapiro 2001; Hofmann 2014).

According to the guidelines for the treatment of post-traumatic disorders (Silver et al. 2008; Schubbe 2009; Flatten et al. 2001; Hofmann 2014), the process should begin with internal and external stabilisation. The EMDR sessions should follow only after this and consist of the initial assessment of symptoms, the central reprocessing phase, anchoring the achieved state and testing residual stress on the bodily level – the so-called body scan. In EMDR just as in any trauma therapy work, there is special emphasis on reaching a good conclusion at the end of the session. At the beginning of the follow-up session, a test is performed to ascertain whether or not the change reached in the last session has remained stable (Silver et al. 2008; Schubbe 2009; Shapiro 2001; Hofmann 2014).

In intercultural trauma-centred psychotherapy, it is important to consider that resources and coping strategies may differ depending on the cultural background of the patient. This pertains in particular to the question of which skills have helped the patient to survive or even to overcome the distressing experiences, which strengths it was necessary to develop, how they have managed to live with their symptoms previous to therapy, and what gives them hope and strength in the therapy process. In trauma-centred psychotherapy, it is not only the post-processing of information which is key, but also the reintegration of resources that were unavailable, blocked by the trauma or bound up with survival strategies and re-enactments of traumatic behaviour patterns (Silver et al. 2008; Schubbe 2009; Hofmann 2014).

Numerous studies have shown that bilateral stimulation through eye movements is associated with a relaxation response (Barrowcliff et al. 2004; Wilson et al. 1995; Hofmann 2014). During deconditioning, the moment of relaxation becomes additionally effective and promotes the therapy process. The relaxation response becomes associated with the memory of the traumatic content, which can then be stored in a much more relaxed way. This effect is called counter-conditioning. Through repeated, controlled exposure to traumatic memories in a protected therapeutic context, the pathological response is weakened (Hofmann 2014; Silver et al. 2008; McNally and Foa 1986). On the cognitive level, the patient's dysfunctional cognitions are also worked with; so too with positive cognitions which the patient develops independently during the EMDR process.

As such, the EMDR process can be distinguished from any other form of free association through its systematic focus on a moment of inner perception at all levels: the part of the traumatic situation which can be narrated, the sensory representation of the worst moment, the generalisation on the cognitive level, the quality and quantity of emotional distress and finally the reactions on the bodily level. The part of the memory which can be narrated forms the introduction; the bodily level, as the deepest level of internal perception, then leads purposefully into the EMDR process that is additionally triggered by the naming of the output image and the associated negative cognition (Schubbe 2009; Hofmann 2014). Reprocessing is at the core of the method and is also referred to as 'processing' or 'EMDR process'.

The therapist begins with bifocal stimulation. In each EMDR session, as many series of stimulations are conducted as necessary in order to eliminate the distress. If necessary, additional strategies (e.g. change of stimulus, cognitive weaving) can be used to continue and support the processing. After each series, the patient is asked which (unprocessed) material entered into consciousness. If the flow of processing falters, Shapiro (2001); Schubbe (2009); Hofmann (2014) recommends cognitive weaving as an EMDR technique to resolve blockages and break out of infinitely repeating cognitive-emotional loops. Since the EMDR process takes place primarily in the patient's inner perception field, cognitive weaving expands the therapeutic options by enabling the therapist to allow certain contents or information to flow into the patient's process. The term 'weaving' is thus related to the therapist's economical and purposeful use of information, offered to the patient in order to allow him or her to connect previously non-associated content. During processing, a close relationship between therapist and patient is formed, in which the therapist steers and accompanies the process with great attention and concentration.

The interposition of a linguistic and cultural mediator in such a process could represent an element of confusion and possibly interrupt the processing. It could be argued that patients could be torn out of the processing and become stuck in the cognitively and emotionally distressing, highly triggered memories that they are exposed to in that moment, in the form of images, sounds and bodily sensations. Since the EMDR process takes place primarily in the patient's inner perception field, there is also a danger of the therapist losing contact with the patient and the process therefore continuing within the patient unchecked. Amongst others, such considerations perhaps explain why there have been no previous publications on intercultural trauma-centred work using the EMDR method with patients with a migration background, with the assistance of a professional linguistic and cultural mediator.

On the other hand, these considerations disregard the fact that through the bilateral stimuli given by the therapist, the EMDR patient can stay in contact with the here and now and can thus maintain the necessary distance to the potentially very stressful and disorientating memories and images. Accordingly, the involvement of a specially trained linguistic and cultural mediator would support the patient's contact with the here and now and possibly slow down the processing in the patient's internal perception. This could lead to the traumatic events being fractionated as they are processed, so to speak, meaning that the reduction of the exposure values would take place more slowly. The distress levels in an individual session would therefore be lower, but a greater number of sessions may be required. Trauma-centred psychotherapy in patients with a migration background using the EMDR method with the assistance of a professional linguistic and cultural mediator thus represents a challenge, but the considerations above and below provide encouraging reasons to take on this challenge.

Final Considerations

Trauma-centred psychotherapy in the native language of people with a migration background generally fails due to the low number of qualified therapists, making intercultural therapy the usual option. Since any one therapist cannot be expected to be knowledgeable of all culture-related issues, nor master the languages of all his/her patients, the involvement of professionally trained linguistic and cultural mediators seems inevitable. Intercultural psychotherapy is hindered not only by language barriers, but also by more complex communication problems, based on different explanations of the causes, characteristics and treatment options for various illnesses. As well as involving the linguistic and cultural mediator, intercultural supervision and intervision can also be useful in the detection, consideration and respectful treatment of culture-specific factors. Although such treatment is fraught with difficulties, people with a migration background deserve access to the same professional care as those being treated in their own cultural context.

The therapist and the linguistic and cultural mediator should not neglect themselves in the midst of considering the factors which have been mentioned. Wellfunctioning stabilisation mechanisms, psychohygiene, supervision and intervision are all crucial when working with traumatised patients, whichever background they are from. This is especially important for professional linguistic and cultural mediators working with traumatised patients with a migration background, because the events which are described can have a strong effect on them as well. Whereas the use of professional linguistic and cultural mediators in intercultural psychotherapy has been well documented (Kluge et al. 2012; Kluge 2011; Qureshi et al. 2008; Qureshi and Collazos 2011; Hsieh 2008; Haenel 2001; Salman 2001; Tuna and Salman 1999; Bhugra et al. 2014; Schouler-Ocak et al. 2015), publications on the inclusion of professional linguistic and cultural mediators in intercultural traumacentred psychotherapy using the EMDR method have not been available until now. Previous publications do not deal with this special setting. Future studies could take on this subject, thereby potentially allowing this very effective method to become available to traumatised patients with a migration background.

References

Al-Safar S, Borga P, Edman G, Hallstrom T (2001) The aetiology of posttraumatic stress disorder in four ethnic groups in outpatient psychiatry. Soc Psychiatry Psychiatr Epidemiol 38(8): 456–462

American Psychiatric Association (2013) Diagnostic and Statistical Manual of Mental Disorders (Fifth ed.). Arlington, VA: American Psychiatric Publishing. ISBN 978-0-89042-555-8

Bahadır S (2009) Müssen alle bikulturellen Krankenhausmitarbeiter dolmetschen (können/wollen)? In: Falge C, Zimmermann G (eds) Interkulturelle Öffnung des Gesundheitssystems. Nomos, Baden-Baden, pp 171–185

Barrowcliff AL, Gray NS, Freeman T, MacCulloch MJ (2004) Eye-movements reduce the vividness, emotional valence and electrodermal arousal associated with negative autobiographical memories. J Forensic Psychiatry Psychol 15(2):325–345

Betancourt JR, Green AR, Carrillo JE, Ananeh-Firempong O 2nd (2003) Defining cultural competence: a practical framework for addressing racial/ethnic disparities in health and health care. Public Health Rep 118(4):293–302

Bhugra D, Mastrogianni A (2004) Globalisation and mental disorders. Br J Psychiatry 184:10–20

Bhugra D, Gupta S, Schouler-Ocak M, Graeff-Calliess I, Deakin NA, Qureshi A, Dales J, Moussaoui D, Kastrup M, Tarricone I, Till A, Bassi M, Carta M (2014) EPA guidance mental health care of migrants. Eur Psychiatry 29(2):107–115

Bhui K, Bhugra D (2002) Explanatory models for mental distress: implications for clinical practice and research. Br J Psychiatry 181:6–7

Birck A, Winter D, Koch F (2001) Diagnostik psychischer Folgen. In: Richtlinien für die Untersuchung von traumatisierten Flüchtlingen und Folteropfer. Deutscher Psychologen Verlag, Bonn, S. 39–53

Breslau N, Davis GC, Andreski P, Peterson E (1991) Traumatic events and posttraumatic stress disorder in an urban population of young adults. Arch Gen Psychiatry 48(3):216–222

Brewin CR, Andrews B, Valentine JD (2000) Meta-analysis of risk factors for posttraumatic stress disorder in trauma-exposed adults. J Consult Clin Psychol 68:748–766

Brucks U, Wahl WB (2003) Über-, Unter-, Fehlversorgung? Bedarfslücken und Strukturprobleme in der ambulanten Gesundheitsversorgung für Migrantinnen und Migranten. In: Borde T, David M (eds) Gut versorgt? Migrantinnen und Migranten im Gesundheits- und Sozialwesen. Mabuse, Frankfurt, pp 15–34

Cantor-Graae E, Selten JP (2005) Schizophrenia and migration: a meta-analysis and review. Am J Psychiatry 162:12–24

Carey PD, Stein DJ, Zungu-Dirwayi N, Seedat S (2003) Trauma and posttraumatic stress disorder in an urban Xhosa primary care population: prevalence, comorbidity, and service use patterns. J Nerv Ment Dis 191:230–236

Crumlish N, O'Rourke K (2010) A systematic review of treatments for post-traumatic stress disorder among refugees and asylum-seekers. J Nerv Ment Dis 198(4):237–251

Ehlers A (1999) Posttraumatische Belastungsstörung. Hogrefe, Göttingen

Ehlers A, Mayou RA, Bryant B (1998) Psychological predictors of chronic posttraumatic stress disorder after motor vehicle accidents. J Abnorm Psychol 107:508–519

Eiser AR, Ellis G (2007) Viewpoint: cultural competence and the African American experience with health care: the case for specific content in cross-cultural education. Acad Med 82(2):176–183

Erim Y (2005) Psychotherapie mit Migranten ± Aspekte der interkulturellen Psychotherapie. In: Senf W, Broda M (eds) Praxis der Psychotherapie. Thieme Verlag, Stuttgart, pp 672–678

Erim Y, Senf W (2002) Psychotherapie mit Migranten. Interkulturelle Aspekte in der Psychotherapie. Psychotherapeutische 47:336–346

Fearon P, Kirkbride JB, Morgan C et al. (2006) AESOP Study Group. Incidence of schizophrenia and other psychoses in ethnic minority groups: results from the MRC AESOP Study. Psychol Med 36(11):1541–50

Federal Statistics Office (2014) Bevölkerung und Erwerbstätigkeit. Bevölkerung mit Migrationshintergrund, Ergebnisse des Mikrozensus 2013. Fachserie 1 Reihe 2.2, Wiesbaden

Fisek G, Schepker R (1997) Kontext-Bewusstsein in der transkulturellen Psychotherapie. Familiendynamik 22:396–413

Flatten G, Hofmann A, Liebermann P, Wöller W, Siol T, Petzhold E (2001) Posttraumatische Belastungsstörung. Schattauer, Stuttgart

Gäbel U, Ruf M, Schauer M, Odenwald M, Neuner F (2006) Prävalenz der Posttraumatischen Belastungsstörung (PTSD) und Möglichkeiten der Ermittlung in der Asylverfahrenspraxis. Z Klin Psychol Psychother 35(1):12–20

Gierlichs HW (2003) Begutachtung psychotraumatisierter Flüchtlinge. Deutsches Ärzteblatt 100(34–35):1098

Gilgen D, Maeusezahl D, Gross C et al (2005) Impact of migration on illness experience and help–seeking strategies of patients from Turkey and Bosnia in primary health care in Basel. Health Place 11(3):261–273

Gomez-Beneyto M, Salazar-Fraile J, Marti-Sanjuan V, Gonzalez-Lujan L (2006) Posttraumatic stress disorder in primary care with special reference to personality disorder comorbidity. Br J Gen Pract 56:349–354

Grosch H, Leenen WR (1998) Materialien zum interkulturellen Lernen. In: Bundeszentrale für politische Bildung (Hg.): Interkulturelles Lernen. Arbeitshilfen für die politische Bildung. Bonn. S. Bundeszentrale für politische Bildung 353–384

Grüsser SM, Becker K (1999) Drogenabhängigkeit und Migration innerhalb der Europäischen Union (EU). In: Gölz J (ed). Moderne Suchtmedizin; Thieme, Stuttgart 5, pp 1–7

Gün AK (2007) Interkulturelle Missverständnisse in der Psychotherapie. Gegenseitiges Verstehen zwischen einheimischen Therapeuten und türkeistämmigen Klienten. Lambertus Verlag, Freiburg im Breisgau

Haenel F (2001) Ausgewählte Aspekte und Probleme der in der Psychotherapie mit Folteropfern unter Beteiligung von Dolmetschern. Curare Sonderband 16:307–316

Heinz A, Kluge U (2011) Ethnologische Ansätze in der transkulturellen Psychiatrie. In: Machleidt W, Heinz A (eds) Praxis der interkulturellen Psychiatrie und Psychotherapie: Migration und psychische Gesundheit. Elsevier, München, pp 27–32

Heinz A, Deserno L, Reininghaus U (2013) Urbanicity, social adversity and psychosis. World Psychiatry 12(3):187–97

Hofmann A (2014) EMDR - Therapie psychotraumatischer Belastungssyndrome, 5., vollst. überarb. u. erweiterte Aufl., Thieme Verlag, Stuttgart, New York

Hofmann A, Liebermann P, Flatten G (2001) Diagnostik der Posttraumatischen Belastungsstörung. In: Flatten G, Hofmann A, Liebermann P, Wöller W, Siol T, Petzhold E (eds) Posttraumatische Belastungsstörung. Schattauer, Stuttgart, pp 71–84

Hsieh E (2008) "I am not a robot!" Interpreters' views of their roles in health care settings. Qual Health Res 18(10):1367–1383

Igel U, Brähler E, Grande G (2010) Der Einfluss von Diskriminierungserfahrungen auf die Gesundheit von Migranten. Psychiatr Prax 37:183–190

Jablensky A, Sartorius N, Ehrenberg G, Anker M, Corten A, Cooper JE, Day R, Bartelsen A (1992) Schizophrenia: manifestations, incidence, and course in different cultures: a World Health Organization ten countries study, vol 20, Psychological medicine, monograph supplement. Cambridge University Press, Cambridge, UK

Katzman MA, Struzik L, Vivian LL et al (2005) Pharmacotherapy of posttraumatic–stress disorder: a family practitioners guide to management the disease. Expert Rev Neurother 5: 129–139

Kirmayer LJ, Rousseau C, Corin E, Groleau D (2008) Training researchers in cultural psychiatry: the McGill-CIHR Strategic Training Program. Acad Psychiatry 32(4):320–326

Kleinman A (1980) Patients and healers in the context of culture: an exploration of the borderland between anthropology, medicine, and psychiatry. University of California Press, Berkeley, Los Angeles

Kleinman A (1988) The illness narratives. Suffering, healing & the human condition. Basic Books, New York

Kluge U (2011) Sprach- und Kulturmittler im interkulturellen psychotherapeutischen Setting. In: Machleidt W, Heinz A (eds) Praxis der interkulturellen Psychiatrie und Psychotherapie: Migration und psychische Gesundheit. Elsevier, München, pp 145–154

Kluge U, Kassim N (2006) »Der Dritte im Raum« – Chancen und Schwierigkeiten in der Zusammenarbeit mit Sprach- und Kulturmittlern in einem interkulturellen psychotherapeutischen Setting. In: Wohlfart E, Zaumseil M (eds) Transkulturelle Psychiatrie und Interkulturelle Psychotherapie – Interdisziplinäre Theorie und Praxis. Springer Medizinverlag, Heidelberg, pp 177–196

Kluge U, Bogic M, Devillé W, Greacen T, Dauvrin M, Dias S et al (2012) Health services and the treatment of immigrants: data on service use, interpreting services and immigrant staff members in services across Europe. Eur Psychiatry 27(Suppl 2):56–62

Koch E, Hartkamp N, Siefen RG, Schouler-Ocak M (2008) Patienten mit Migrationshintergrund in stationär-psychiatrischen Einrichtungen – Pilotstudie der Arbeitsgruppe "Psychiatrie und Migration" der Bundesdirektorenkonferenz. Nervenarzt 79(3):328–339

Lindert J, Priebe S, Penka S, Napo F, Schouler-Ocak M, Heinz A (2008) Mental health care for migrants. Psychother Psychosom Med Psychol 58:123–129

Machleidt W (2011) Das gedoppelte Stigma: Psychisch krank und Migrant – Perspektiven der Ethnopsychiatrie. In: Machleidt W, Heinz A (eds) Praxis der Interkulturellen Psychiatrie und Psychotherapie. Elsevier, München

McFarlane AC, Yehuda R (2000) Widerstandskraft, Vulnerabilität und der Verlauf posttraumatischer Reaktionen. In: Van der Kolk B, McFarlane C, Weisaeth L (eds) Traumatic stress. Jungfermann, Paderborn, pp 141–168

McNally RJ, Foa EB (1986) Preparedness and resistance to extinction to fear-relevant stimuli: a failure to replicate. Behav Res Ther 24(5):529–535

Morina N, Maier T, Schmid M (2010) Lost in translation? Psychotherapie unter Einsatz von Dolmetschern. Psychother Psych Med 60:104–110

Munro CG, Freeman CP, Law R (2004) General practitioners' knowledge of posttraumatic stress disorder: a controlled study. Br J Gen Pract 54:843–847

Odawara E (2005) Cultural competency in occupational therapy: beyond a cross-cultural view of practice. Am J Occup Ther 59(3):325–334

Oesterreich C, Hegemann T (2010) Interkulturelle Systemische Therapie und Beratung. PiD Psychotherapie im Dialog 11(4):319–325

Ozer EJ, Best SR, Lipsey TL, Weiss DS (2003) Predictors of posttraumatic stress disorder and symptoms in adults: a meta-analysis. Psychol Bull 129(1):52–73

Özkan I (2002) Problembereiche in der traumazentrierten Arbeit mit ethnischen Minoritäten. In: Sachsse U, Özkan I, Streeck-Fischer A (eds) Traumatherapie – Was ist erfolgreich? Vandenhoeck & Ruprecht, Göttingen, pp 72–82

Penka S, Heimann H, Heinz A, Schouler-Ocak M (2008) Explanatory models of addictive behaviour among native German, Russian-German, and Turkish youth. Eur Psychiatry 23(Suppl 1):36–42

Penka S, Schouler-Ocak M, Heinz A, Kluge U (2012) Interkulturelle Aspekte der Interaktion und Kommunikation im psychiatrisch/psychotherapeutischen Behandlungssetting – Mögliche Barrieren und Handlungsempfehlungen. Bundesgesundheitsblatt 55(9):1168–1175

Pette M, Borde T, David M (2004) Kenntnis über die Diagnose und Therapie ihrer Erkrankung bei deutschen und türkischstämmigen Patientinnen vor und nach einem Krankenhausaufenthalt. J Turk Ger Gynecol Assoc 5(4):130–137

Pross C (2009) Verletzte Helfer – Umgang mit dem Trauma: Risiken und Möglichkeiten sich zu schützen. Klett-Cotta Verlag, Stuttgart

Qureshi A, Collazos F (2011) The intercultural and interracial therapeutic relationship: challenges and recommendations. Int Rev Psychiatry 23(1):10–19

Qureshi A, Collazos F, Ramos M, Casas M (2008) Cultural competency training in psychiatry. Eur Psychiatry 23:49–58

Razum O, Zeeb H, Schenk L (2008) Ähnliche Krankheiten, unterschiedliche Risiken. Migration und Gesundheit Deutsches Ärzteblatt 47:A2520–A2521

Reddemann L, Sachsse U (1997) Traumazentrierte Psychotherapie. PTT Persönlichkeitsstörungen 2:11–45

Sachsse U (2004) Traumazentrierte Psychotherapie. Theorie, Klinik und Praxis. Schattauer GmbH, Stuttgart

Sack M (2004) Diagnostische und klinische Aspekte der komplexen posttraumatischen Belastungsstörung. Nervenarzt 75:451–459

Salman R (2001) Sprach- und Kulturvermittlung – Konzepte und Methoden der Arbeit mit Dolmetschern in therapeutischen Prozessen. In: Hegemann T, Salman R (eds) Transkulturelle Psychiatrie-Konzepte für die Arbeit mit Menschen aus anderen Kulturen. Psychiatrie-Verlag, Bonn, pp 169–190

Saß H, Wittchen H-U, Zaudig M, Houben I (2003) Diagnostisches und Statistisches Manual Psychischer Störungen – Textversion – DSM-IV-TR. Anhang F: Leitfaden zur Beurteilung kultureller Einflussfaktoren und ein Glossar kulturabhängiger Syndrome. Hogrefe, Göttingen, pp 929–936

Schlippe von A, El Hachimi M (2000) Systemische Therapie und Supervision in multikulturellen Kontexten. Syst Fam 13(1):3–13

Schomerus G (2009) Obstacles in the way – stigma and help-seeking. Psychiatr Prax 36:53–54

Schouler-Ocak M (1999) Posttraumatische Belastungsstörung – Bedeutung in der Begutachtung im interkulturellen Feld. In: Collatz J, Hackhausen W, Salam R (eds) Begutachtung im interkulturellen Feld. Zur Lage der Migranten und zur Qualität ihrer sozialrechtlichen und sozialmedizinischen Begutachtung in Deutschland, vol 1, Forum Migration Gesundheit Integration. VWN – Verlag für Wissenschaft und Bildung, Berlin, pp 233–242

Schouler-Ocak M (2011) "Ich habe mir den Kopf erkältet": Die Angst, verrückt zu werden. Deutsch-türkische Nachrichten, 14.11.2011. URL: http://www.deutsch-tuerkische-nachrichten. de/2011/10/217671/ich-habe-mir-den-kopf-erkaeltet-die-angst-verrueckt-zu-werden/(Stand: 09.03.2012)

Schouler-Ocak M, Reiske S-L, Rapp M, Heinz A (2008) Cultural factors in the diagnosis and treatment of traumatised migrant patients from Turkey. Transcult Psychiatry 45(4):652–670

Schouler-Ocak M, Graef-Calliess IT, Tarricone I, Qureshi A, Kastrup M, Bhugra D (2015) EPA Guidance on Cultural Competence Training. Eur Psychiatry 30(3):431–40

Schubbe O (2009) Eye-movement desensitization and reprocessing (EMDR). In: Maercker A (ed) Posttraumatische Belastungsstörung, 3rd edn. Springer, Berlin/Heidelberg, pp 285–300

Schützwohl M (1997) Diagnostik und Differentialdiagnostik. In: Maerker (ed) Therapie der posttraumatischen Belastungsstörungen. Springer, Berlin

Selten JP, Cantor-Graae E, Kahn RS (2007) Migration and schizophrenia. Curr Opin Psychiatry 20(2):111–115

Selten JP, Laan W, Kupka R, Smeets HM, van Os J (2012) Risk of psychiatric treatment for mood disorders and psychotic disorders among migrants and Dutch nationals in Utrecht, The Netherlands. Soc Psychiatry Psychiatr Epidemiol 47(2):271–8

Shapiro F (2001) Eye movement desensitization and reprocessing. Guilford, New York

Silver SM, Rogers S, Russell M (2008) Eye movement desensitization and reprocessing (EMDR) in the treatment of war veterans. J Clin Psychol 64(8):947–957

Tagay S, Zararsiz R, Erim Y, Düllmann S, Schlegl S, Brähler E, Senf W (2008) Traumatische Ereignisse und Posttraumatische Belastungsstörung bei türkischsprachigen Patienten in der Primärversorgung. Psychother Psych Med 58:155–161

Tuna S, Salman R (1999) Phänomene interkultureller Kommunikation im Begutachtungsprozess. In: Collatz J, Hackhausen W, Salman R (eds) Begutachtung im interkulturellen Feld. Zur Lage der Migranten und zur Qualität ihrer sozialgerichtlichen und sozialmedizinischen Begutachtung in Deutschland, vol 1, Reihe Forum Migration Gesundheit Integration. VWB – Verlag für Wissenschaft und Bildung, Berlin, pp 169–178

Vardar A, Kluge U, Penka S (2012) How to express mental health problems- Turkish immgrants in Berlin compared to native Germans in Berlin and Turks in Istanbul. Eur Psychiatry 27(Suppl 2):50–56

Veling W, Susser E, van Os J, Mackenbach JP, Selten JP, Hoek HD (2008) Ethnic density of neighborhoods and incidence of psychotic disorders among immigrants. Am J Psychiatry 165(1):66–73

Wesselmann E (2000) Sprachmittlung im Krankenhaus durch den hausinternen Dolmetscherdienst. In: Gesundheitliche Versorgung von Personen mit Migrationshintergrund, Dokumentation Experten-Workshop am 5. Mai 2009 im Ministerium für Arbeit und Soziales, Berlin

Wilson SA, Becker LA, Tinker RH (1995) Eye movement desensitization and reprocessing (EMDR). Treatment for psychologically traumatized individuals. J Consult Clin Psychol 63(6):928–937

Wohlfart E, Zaumseil M (eds) (2006) Transkulturelle Psychiatrie –interkulturelle Psychotherapie. Interdisziplinäre Theorie und Praxis. Springer Medizin, Heidelberg

Wöller W, Siol T, Liebermann P (2001) Traumaassiziierte Störungsbilder neben der PTSD. In: Flatten G, Hofmann A, Liebermann P, Wöller W, Siol T, Petzhold E (eds) Posttraumatische Belastungsstörung. Schattauer, Stuttgart

Yeo, S (2004) Language barriers and access to care. Annual review of nursing research [serial on the Internet]. 22. URL: http://www.springerpub.com/samples/9780826141347_chapter.pdf

Resilience-Oriented Treatment of Traumatised Asylum Seekers and Refugees

Cornelis J. Laban

Introduction

Many mental health workers think their ability to treat asylum seekers and refugees is limited. They are often overwhelmed with feelings of powerlessness when they are confronted with the complexity of psychiatric problems, the past traumatic experiences and the present living problems. However, there is no need for such feelings. In the last decades, a lot of progress has been made, and both theoretical concepts and practical approaches are developed, which show accessible ways of helping this group of patients. That does not mean there are no obstacles and improvement is easy to reach. Many patients have more than one psychiatric disorder, they have a lot of concomitant somatic health problems and complaints, they have a high rate of disability and low quality of life and besides that they experience a lot of post-migration living problems. This complexity of the problems of asylum seekers and refugees reduces the applicability of routine treatment protocols.

In this chapter, we will discuss the concept of resilience and describe a resilience-oriented diagnostic and treatment model. Subsequently, we will discuss some resources of resilience and illustrate the applications in clinical practice. The main purpose of this chapter is to show that, although the limitations in the treatment of asylum seekers and refugees are substantial, it is nevertheless possible and sensible to offer mental healthcare for this group.

Resilience: the ability to sustain, to recover and to grow.

The term 'resilience' is related to the Latin words 'salire' which means jump, bounce and also splash (of water) and 'resilire' which means to bounce back or to

C.J. Laban, MD, PhD
De Evenaar, North Netherlands Centre for Transcultural Psychiatry,
Institute of Community Mental Health Care Drenthe, Altingerweg 1,
Beilen 9411PA, The Netherlands
e-mail: kees.laban@ggzdrenthe.nl

© Springer International Publishing Switzerland 2015
M. Schouler-Ocak (ed.), *Trauma and Migration:*
Cultural Factors in the Diagnosis and Treatment of Traumatised Immigrants,
DOI 10.1007/978-3-319-17335-1_13

splash again (like in a fountain). Scientific findings (Bonanno 2004) show that many individuals survive all sorts of hardships with minimal distress, or with the ability to tolerate their distress, and move on with their lives in a positive manner. Interest in the phenomenon of resilience has grown tremendously in the last decades. It was the leading theme at the annual meeting 2013 of the International Society for Traumatic Stress Studies (ISTSS), and many authors contributed publications in recent books (Southwick et al. 2011; Kent et al. 2014).

There is no single agreed-upon definition of resilience. In a review of the published literature on risk, vulnerability, resistance and resilience, Layne et al. (2007) identified at least eight distinct meanings for the term 'resilience'. One distinction between definitions of resilience is the focus on outcome, e.g. symptom-free functioning after adversities, and the focus on process, which includes cognitions, emotional reactions and behaviours that are adaptive in response to stress and trauma, for example, active coping and seeking social support. The American Psychological Association (2010) has defined resilience as 'the process of adapting well in the face of adversity, trauma, tragedy, threats or even significant sources of threat'.

Resilience and a diverse range of resources of resilience have been the subject of theoretical, psychological as well as biological studies (Rutter 1987, 2006; Masten et al.1990; Luthar et al. 2000; Charney 2004; Southwick et al. 2005; Yehuda et al. 2006; Ozbay et al. 2007; Feder et al. 2011).

Southwick and Charney (2012) summarise the psychosocial factors that have been associated with resilience. They conclude these factors from interviews with a variety of groups of trauma survivors. The factors include positive emotion and optimism, loving caretakers and sturdy role models, a history of mastering challenges, cognitive flexibility including the ability to cognitively reframe adversity in a more positive light, the ability to regulate emotions, high coping self-efficacy, strong social support, disciplined focus on skill development, altruism, commitment to a valued cause or purpose, capacity to extract meaning from adverse situations, support from religion and spirituality, attention to health and good cardiovascular fitness and the capacity to rapidly recover from stress.

The literature on resilience-oriented interventions in treatment programmes are scarce but growing (Layne et al. 2007; Southwick and Charney 2012; Kent et al. 2011, Kent and Davis 2014).

With regard to asylum seekers and refugees, we propose the following definition of resilience: *the capacity to maintain or regain health and function ability despite past experiences and to endure stressors of the asylum procedure and all daily living hassles (post-migration living problems)*.

Trauma-Focused and Resilience-Focused Interventions

Epidemiological research shows high prevalence rates of psychopathology among asylum seekers and refugees (Porter and Haslam 2005: Fazel et al. 2005; Laban et al. 2005; Gerritsen et al. 2006; Ryan et al. 2008). Next to their traumatic experiences in their country of origin, they face many challenges, disappointments and adversities in the host country. Research among asylum seekers (Laban et al. 2004) has shown that the length of the asylum procedure and the related post-migration living problems had a higher risk for psychopathology compared to the risk of the traumatic experiences in the past. In both asylum seekers and refugees, the acculturation process, intergenerational difference in this process, language problems, discrimination, financial problems, worries about the family back home, lack of a solid social network and in many cases unemployment are issues which all interfere with the treatment. In searching to find the most effective and suitable therapy, these day-to-day stressors cannot be neglected. The debate of what kind of treatment should be given to asylum seekers and refugees is still going on. Nickerson et al. (2011) observe two contrasting approaches, namely, trauma-focused therapy and multimodal intervention. They conclude that 'trauma-focused approaches may have some efficacy in treating PTSD in refugees, but limitations in the methodologies of studies caution against drawing definitive inferences'. In their recommendations for further studies, they emphasise the importance of recognising the context of treatment delivery in terms of ongoing threats, the feelings of grief, anger over past injuries and a myriad of psychosocial difficulties with the resettlement process.

Layne et al. (2007) discuss the implications for interventions of resilience-based theories and suggest that trauma- and resilience-focused interventions may complement one another. We support this vision, and in this chapter, we follow that line: in a resilience-focused treatment programme, tailored to the individual and contextual situation and needs, trauma-focused specialised therapies can be used as a module, if needed, acceptable and possible.

The ROTS Model

The here presented model, the so-called 'resilience-oriented therapy and strategies' model (ROTS), brings together the concepts of vulnerability and stress and two aspects of resilience, i.e. personal strength (e.g. coping) and social support. The model was first described by De Jonghe et al. (1997). It recognises the multifactorial aetiology of psychopathology and puts emphasis on the importance of personal strength and potentials of recovery. To emphasise the importance of resilience in the model, we decided to change the name to resilience-oriented therapy and strategies (ROTS).

The model is an expansion of the well-known stress-vulnerability model developed by Zubin and Spring (1977), De Jong (2002) and Ingram and Luxton (2005). The hypothesis in this model is that health complaints will occur when the level of stress exceeds the (biological or psychological) capability of a patient. In the ROTS model, the factors social support and personal strength are added. Social support can be divided into several categories (see later). Personal strength implies all abilities to bear, cope, solve and live on after adverse life events. Both factors can eliminate or reduce the impact of stress and vulnerability and are considered resilience factors. Consequently, the ROTS model (Fig. 13.1) is based on the aforementioned concepts of vulnerability and stress as risk factors and personal strength and social support as resilience factors.

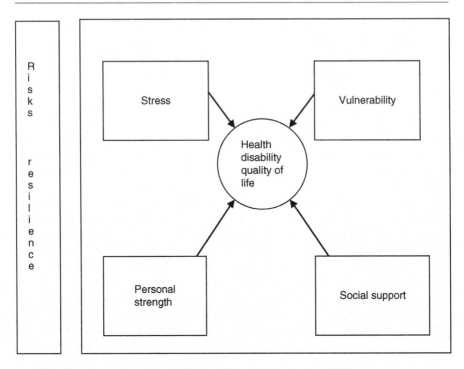

Fig. 13.1 Resilience-oriented model (Adapted from De Jonghe et al. 1997)

Vulnerability and strength are considered personal characteristics (internal factors), and stress and social support are considered ecosocial characteristics (external factors). It is assumed that a dynamic equilibrium between these factors is required to remain or become a healthy person. Health, disability and quality of life are affected by all four factors. The rectangle around the core model reflects the interactions between the factors. However, for the sake of practical use, we did not include more lines in the picture of the model. In our view, the model has some important advantages:

1. It emphasises the healing ability (resilience) of the patient, instead of focusing solely on stressors and complaints.
2. It helps in finding protective, supporting and strengthening factors (resources of resilience).
3. It challenges to investigate a broad scope of interventions tailored to the individual situation and characteristics of the patient.
4. It is very easy to explain to staff members as well as to patients and their families.
5. It gives a shared frame of reference.
6. It heavily involves the patient in his or her own healing and/or surviving process.

The fundamental issues in relation to formulate an adequate treatment plan are what can be done to lower the stress and vulnerability and what can be done to increase resilience (i.e. social support and personal strength).

The final goal is to improve health, to lower disability and to increase quality of life.

Resources of Resilience

The resources of resilience which are discussed below are based on findings in the literature and on our own clinical experience. The resources are often related to one another, but for the sake of clarity, we classify them according to the bio-psychosocial model: *biological* (physical exercise, understanding the body, relaxation, treatment of medical illnesses), *psychological* (positive emotions and humour, acceptance, cognitive flexibility, empowering self-esteem, active coping), *social* (social related-ness, reconnecting the family, creating social support), *cultural* (cultural identity, acculturation, language skills) and *religious/spiritual* resources.

Biological Resources

Understanding the Body

Educating/informing patients about the physical symptoms of and reactions to (traumatic) stress is an important first step towards control and reduction of fear, and its value has been recognised widely (Levine 1997, 2010; Van der Kolk 1996, 2006; Horowitz 2005; Rothschild 2000). Patients are offered an explanatory biological and psychological model of their symptoms to understand their own symptoms and reactions in order, subsequently, to get a grip on their own healing and resilience process. Although the effectiveness of this type of education is not yet studied (probably because it is always seen as complementary to the 'official' treatment), combining education and body-oriented activities in one programme appears to be essential to bring along changes in relatively fixed action patterns/routine ways of dealing with past and present stress.

Physical Exercise

Research has been done on the effectiveness of physical exercise training in the treatment of depression (Stathopoulou et al. 2006; Babyak et al. 2000; Blumenthal et al. 1999) and, to a lesser extent, of PTSD (Manger and Motta 2005). Blumenthal et al. (1999) reported significant reductions in depression scores among subjects treated with 16 weeks of aerobic exercise. The reduction was similar to sertraline or a combination of aerobic exercise and sertraline. Six months after the interventions, patients who had aerobic training had better results than patients from the other groups, especially the ones that continued to exercise at home (Babyak et al. 2000). In a meta-analysis with 11 studies, (Stathopoulou et al. 2006) concluded that physical exercise was a powerful intervention in depressive disorders. A preliminary study (Manger and Motta 2005) assessed the impact of a 12-session aerobic exercise programme on symptoms of PTSD, anxiety and depression and found positive results. Arnson et al. (2007) show that physical exercise in male patients with combat-related PTSD provides protection from future development of somatoform disorder. In an epidemiological cross-representative sample of Vietnamese living in the Mekong Delta region of Vietnam, Rees et al. (2012) found that high physical activity was significantly associated with low levels of psychological distress. Neurobiological research has shown that exercise induces expression of multiple genes known to be involved in plasticity and neurogenesis in the hippocampus (Cotman and Berchtold 2002; Elder et al. 2006).

In conclusion, educating patients on the importance of exercises, making training schedules for them and organising a guided exercise programme (by physiotherapists and movement therapists) are all means to increase positive effects of exercise on the process of resilience.

Stress Management/Relaxation

Bisson and Andrew (2007) found that stress management (SM) and trauma-focused cognitive behaviour therapy/exposure therapy (TFCBT) were equally effective in the treatment of PTSD. Stress management interventions vary widely in content and duration and may include progressive muscle relaxation (Jacobson 1965; Ehrenreich 1999). This type of SM is still widely used and considered to be a safe and accessible technique to reduce mental stress. As many traumatised patients are not aware of their bodily sensations, the technique is a nice start to connect the body and mind. Recently, meditation and mindfulness have been shown effective in reducing stress, as indicated by lowering of cortisol levels (Baer 2003). CBT mindfulness reduced the risk of a relapse of depression (Teasdale et al. 2000) and alleviated anxiety and depressive complaints (Santorelli 1992; Reibel et al. 2001). Mindfulness focuses on being completely in touch with and aware of the present moment, as well as taking a nonevaluative and non-judgmental approach to inner experiences. Although traumatised individuals tend to feel overwhelmed or deny an inner sense of themselves, elements of these techniques can readily be used: learning the difference between emotions and bodily sensations and between various emotions (anger, fear, sadness), learning techniques (breathing, movements, thoughts, etc.) on how to deal with stress, and experiencing that remembering the past does not inevitably result in overwhelming emotions. All these aspects increase the person's ability to cope with stress, which is an important element related to resilience.

Medication

Specific aspects of pharmacotherapeutic interventions in refugee populations are described (e.g. Kinzie and Friedman 2004). However, in daily practice, in the treatment of asylum seekers and refugees, it is not always easy to find effective medication for the individual patient. Co-morbidity, a wide variety of symptoms, high sensitivity to side effects, different genotypes and compliance problems are all factors to deal with (Kortmann and Oude Voshaar 1998; Han and Liu 2005). In order to lower the resistance to using medication and to improve intake, it might be helpful to discuss medication in the context of resilience. Special focus on the most wearing symptoms (e.g. sleeping problems, nightmares, pain) and the supportive (but often non-curative) character of the medicine is important, next to adequate monitoring and explaining the working mechanism and potential side effects.

Treatment of Nonpsychiatric Illnesses

Several studies show high rates of physical diseases and complaints in asylum seekers (Laban et al. 2008; Gerritsen et al. 2006). Chronic physical health problems have a negative impact on functioning and quality of life (Laban et al. 2008). The relationship between physical complaints and depression is well established (e.g. Simon et al. 1999). PTSD appears to be a particular risk factor for several chronic diseases (Weisberg et al. 2002). These diseases are a threat to the resilience process. In order to limit their impact, adequate diagnoses and treatment of these nonpsychiatric illnesses are important.

Psychological Resources

Positive Emotions and Humour

Negative emotions narrow one's momentary thought-action repertoire by preparing one to behave in a specific way (e.g. attack when angry, escape when afraid). In contrast, positive emotions (e.g. joy, interest, satisfaction, pride, love) broaden one's thought-action repertoire and improve coping mechanisms such as positive reappraisal and goal-directed problem-focused coping (Folkman and Moskowitz 2000; Frederickson 2001; Tugade and Fredrickson 2004). Positive emotions also broaden one's focus of attention in reliance to creativity, exploration and flexibility in thinking. In a study among refugees after an earthquake, Vazquez et al. (2005) interviewed 115 victims living in shelters. Surprisingly, they found that even such extraordinarily difficult circumstances, most of them revealed a consistent pattern of positive reactions and emotions. Also humour has been described as a source of resilience (Southwick et al. 2005). Humour appears to reduce the threatening nature of a situation through cognitive reappraisal (Juni and Katz 2001). Positive emotions as well as humour tend to decrease autonomic arousal. Mobbs et al. (2003) showed that humour engages a network of subcortical regions including the nucleus accumbens and the amygdalae, which plays a well-known role in fear and fear-related behaviour. Helping asylum seekers and refugees find distracting activities, areas of pride and episodes of joy might not only reduce stress but also improve coping. Examples of these activities within the reach of most mental health institutions are occupational, music and movement therapy. Otherwise, local opportunities (e.g. voluntary work, a local theatre project) can be used. Also, in all conversations with asylum seekers and refugees, the mental health worker should look for opportunities to enhance positive emotions: positive feedback, empowering remarks and something to laugh about. If children are around, this may assist in bringing about the desired emotions.

Cognitive Flexibility

Cognitive flexibility is exemplified by positive reframing, or reappraisal, and refers to the ability to reinterpret an adverse or negative event so as to find meaning and opportunity (Yehuda et al. 2006). A recent brain imaging study has shown that cognitive reappraisal brings about decreased activation of the amygdalae (Ochsner et al. 2002). Cognitive behaviour therapy (CBT) provides an evidence-based therapy for depression, and trauma-focused CBT has been proven effective in PTSD treatment in various populations (Bradley et al. 2005). A systematic review of treatments for PTSD among refugees and asylum seekers (Crumlish and O'Rourke (2010) concluded that no treatment was firmly supported, but there was evidence for narrative exposure therapy (NET) and CBT. And the study of d'Ardenne et al. (2007) show that CBT was also applicable in these specific populations when the therapy is done with the help of an interpreter.

However, in many cases, asylum seekers and refugees do not fulfil the criteria for these therapies (e.g. safe life situation/environment) or do not have the ability to tolerate exposure. Therefore, it is necessary to find other ways to increase cognitive flexibility and reappraisal related to events in the past as well as events in the present. In our experience, several methods can be applied: analysing daily stressors individually or sharing them in a group setting creates the opportunity to learn to look at events from different angles and to reflect on the attributional styles (e.g. to place the blame where it realistically belongs). Furthermore, learning to find words for the variety of emotions and discovering the relationships between emotions, thoughts and behaviours (the basis of CBT) can be taught in a group and in an individual treatment setting. Patients can be asked to work out examples in their daily life and subsequently train themselves to change unhealthy patterns. A daily exercise is to distract yourself from negative thoughts by thinking or doing something else. All these activities are resilience oriented: they emphasise helping thoughts and behaviour.

Empowering Self-Esteem

Esteem needs of every human being are, for instance, to achieve, be competent and gain approval and recognition (Maslow 1954). Self-esteem has been defined as 'The experience of being capable of meeting life's challenges and being worthy of happiness' (Reasoner 2004). Many people that are suffering from a psychiatric disorder have a low self-esteem (Silverstone and Salsali 2003). The authors suggest that there is a vicious circle: low esteem increases the risk of a psychiatric disorder and a disorder leads to a low self-esteem. Asylum seekers and refugees are at risk for a low self-esteem. Carballo et al. (2004) found in a study among Bosnian war survivors that there was an 'overwhelming loss of perceived power and self-esteem'. Over 25 % of displaced people, for example, said they no longer felt they were able to play a useful role; even in non-displaced populations, approximately 11 % of those interviewed said that they had lost their sense of worth. The cumulative effect of the stressors during the asylum procedure may constitute an important risk for a low self-esteem. These experiences often lead to cognitive appraisals such as 'I am not worthwhile', etc. An overall positive therapeutic attitude is as important as more specific activities directed towards the improvement of self-esteem. Being taken seriously, being welcome in therapy, receiving positive feedback by an individual therapist or a team and being embedded in a coherent, reliable, predictable interaction can all lead to corrective emotional experiences during which self-esteem can be restored and improved. More specific treatment interventions can be working with patients to search for and set new (achievable) goals, to stop activities that decrease self-esteem, to recognise and change cognitions which undermine self-esteem (guilt, shame), to learn to be creative, to learn new things (e.g. a language, playing music), to be proud of what can be achieved in difficult situations, to find things to do for other people within or outside the family, to ask for feedback and to learn how to receive positive and negative feedback, to be assertive, to learn from experiences (instead of blaming oneself), etc. Also in the trauma-focused therapy sessions, every opportunity should be used to emphasise strength and adequate coping to correct, restore and increase self-esteem.

Coping

Coping has been defined as conscious attempts to manage internal or external stressors (Folkman et al. 1986). It can be divided into active, approach-based coping (resolving or conquering the stressor) and passive, avoidance-based coping (Moos 1995). The way an individual copes with stress is thought to mediate the possible negative influence of stress on physical and mental health. In general, resilient individuals have been described as using active coping mechanisms when dealing with stressful life situations (LeDoux and Gorman 2001). Possibly, if circumstances cannot be changed, a more passive coping style might be more adequate and healthy. Consequently, the most important ability is to be able to vary in coping styles, depending on the situation. Asylum seekers and refugees have to cope with many stressors. Working on resilience is working on coping. The difference between the two concepts is that the starting point in the resilience-oriented approach is one's motivation, drive and personal strength rather than the more technical behaviour in the coping-oriented approach. This approach is very much in line with the documents of many survivors of adverse and horrible events. Frankl (1959) and Lindhout and Corbett (2013) learned that having a purpose in life literally keeps us alive. The resilience-oriented approach involves trying to create the conditions in which a more adequate coping can emerge and, subsequently, discussing with the patient which techniques can be used that fit the circumstances and the personal style.

Social Resources

Social Relatedness/Connectedness to the Family

Family resilience has been examined in various studies (e.g. Sossou et al. 2008). According to Walsh (2007, 2012), the resilience of families has a particular dynamic that is different from the combined resilience of separate individuals. She developed a 'family resilience framework' consisting of three domains: *family beliefs* (the extent in which a common view of reality exists), *organisational patterns* (the manner in which the family is organised) and *communication/problem solving* (the ways of communication and searching for solutions to problems). Among asylum seekers and refugees' families, usually, problems in more than one of these domains are observed. Analysing the above-mentioned domains with the help of the ROTS model leads to questions as: *Stress*: what are the problems and how are these assessed by each member of the family? *Vulnerability*: what should be the focus to avoid problems becoming bigger? *Social support*: who assists in solving the problems, which members of the family receive such support and which not? *Strength*: how does the family try to solve the problems; what helped in the past; who helps whom in the family, what makes the family a family and what are they proud of as a family? Such an analysis also makes clear in what way a family is organised and embedded in its environment (asylum seeker centre, neighbourhood, countrymen, church, school, assistance, etc.). In resilience-oriented systemic family therapy, the resilience potential of each individual member and of the family as a whole is continuously monitored, and strengthening and healing mechanisms and activities are stimulated. In our experience, the model offers a good opening to discuss or observe all domains of Walsh's framework. The model leaves room for including the complex social-societal context of the families. It can be tempting to forget this context and concentrate solely on solutions within the family; however, the 'outside world' can yield a lot of stress, which one cannot avoid. Talking about, for instance, life in the asylum seeker centre, a negative decision in the asylum procedure, discrimination or lack of money should not be seen as an interruption of the actual therapy. Family therapy with this group is often a search, in which one should take into account unexpected and sometimes unknown stressors. The joint learning on how to deal with these stressors can make this family grow.

Social Support

The feeling of belongingness, being affiliated with others and being accepted and loved is one of people's basic needs (Maslow 1954; Sandler 2001). Asylum seekers and refugees have lost many of their social contacts, and building up a new social network is difficult, for example, due to frequent moves, lack of money, language problems and cultural problems. Extensive research has been done on the influence of social support on health. The division in emotional, practical, informational and 'esteem' support (Schwarzer and Leppin 1999) is often used and makes sense in practice. Positive relations have been found in the general population (e.g. Schwarzer and Leppin 1999; Southwick et al. 2005) as well as in refugee populations (Gorst-Unsworth and Goldenberg 1998; Ahern et al. 2004; Stewart et al. 2011). The lack of social support, on the other hand, increases the chance of psychiatric problems (Southwick et al. 2005). In neurobiological research (Heinrichs et al. 2003), it appears that social support interacts with oxytocin (a neuropeptide affecting attachment) in lowering the cortisol levels and decreasing the response to psychological stress. Interventions should start with an analysis of the extent and nature of social support. Many patients only have a vague idea about their own wishes with regard to social support; they do not know what type of support they can get from whom and where they can access this particular type. They therefore ask or expect a particular type of support from the wrong people (e.g. practical support from a psychiatrist and emotional support from a traumatised spouse). Some patients feel ashamed to ask for help. They must learn that even though one's own strength is always necessary, asking for support is not shameful and receiving support sometimes even is right. Other patients ask for help in an inadequate manner. Here also cultural aspects can play a role: in some cultures, you can only receive support if you act like you are completely powerless and treat the other as being superior. In the Netherlands, such an attitude will only cause irritations; your chances of being supported are larger if you tell someone what you have already tried yourself and what you would require the other to do. In conclusion, there are all sorts of possibilities for increasing (a chance on better) social support, and this is of great importance with regard to resilience.

Meaningful Activities

One of the most important risk factors for a psychiatric illness among asylum seekers is worrying about not having work (Laban et al. 2005). In an earlier study among refugees and native Canadians, Beiser et al. (1993) found a significant relationship between unemployment and depression. The same connection was also found later in a longitudinal study (Beiser and Hou 2001), in which depression followed unemployment, especially among men. Unfortunately, in many countries, entering the labour market is not easy for many refugees. The unemployment rates are high and discrimination seems to be part of the problem (Nievers and Andriessen 2010). Cooperative programmes of governments, businesses and refugees agencies are needed. Asylum seekers in the Netherlands can only work a limited number of weeks per year, and because of many practical problems or limitations arising from psychological problems, only a few succeed to do that. Doing volunteer work is possible for asylum seekers; however, volunteering is an unknown phenomenon among many of them. Explanation and cooperation are thus necessary. Many mental healthcare institutions offer all sorts of activity therapy and can refer to Day Activity Centres (DAC). The value of participation in such activities should not be underestimated. People feel better being able to perform, they come in contact with others, they simply are in another environment, etc. The main purpose of this type of activity is breaking through the feelings of powerlessness and isolation and derives meaning from the activities. However, it is clear that in the end, full participation in the job market should follow on these activities. Unfortunately, there are often many obstacles to overcome and drop out, and medicalisation of social problems is a real threat.

Religious/Spiritual Resources

Religion as well as spirituality concerns feelings, thoughts with regard to the meaning of life and connectedness to a higher power or a higher dimension (Latin: *religare* means 'to connect'). The word religion usually points to a more rigid, organised form of spirituality. Because the term spirituality is more difficult to define, scientific research has focused nearly exclusively on religion. The interest in the relation between religion and health has increased tremendously over the last decades, with regard to the prevention, the coping with as well as the recovering from (physical and psychological) illnesses. Review articles (e.g. Harrison et al. 2001) show that religion in general has a positive influence on all these aspects. Research has also been done in the Netherlands on this topic (Pieper and Van Uden 2005). However, little research is available on the possible protective and supportive role of religion for asylum seekers/refugees. Schweitzer et al. (2007) examined coping and resilience in a small group (13) of Sudanese refugees and found that besides social support, religion was the most important source of resilience. This finding was confirmed in a qualitative study among 23 Sudanese refugees in Australia (Khawaja et al. 2008). In our study among almost 300 Iraqi asylum seekers, we found that 77.6 % of them considered religion to be moderately to very important (not published data). Compared to the period before the flight, 63.9 % of respondents trusted in God/Allah in an equal manner and 29.6 % had higher trust. Engelhard and Goorts (2005) interviewed 120 asylum seekers and refugees. One third of the respondents saw their problems as a test of God/Allah, and half considered God/Allah the originator of their problems. Most respondents from both groups however mentioned that God/Allah had been a source of support and comfort. The authors did not find a difference between Christians and Muslims. Some respondents identified themselves with persons described in holy texts, like the figure of Job in the Bible.

In the mental health practice for asylum seekers and refugees, it makes sense to talk about religion in a standardised way, as part of the diagnostic process as well as during treatment. Most of them come from countries where religion is an integral part of life, and in general, they think it is normal to be asked questions about this subject. In many ways, religion can play a role in their life. For instance, religion can be the cause of their flight (e.g. Christians from Iraq), can strongly influence their lifestyle (food habits, manners, clothing), can be a 'troublemaker' (e.g. when a patient continuously wonders whether God/Allah is for or against him/her), can be an explanation for their feeling unwell (break of taboos, having been disobedient, etc.), can play a role in mutual conflicts and can contribute to getting into contact with new people or not. In connection to resilience, religion can be considered an interpretation frame, it can strengthen one's 'connection to life' (and become for instance a protective factor against suicide), it can give the feeling to be part of a greater union and it can give emotional support and also social support of co-religionists and communities. In short, religion can be an important source of resilience, and therefore, it is imperative to pay attention to it continuously.

Cultural Resources

Even though the literature about culture and psychiatry has grown quickly over the last decades, there are only a few publications about culture as a resource for resilience in patients (Peddle 2007; Tummala-Narra 2007). The focus of culture and psychiatry is mainly on the necessity of knowing the elements of the culture of the patient, recognising culture-specific syndromes, paying attention to differing explanations for being ill, and of being able to take into account cultural elements during contacts and conversations in the diagnostic and in the treatment phase. These are all very relevant points of attention; however, it would be wrong to disregard culture as a source of resilience. Tummala-Narra (2007) identified a number of important points concerning trauma and resilience in a multicultural context: (1) resilience is not an individual process but always takes shape in interaction with the family and wider environment, especially in group-oriented cultures; (2) recovery of trauma means among other things that you redefine the image you have of yourself; this is also true for the acculturation process; thus, it concerns in fact a double-identity adaptation; (3) fear related to trauma can be increased through negative confrontations in the guest country (discrimination, lack of understanding, hostility); and (4) many people come to a new country with the hope of a better life. Even though some expectations need to be adjusted, many people remain hopeful. This can be a source of resilience, especially if this hope is being shared with others. (5) Artistic expressions (e.g. writing, painting, making music) can be important in the recovery phase as well as in the acculturation process, to bridge the gap between 'then and now' and 'there and here'. Dutch studies (Kamperman et al. 2005; Knipscheer and Kleber 2007) show that the right balance between holding on to their own culture and opening up to and participating in the new culture gives the best chance on a good health. In conclusion, attention paid to the process of acculturation and identity is of large interest to the treatment, especially if one looks for cultural aspects (values, norms, customs, skills, etc.) that can be a source of resilience for the patients and their families. One of the ways to discover these aspects is by discussing the following topics:

- Meaning of the trauma in the cultural/social context of then and now
- Political reality/development in comparison to the individual story of the patient
- Looking for aspects of the cultural identity that increase coping (e.g. music) and self-esteem
- Possibilities for participation in (e.g. refugee) organisations
- Meaning of and possibilities for cultural celebrations in the family/group
- Which rituals, stories and metaphors, proverbs with regard to resilience are important
- Importance of integration with regard to health

The forms in which these subjects can be discussed can differ. Using the Cultural Formulation of Diagnosis and the Cultural Interview (Rohlof et al. 2002; Groen 2008; APA 2013) is a good start. Further exploration can take place in individual sessions, but preferably also in group discussions. Exchange of cultural customs, norms, values, etc. may help someone to get to know his/her own culture better and may increase one's understanding of the extent to which one is different. Only then can someone reflect on which elements one would like to keep and which aspects can help him/her in the present life. A lot depends also on the hospitality of the new country and which new cultural resources someone is offered there.

Conclusion

The problems of asylum seekers and refugees are numerous, and a high percentage has or develops physical and mental health problems. They perceive serious disabilities and a low quality of life. Treatment possibilities are limited due to the experienced complex trauma, the ongoing stress and the existence of co-morbidity of stress-related psychiatric disorders. Notwithstanding these limitations, however, treatment is possible. We described a resilience-oriented diagnostic and treatment model in which the concepts of stress, vulnerability and resilience (distinguished in personal strength and social support) are incorporated. In our opinion, this model is very well applicable in all treatment modalities with asylum seekers and refugees. For humanitarian reasons, this group needs our attention, and there is no professional reason to deny this group from mental healthcare. So all financial and logistic facilities should be created and ensured to enable asylum seekers and refugees to get the help they often so desperately need.

References

Ahern J, Galea S, Fernandez WG, Koci B, Waldman R, Vlahov D (2004) Gender, social support, and posttraumatic stress in postwar Kosovo. J Nerv Ment Dis 192:762–770

American Psychiatric Association (2013) Diagnostic and statistical manual of mental disorders, 5th edn. DSM-5, Arlington

d'Ardenne P, Ruaro L, Cestari L, Fakhoury W, Priebe S (2007) Does interpreter-mediated CBT with traumatized refugee people work ? A comparison of patient outcomes in East London. Behav Cogn Psychother 35:293–301

Arnson Y, Amital D, Fostick L, Silberman A, Polliack ML, Zohar J, Rubinow A, Amital H (2007) Physical activity protects male patients with post-traumatic stress disorder from developing severe fibromyalgia. Clin Exp Rheumatol 25(4):529–533

Babyak M, Blumenthal JA, Herman S (2000) Exercise treatment for major depression: maintenance of therapeutic benefit at 10 months. Psychosom Med 62:633–638

Baer R (2003) Mindfulness training as a clinical intervention: a conceptual and empirical review. Clin Psychol Sci Pract 10(2):125–142

Beiser M, Hou F (2001) Language acquisition, unemployment and depressive disorder among Southeast Asian refugees: a 10-year study. Soc Sci Med 53:1321–1334

Beiser M, Johnson PJ, Turner RJ (1993) Unemployment, underemployment and depressive affect among Southeast Asian refugees. Psychol Med 23:731–743

Bisson J, Andrew M (2007) Psychological treatment of post-traumatic stress disorder (PTSD). Cochrane Database Syst Rev.;(3):CD003388

Blumenthal JA, Baybak MA, Moore KA, Craighead WE, Herman S et al (1999) Effects of exercise training on older patients with major depression. Arch Intern Med 159:2349–2356

Bonanno S (2004) Loss, trauma, and human resilience; have we underestimated the human capacity to thrive after extremely aversive events? Am Psychol 59:20–28

Bradley R, Greene J, Russ E (2005) A multidimensional meta-analysis of psychotherapy for PTSD. Am J Psychiatry 162:214–227

Carballo M, Smajkic A, Zeric D, Dzidowska M, Gebre-Medhin J, van Halem J (2004) Mental health and coping in a war situation: the case of Bosnia and Herzegovina. J Biosoc Sci 36:463–477

Charney DS (2004) Psychobiological mechanisms of resilience and vulnerability: implications for successful adaption to extreme stress. Am J Psychiatry 161:195–216

Cotman CW, Berchtold MC (2002) Exercise: a behavioural intervention to enhance brain and plasticity. Trends Neurosci 25:295–301

Crumlish N, O'Rourke K (2010) A systematic review of treatment for PTSD among refugees and asylum seekers. J Nerv Ment Dis 198:237–251

de Jonghe F, Dekker J, Goris C (1997) Steun, stress, kracht en kwetsbaarheid in de psychiatrie. Van Gorcum, Assen

Ehrenreich JH (1999) Coping with disaster: a guidebook to psychosocial intervention. http://www.mhwwb.org/contents.htm

Elder GA, de Gasperi R, Gama Sosa MA (2006) Research update: neurogenesis in adult brain and neuropsychiatric disorders. Mt Sinai J Med 73:931–940

Engelhard D, Goorts I (2005) God will take care of me. Religious coping among refugees with health problems (in Dutch: God zal voor mij zorgen. Religieuze coping van vluchtelingen met gezondheidsproblemen). Pharos, Utrecht

Fazel M, Wheeler J, Danesh J (2005) Prevalence of serious mental disorder in 7000 refugees resettled in western countries: a systematic review. Lancet 365:1309–1314

Feder A, Charney D, Collins K (2011) Neurobiology of resilience. In: Southwick SM, Litz BT, Charney D, Friedman MJ (eds) Resilience and mental health: challenges across the lifespan. Cambridge University Press, Cambridge

Folkman S, Moskowitz JT (2000) Positive affect and the other side of coping. Am Psychol 6:647–654

Folkman S, Lazarus RS, Dunkel-Schetter C, DeLongis A, Gruen RJ (1986) Dynamics of a stressful encounter: cognitive appraisal, coping, and encounter outcomes. J Pers Soc Psychol 3:571–579

Frankl V (1959) Man's search for meaning. Pocket books, New York

Fredrickson BL (2001) The role of positive emotions in positive psychology: the broaden-and-build theory of positive emotions. Am Psychol 56:218–226

Gerritsen AA, Bramsen I, Devillé W, van Willigen LH, Hovens JE, van der Ploeg HM (2006) Physical and mental health of Afghan, Iranian and Somali asylum seekers and refugees living in the Netherlands. Soc Psychiatry Psychiatr Epidemiol 41:18–26

Gorst-Unsworth C, Goldenberg E (1998) Psychological sequelae of torture and organized violence suffered by refugees from Iraq: trauma-related factors compared with social factors in exile. Br J Psychiatry 172:90–94

Groen SPN (2008) A new version of the cultural interview. Application and evaluation of a questionnaire for cultural sensitive diagnostics in mental health care. Cultuur, Migratie en Gezondheid. 5:96–103

Han E, Liu GG (2005) Racial disparities in prescription drug use for mental illness among population in US. Ment Health Policy Econ 8:131–143

Harrison MO, Koenig HG, Hays JC, Eme-Akwari AG, Pargament KI (2001) The epidemiology of religious coping: a review of recent literature. Int Rev Psychiatry 13:86–93

Heinrichs M, Baumgartner T, Kirshbaum C, Ehlert U (2003) Social support and oxytocin interact to suppress cortical and subjective responses to psychological stress. Biol Psychiatry 54:1389–1398

Horowitz MJ (2005) Treatment of stress response syndromes. American Psychiatric Publishing, Washington, DC

Ingram RE, Luxton DD (2005) Vulnerability-stress models. In: Hankin BL, Abela JRZ (eds) Development of psychopathology: a vulnerability stress perspective. Sage, New York

Jacobson E (1965) Progressive relaxation; a physiological and clinical muscular states. Chicago Press, Chicago

Jong de JTVM (2002) Public mental health, traumatic stress and human rights violations in low-income countries: a culturally, appropriate model in times of conflict, disaster and peace. In: Jong de JTVM (ed) Trauma, war, and violence: public mental health in socio-cultural context. Kluwer Academic Plenum Publishers, New York

Juni S, Katz B (2001) Self-effacing wit as a response to oppression: dynamics in ethnic humor. J Gen Psychol 128:119–142

Kamperman AM, Komproe YH, Jong JTVM de (2005) The relationship between cultural adaptation and mental health in first generation migrants. In: AM Kamperman (ed) Deconstructing ethnic differences in mental health of Surinamese, Moroccan and Turkish migrants in The Netherlands. PhD thesis, Vrije Universiteit Amsterdam

Kent M, Davis MC, Reich JW (2014) The resilience handbook: apporaches to stress and trauma. Routledge, New York

Kent M, Davis MC (2014) Resilience training for action and agency to stress and trauma; becoming the hero of your life. In: Kent M, Davis MC, Reich JW (eds) The resilience handbook; approaches to stress and trauma. Routledge, New York, pp 227–244

Kent M, Davis MC, Stark SL, Stewart LA (2011) A resilience-oriented treatment for post traumatic stress disorder: results of a preliminary randomized clinical trial. J Trauma Stress 24:591–595

Khawaja NG, White KM, Schweitzer R, Greenslade JH (2008) Difficulties and coping strategies of Sudanese refugees: a qualitative approach. Transcult Psychiatry 45:489–512

Kinzie D, Friedman MJ (2004) Psychopharmacology for refugees and asylum seeker patients. In: Wilson JP, Drozdek B (eds) Broken spirits: the treatment of traumatized asylum seekers, refugees, war and torture victims. Brunner-Routledge, New York

Knipscheer JW, Kleber RJ (2007) Acculturation and mental health among Ghanaians in the Netherlands. Int J Soc Psychiatry 53:369–383

Kortmann FAM, Oude Voshaar RC (1998) Aspects of pharmacotherapy in ethnic minorities (in Dutch, summary in English). Tijdschr Psychiatr 3:143–155

Laban CJ, Gernaat HBPE, Komproe IH, Schreuders GA, De Jong JTVM (2004) Impact of a long asylum procedure on the prevalence of psychiatric disorders in Iraqi asylum seekers in the Netherlands. J Nerv Ment Dis 192:843–852

Laban CJ, Gernaat HBPE, Komproe IH, Van Tweel I, De Jong JTVM (2005) Post migration living problems and common psychiatric disorders in Iraqi asylum seekers in the Netherlands. J Nerv Ment Dis 193:825–832

Laban CJ, Komproe IH, Gernaat HBPE, De Jong JTVM (2008) Impact of a long asylum procedure on quality of life, disability and physical health in Iraqi asylum seekers in the Netherlands. Soc Psychiatry Psychiatr Epidemiol 43:507–515

Layne CM, Warren JS, Watson PJ, Shalev AY (2007) Risk, vulnerability, resistance, and resilience toward and integrative conceptualization of posttraumatic adaptation. In: Friedman MJ, Keane TM, Resick PA (eds) Handbook of PTSD: science and practice. Guilford Press, New York, pp 497–520

LeDoux JE, Gorman JM (2001) A call to action: overcoming anxiety through active coping. Am J Psychiatry 158:1953–1955

Levine P (1997) Waking the tiger; healing trauma. North Atlantic Books, Berkeley

Levine P (2010) In an unspoken voice. North Atlantic Books, Berkeley

Lindhout A, Corbett S (2013) A house in the sky. Scribner, New York

Luthar SS, Cicchetti D, Becker B (2000) The construct of resilience: a critical evaluation and guidelines for future work. Child Dev 3:543–562

Manger TA, Motta RW (2005) The impact of an exercise program on posttraumatic stress disorder, anxiety, and depression. Int J Emerg Ment Health 7(1):49–57

Maslow AH (1954) Motivation and personality. Harper, New York

Masten A, Best K, Garmezy N (1990) Resilience and development: contributions from the study of children who overcome adversity. Dev Psychopathol 2:425–444

Mobbs D, Greicius MD, Abdel-Azim E, Menon V, Reiss AL (2003) Humor modulates the meso-limbic reward centers. Neuron 40:1041–1048

Moos RH (1995) Development and application of new measures of life stressors, social resources, and coping responses. Eur J Psychol Assess 11:1–13

Nickerson A, Bryant RA, Silove D, Steel Z (2011) A critical review of psychological treatments of posttraumatic stress disorder in refugees. Clin Psychol Rev 31:399–417

Nievers E, Andriessen I (2010) Discrimination monitor 2010: non-western migrants on the Dutch labour market. The Netherlands Institute for Social research. The Hague

Ochsner KN, Bunge SA, Gross JJ, Gabrieli JD (2002) Rethinking feelings: an fMRI study of the cognitive regulation of emotion. J Cogn Neurosci 14:1215–1229

Ozbay F, Johnson DC, Dimouglas E, Morgan CA, Charney D, Southwick S (2007) Social support and resilience to stress: from neurobiology to clinical practice. Psychiatry 4:35–40

Peddle N (2007) Assessing trauma impact, recovery and resiliency in refugees of war. J Aggress Maltreat Trauma 14:185–204

Pieper JZT, van Uden MHF (2005) Religion and coping in mental health care. Rodopi, Amsterdam

Porter M, Haslam N (2005) Predisplacement and postdisplacement factors associated with mental health of refugees and internally displaced persons: a meta-analysis. JAMA 294(5):602–612

Reasoner R (2004) The true meaning of self-esteem. NASE (National Association for Self-Esteem), Fulton, http://www.self-esteem-nase.org/whatisselfesteem.shtml

Rees S, Silove D, Chey T, Steel Z, Bauman A, Phan T (2012) Physical activity and psychological distress amongst Vietnamese living in the Mekong Delta. Aust NZ J Psychiatry 46:966–971

Reibel D, Greeson J, Brainard G, Rosenzweig S (2001) Mindfulness-based stress reduction and health-related quality of life in a heterogeneous patient population. Gen Hosp Psychiatry 23:183–192

Rohlof H, Loevy N, Sassen L, Helmich S (2002) Het culturele interview, Nederlandse versie. In: Borra R, van Dijk R, Rohlof H (eds) Cultuur, classificatie en diagnose, cultuursensitief werken met de DSM IV. Bohn Stafleu Van Loghum, Houten

Rothschild B (2000) The body remembers. The psychophysiology of trauma and trauma treatment. W.W. Norton & Company, New York, pp 95–96

Rutter ME (1987) Psychosocial resilience and protective mechanisms. Am J Orthopsychiatry 67:316–331

Rutter M (2006) Implications of resilience concepts for scientific understanding. Ann N Y Acad Sci 1094:1–12

Ryan DA, Benson CA, Dooley BA (2008) Psychological distress and the asylum process a longitudinal study of forced migrants in Ireland. J Nerv Ment Dis 196:37–45

Sandler I (2001) Quality and ecology of adversity as common mechanism of risk and resilience. Am J Community Psychol 29:19–55

Santorelli SF (1992) Effectiveness of a meditation-based stress reduction program in the treatment of anxiety disorders. Am J Psychiatry 149:936–943

Schwarzer R, Leppin A (1999) Social support and health: a theoretical and empirical overview. J Soc Pers Relatsh 8:99–127

Schweitzer R, Greenslade J, Kagee A (2007) Coping and resilience in refugees from the Sudan: a narrative account. Aust NZ J Psychiatry 41:282–288

Silverstone PH, Salsali M (2003) Low self-esteem and psychiatric patients: part 1 – the relationship between low self-esteem and psychiatric diagnosis. Ann Gen Hosp Psychiatr. 2.2 [open access]. http://www.general-hospital-psychiatry.com/content/2/1/2

Simon GE, VonKorff M, Piccinelli M, Fullerton C, Ormel J (1999) An international study of the relationship between somatic symptoms and depression. N Engl J Med 341(18):1329–1335

Sossou MA, Craig CD, Ogren H, Schnak M (2008) A qualitative study of resilience factors of Bosnia refugee women resettled in the southern United States. J Ethn Cult Divers Soc Work 17(4):365–385

Southwick SM, Charney DS (2012) Resilience: the science of mastering life's greatest challenges. Cambridge Univ. Press, New York

Southwick SM, Vythilingam M, Charney DS (2005) The psychobiology and resilience to stress: implications for prevention and treatment. Annu Rev Clin Psychol 1:255–291

Southwick SM, Litz BT, Charney D, Friedman MJ (eds) (2011) Resilience and mental health: challenges across the lifespan. Cambridge Univ. Press, New York

Stathopoulou G, Powers MB, Berry AC, Smits JAJ, Otto MW (2006) Exercise Interventions for Mental Health: A Quantitative and Qualitative Review. Clin Psychol Sci Pract 13:179–193

Stewart M, Simich L, Beiser M, Makumbe K, Makwarimba E, Shizha E (2011) Impacts of a social support intervention for Somali and Sudanese refugees in Canada. Ethn Inequal Health Soc Care 4:186–199

Teasdale JD, Segal ZV, Williams JMG et al (2000) Prevention of relapse/recurrence in major depression by mindfulness-based cognitive therapy. J Consult Clin Psychol 68:615–623

Tugade MM, Fredrickson BL (2004) Resilient individuals use positive emotions to bounce back from negative emotional experiences. J Pers Soc Psychol 2:320–333

Tummala-Narra P (2007) Conceptualizing trauma and resilience across divers contexts: a multicultural perspective. In: Harvey MR, Tummala-Narra P (eds) Sources and expressions of resiliency in trauma survivors. Haworth Maltreatment and Trauma Press, New York

van der Kolk BA (1996) The body keeps the score: approaches to psychobiology of post traumatic stress disorder. In: van der Kolk BA, McFarlane A, Weisaeth L (eds) Traumatic stress: the effects of overwhelming experience of mind, body and society. The Guilford Press, New York

van der Kolk BA (2006) Clinical implications of neuroscience research in PTSD. Ann N Y Acad Sci 1071:277–293

Vazquez C, Cervellon P, Perez-Sales P, Vidales D, Gaborit M (2005) Positive emotions in earthquake survivors in El Salvador (2001). Anxiety Disord 19:313–328

Walsh F (2007) Traumatic loss and major disasters: strengthening family and community resilience. Fam Process 46:207–227

Walsh F (2012) Family resilience; Strengths forged through adversity. In : Walsh F (ed.) Normal Family Processes (4th ed. pp. 399–427), New York, Guilford Press

Weisberg RB, Bruce SE, Machan JT, Kessler RC, Culpepper L, Keller MB (2002) Nonpsychiatric illness among primary care patients with trauma histories and posttraumatic stress disorder. Psychiatr Serv 53:848–854

Yehuda R, Flory JD, Southwick S, Charney DS (2006) Developing an agenda for translational studies of resilience and vulnerability following trauma exposure. Ann N Y Acad Sci 1071:379–396

Zubin J, Spring B (1977) Vulnerability: a new view of schizophrenia. J Abnorm Psychol 86:103–126

Traumatised Immigrants in an Outpatient Clinic: An Experience-Based Report

14

Johanna Winkler

Introduction

The psychiatric outpatient clinic (PIA) treats patients with serious psychiatric disturbances and for whom appropriate treatment is not otherwise available at psychiatric or psychotherapy outpatient clinics. This applies to a specific catalogue of indications of particularly serious psychiatric disorders which show chronic progression. Such treatment takes place very frequently and is carried out by a multiprofessional team (Memorandum of the BDK – German Federal Conference of Psychiatric Hospital Directors 2011).

In Germany, there are now more than 450 such psychiatric outpatient clinics. In 2008, an average of 32.5 % of the patients who were treated at these PIAs had a background of migration (Schouler-Ocak et al. 2010); in the same year, a total of 15,566 million people with a migration background were living in Germany, representing just under 19 % of the total population (Federal Statistical Office 2008). The proportion of people with a background of migration receiving treatment at the PIAs is thus above average.

The PIA of Charité University Psychiatric Clinic at St. Hedwig Hospital in Berlin offers several areas of treatment. The catchment area of the hospital encompasses the districts of Wedding and Tiergarten in central Berlin, home to an especially high number of people with experiences of migration. In 2013, the percentages of people with a background of migration were between 30.8 and 57.6 %, depending on the subdistrict (Migration and Health in the District of Central Berlin 2011).

J. Winkler
Department of Psychiatry and Psychotherapy of the Charité,
St. Hedwig Hospital, Berlin, Germany
e-mail: Johanna.winkler@charite.de

The Concept of the Psychiatric Outpatient Clinic (PIA)

On the basis of statutory provisions in the German Social Security Code (Book V, §118), the PIAs fulfil a specific mandate to provide care for those with a mental illness who, because of the nature, severity or duration of their illness, require treatment services which are close to those provided in hospitals. Such treatment is for patients who are not adequately catered for by any of the German 'vertragsärztliche' ambulatory medical care services (Koch-Stoecker 2011).

As part of the concept of intercultural openness at the PIA at Charité University Psychiatric Clinic at St. Hedwig Hospital, all the employees work with patients with a migration background as part of their role as reference therapist. Regular intervision, case discussions with other therapists, team meetings and supervision in individual cases all ensure that the therapeutic treatment is regularly reviewed, that problematic areas are named and shed light upon and that future courses of action are clarified. Such teamwork offers an opportunity for the discussion of social aspects and elements which are specific to certain cultures or to migration as a whole. Every patient, regardless of origin or nationality, is looked after by two members of the multi-professional team, one physician and at least one other healthcare professional. This is in order to prevent discontinuity in the therapeutic relationship when one of them is absent due to annual leave or illness. Each patient therefore has two points of reference who regularly exchange information and impressions about the current situation and cooperate closely in crisis situations – an example of interprofessional teamwork (Schouler-Ocak 2000) in action!

When engaging in an intercultural treatment process, therapists cannot be expected to speak all the languages of their patients or to know the migration-specific, disease-specific and cultural aspects of each of their patients. However, they should possess knowledge and understanding of intercultural competence so as not to slip into stereotyped thinking (Schouler-Ocak 2000).

Patients with a Migration Background in Psychiatric Outpatient Institutions

A nationally representative survey, carried out in 2008 on the utilisation of PIA services by patients with a migration background, found, as mentioned above, that this population group represented 32.5 % of PIA patients, a larger percentage than their representation in the overall German population. Additionally, on average, they were younger and had more children than patients without a migration background. Neurotic, stress-related and somatoform disorders were diagnosed with a significantly higher frequency among patients with a background of migration than among those without such a background (Schouler-Ocak et al. 2010).

In 2012, Berlin had around 3.38 million inhabitants, of whom 12,084 had an uncertain residential status. Of these, 2,643 had applied for asylum and were still waiting for the official decision about their desire, and 9,441 were required to leave the country – for example, due to the fact that their applications for asylum were already rejected officially. Together, they accounted for approximately 0.36 % of the population of Berlin (Federal Statistical Office 2012). Nationwide, 127,023 asylum applications were made in Germany in 2013, 24.9 % of which were recognised due to various legal requirements, 38.5 % of which were rejected and 36.7 % of which were decided (negatively) upon on the basis of formal criteria – such as Dublin II order – without a hearing.

Around three-quarters of asylum seekers thus remained in unsatisfactory, precarious living conditions and faced a lack of participation in social life if they do not leave the country (Federal Statistical Office 2012; Federal Office for Migration and Refugees 2014). This social insecurity increases the vulnerability and morbidity of people with a migration background. Heeren et al. (2014) found post-traumatic stress disorder (PTSD) rates of 41.4 % and 54.0 % among asylum seekers and refugees, respectively, and symptoms of anxiety and depression in 84.6 % and 63.1 % of the same groups. They concluded that mental health is significantly associated with residency status (Heeren et al. 2014). In other studies, high rates of mental disorders have been described among refugees, in particular PTSD, found in 20–40 % of the refugees, and comorbid disorders which often remain undiagnosed (von Lersner et al. 2008; Gierlichs 2003). Observations made in our PIA confirm these results.

Therapeutic Approach to Treating Traumatised Refugees and Asylum Seekers in Our PIA

When traumatised patients with a background of migration (primarily refugees and asylum seekers) attend their first appointment, often with an unclear insurance and residency status, they usually come across as apathetic, hopeless, lacking in drive and showing little affect. A detailed history is very difficult to collect at the beginning, and the patients very often report bodily symptoms such as physical pain or emotional states which conventional medicine does not always recognise as a known symptom of dysfunction (Pourgourides 2006). Schubert and Punamäki (2011) also documented this very clearly in Finland through their survey of 78 asylum seekers who had survived severe trauma such as torture; they observed that the secondary symptoms seemed to lead to either reports of *psychiatric* symptoms such as those of PTSD and depressive or anxiety disorders or complaints about *physical* symptoms, depending on the patient's culture of origin. They concluded that depending on the person's cultural background, the way symptoms of psychological distress manifested could be often misunderstood as physical illness in medical facilities of Western orientation (Schubert and Punamäki 2011), an issue that we also often observe in the career of our patients.

Before the actual therapy can begin, often a basic foundation for working together must first be created. Depending on the patient's cultural and social background, it may not work, for example, if the treatment concept and planned treatment steps are not explained first. Subjects such as why regular medication is necessary, where to obtain this medication, how to register in the PIA and how punctual one must be to appointments all necessitate very different explanations depending on cultural background.

In most cases, it is just as important to help in making the alien environment more easy to understand, influence and manage. Sometimes, practical support from the social services department can be very beneficial for the patient. In individual cases, mental stabilisation can also be aided through practical support such as is sometimes offered through counselling centres; such support can enable the patient to find their way as far as possible in the new environment (Chu et al. 2013). Occasionally, it is possible to intervene usefully in the interests of the patient's health in dealings with the appropriate authorities; in so doing, stressful living conditions can, for example, be improved. In most cases, the support of a lawyer is necessary; some patients need to have the asylum procedure explained so that those incalculable risks to which they are exposed can be made as controllable, predictable and transparent as possible.

In so doing, the foundations for therapeutic work together can be laid, and the stabilisation of the patient's social situation can at the same time be supported. Now the actual therapeutic work can begin:

Patients who suffer from PTSD typically experience such phenomenon as flashbacks, vivid nightmares, free-floating anxiety, the feeling of being observed and restlessness. However, if we are talking about refugees with uncertain residency status, empirically, these symptoms cannot initially be treated because the stress experienced from day to day is clearly in the foreground. A stabilisation period of several months is required, during which effort is made to diminish the stress of everyday life to a minimum and in which those acute symptoms which are medically controllable are sought to be reduced. Drug treatments are usually necessary and effective in improving sleep quality or mood, and psychoeducation is necessary to cope better with some symptoms. In addition, nonverbal therapies such as those offered in our PIA – occupational therapy, sports and cooking groups – can be employed. Patients with a background of migration can usually be stabilised sufficiently within a few weeks such that further psychiatric diagnosis and therapy are possible.

It is often at this point that therapeutic work must be done on the patient's hopelessness, anxiety, instability and suicidal tendencies, meaning that a considerable amount of time sometimes passes before a detailed anamnesis can be taken. Whereas the complete case history is not only important to bring the best treatment to the patient, it might be also important to help to prevent a rejection of the asylum application and therefore help to stabilise the social environment. This time delay can be very stressful, since in our experience, any support network the patient may have, lawyers or employees of the federal authorities, often has high expectations that detailed statements will be produced quickly in order to help in the asylum process.

As the therapeutic process continues, confusion, anxiety and feelings of helplessness may repeatedly recur, for example, if the authorities conduct an interrogation or the patient's asylum application is rejected; symptoms will sometimes worsen consecutively (Haenel 2002). Some patients express a strong bitterness and lack of understanding about the fact that they are not allowed to work or to attend a German course and that going in contact with the native German people turns out to be so difficult. The goal of becoming a citizen with equal rights seems infinitely distant. Resentment is often expressed about having to stay in an assigned asylum centre, not being allowed to visit relatives and acquaintances outside the enforced residential districts and, occasionally, having to live in a different federal state than their spouse if they were unable to bring a marriage certificate when they migrated (Coffey et al. 2010). As part of the psychotherapeutic treatment, it is of course necessary to clarify these issues and to discuss the resulting feelings of resentment, despair and anger in order to develop coping strategies where necessary.

This therapeutic phase of stabilisation and support, aiming for at least partial reconciliation with a life situation which is usually precarious, socially unsatisfactory and deprived, with uncertain future prospects and often additional homesickness or concern about and missing of relatives, is slightly different than is seen in classic trauma-centred psychotherapy; it is upstream, so to speak. An actual 'resource-oriented trauma psychotherapy', as Reddemann (2002) describes it, is either not yet possible or only partly so, during this period of social instability in the host country which can be ongoing for several months and sometimes years. Only once external stability has been reached can the phases that are recommended by Reddemann be progressed through, namely, internal stabilisation, learning to have a healing relationship with one's own body, confrontation with the trauma, acceptance and integration (Reddemann 2002).

If they are stabilised sufficiently to be prescribed specific trauma psychotherapy, traumatised patients who speak German can be sent to external outpatient disorder-specific psychotherapy; in recent years, this was possible after 2–8 months. Should more intensive treatment be required, the Centre for Intensified Psychotherapy and Counselling in Berlin at Charité University Psychiatric Clinic at St. Hedwig Hospital offers highly specialised and specific therapy services for German-speaking patients with trauma disorders.

Patients with a background of migration who speak insufficient German cannot participate in such treatment, and the 'Treatment Centre for Victims of Torture' Association in Berlin can see only a small percentage of them. Treatment or at least a reduction in the suffering of these patients, some of whom are seriously traumatised, is only made possible through mediated therapy with the help of an interpreter or professionally qualified translator (Schouler-Ocak 2014; Morina et al. 2010). For these patients, we have developed a specific therapy service, as follows.

Special Group Concept

As part of our PIA, we have developed a specialised multicultural interpreter-aided psychotherapy group, in which specialised group therapy takes place. This involves psychotherapeutic group therapy which is based primarily on mentalising and which takes place in alternation with psychoeducational elements and trauma-specific sessions. Alongside this, the patients also participate in outdoor activities in the local environment guided by an occupational therapist; these often allow patients to gain a whole new understanding of the culture and surroundings. In addition, patients who are particularly stressed or isolated are involved in other occupational therapy groups offered by the standard health-care providers.

In the Netherlands, Drožđek and Bolwerk (2010) also reported that trauma-focused group therapy in combination with nonverbal therapy sessions resulted in a significantly greater reduction of symptoms compared to purely supportive group therapy. They also reported that the more nonverbal therapy sessions the patients engaged in per week, the more successful the treatment (Drožđek and Bolwerk 2010).

In one of our psychotherapy group, therapists, patients and interpreters all sit in a circle together. When several patients from different language groups attend a therapy group, several interpreters are required: one interpreter interprets for one to four patients. In practical terms, this can work as follows:

Patient A speaks in Arabic, and the corresponding interpreter (a) translates this into German, while interpreters (b), (c) and (d) translate it into Armenian, Tamil and Chechen. Patient D responds in Chechen, and interpreter (d) translates this into German, etc. Practice is certainly needed on the part of patients, therapists and interpreters in order to comply with this conversation mode. The therapist must take in and hold not only the patients and the group matrix, as Foulkes (1992) calls it, but also the interactions of the interpreters, which require certain training.

In fact, from my own experience of working in this setting with multiple language groups, such a process enables the therapist to accurately grasp what has been said, as well as to respond to it; this is because the interpreter translates very quickly and in short sections; while the majority of the group perceives the speaker's non-verbal statement and must then wait for the translation, only a few of them can already understand and respond to the spoken language at this point. We prefer this kind of setting, whereas when a large group of patients all speak the same language, a relatively large number of short observations and comments, which are reactions to what has been said, will be exchanged quickly during the process of translating into German and therefore cannot be translated in their entirety. It can be very beneficial to understand what has meanwhile been said – so to speak, to understand when or before the spoken word enters the official 'language space' of the group. More precisely, understanding the translated word is actually necessary to retain control of the entire group process as much as possible, especially when working with patients who are easily flooded by traumatic material and tending towards dissociation as soon as they are confronted with material which is reminiscent of the trauma.

Interpreting techniques used in a group such as this differ in some ways from those used when interpreting an individual psychotherapy. In order to keep such group therapy anchored in the reality of group therapy without an interpreter as much as possible, as well as to make it easier for the interpreter to maintain their mediating role, even in moments of dramatic group dynamics, we have developed some useful techniques along with the interpreters over the course of several years of such group therapy.

The additional therapy which takes place alongside this verbal psychotherapy group remained largely nonverbal, with communication taking place through looks, gestures and symbols. This group is run by an occupational therapist and consists solely of the same refugees who know each other from the psychotherapy group. Outings together in the local area, to museums, zoos, parks, local attractions and cultural sites such as castles and churches, turned out to be a very useful therapeutic intervention: patients experience a different society than the one they encounter in their daily lives through the limitations of the asylum centre, social services and immigration authorities. Some report gaining hope and strength and others short-term distraction from their worries; either way, all of them benefit from a change in perspective.

If symptoms such as flashbacks and trauma-specific nightmares continue, despite all of these measures, and it is not possible to prescribe specialised individual therapy as a follow-up, we try to estimate whether a relatively short period of intense individual psychotherapy might at least alleviate these symptoms. We then try, alongside group therapy, to work towards the reorganisation of the traumatic material and its integration into memory; this is done through weekly or biweekly individual therapy sessions that build sequentially upon one another and involve detailed discussion of isolated traumatic events in minimally small sequences.

Working with Interpreters

Treatment with interpreters, professionally qualified translators (henceforth referred to simply as 'interpreters'), sounds very complicated. In practice, in a consistent course of treatment by an interpreter/therapist team who are used to working together, it seems as if the interpreted conversation between the patient and therapist is taking place like a normal conversation. The interpreter's mediation is of course always noticeable but definitely slips into the background (Wenk-Ansohn and Gurris 2011). The mediated conversation certainly requires twice as much time as a non-interpreted conversation but does however offer the possibility of listening more closely to what is said and to consider intervention strategies while the interpreting is going on. It also offers the additional opportunity, through debriefing sessions with the interpreter, to discuss or clarify perceptions as well as statements which may have been contradictory or unintelligible.

The interpreter-mediated therapeutic process requires special technical skills and competences from both the therapist and interpreter. The therapist preferably uses short phrases or subsets and avoids sayings or abstract transcriptions possibly without equivalent in the interpreted language. Meanwhile, the therapist has to overview the entire process to be capable of resuming his or her therapeutic responsibility. He or she has to overview not only the patient's actual being but also the interpreter's situation. The therapist also should be aware about the interpreter's abilities and limitations.

Qualified and trained interpreters are currently available in many larger cities across Germany via the community interpreting services established in these places. It is useful for therapists to be aware that the level of training of individual interpreters can vary dramatically. While some of the linguists working there are very experienced interpreters in the therapeutic setting, others are less trained or are used to interpreting in the field of social counselling, which is a different setting than the psychotherapeutic context. It is important that interpreters have very finely honed language skills, preferably with one of the interpreted languages as their native language. This is very useful, for example, when the patient is describing difficult experiences such as abuse and sexual assault; being able to estimate the emotional and moral connotations of each word often requires native-speaking competence (Haus 2012).

Another precondition for this work, and something which is checked as a rule by community interpreting services prior to employment, is sufficient mental/emotional stability on the part of the interpreter. For interpreters, the emotional processing of what they feel or experience while interpreting can be quite stressful. This may include situations in which the patient is silent, and when during this silence, the interpreter's own thoughts, fears and other feelings occur, or the feelings perceived in the atmosphere or through transference can creep into conscious awareness. In a conversation about traumatic experiences, these are often mixed with aggressive impulses and can be difficult to bear.

In addition, the patient may report certain traumatic events that touch so closely on the interpreter's own biographical memories that would re-traumatise the interpreter if he or she would have to translate these. In such cases, it is important to find common ground. It may be helpful if the therapist and interpreter can communicate about such unpleasant feelings and concerns. The therapist shows a willingness to take on some responsibility for the mental hygiene of the interpreter by being sensitive towards such processes and paying them due attention. A professional interpreter who works frequently in psychotherapeutic settings will tell the therapist if he or she cannot translate certain utterances about a specific event. We experienced this, for example, when a patient began to talk about the rape of her son and this touched on the biographical material of the interpreter.

Very dramatic descriptions of war scenes, torture methods or corpses can trigger strong feelings of horror. Patients reporting these tend to give intrusive reports of traumatic experiences, typically speaking incessantly in a monotonous tone of voice, and are difficult to interrupt. In the therapeutic setting, it can make sense for the therapist to limit the utterances of the patient and interrupt the uncontrollable and constant repetition of traumatic material, in order to divide it into sections – to control it, so to speak, as this can also be of benefit to the patient. If this intervention is successful, the discussion is often easier for the interpreter to translate. For high-quality, successful therapy, a trusting relationship between the therapist and linguist is very important (Mirdal et al. 2012). In debriefing sessions, which should take place regularly and should not be omitted due to time constraints, explicitly addressing these issues and if necessary debriefing about highly stressful moments are all part and parcel of working with interpreters. Regardless of these debriefings, ongoing external supervision is also an essential precondition for the work of the interpreter.

In the therapeutic setting, good communication between interpreters and therapist is essential. While it can sometimes be useful in the somatic field for interpreters to not only translate but to actually mediate the language and also the situation, thus conveying to the patient what the doctors and nurses expect of them or how the normal treatment scenario works, it is a different situation in the psychiatric and especially in the psychotherapeutic area. Indeed, in such a setting, the therapist can only ensure that full responsibility is taken for what has been said and decide on further treatment if he or she can build up a therapeutic relationship with the patient and receive a precise translation of the contents of what the patient has said. Content, here, means an absolutely literal translation in languages that are closely related or as accurate as possible a translation based on the wording when the two languages are not related.

Inexperienced or lay interpreters tend to convey what they suspect the patient meant to say. They therefore make a preconscious decision not to reflect the exact wording but rather to convey the (logical) sense as they understand it (Bauer and Alegria 2010). In simple consultations, this can be appropriate, but with psychotic patients, for example, with someone suffering from significant dissociative restrictions or speaking in a convoluted way, then what the patient actually says and what the interpreter suspects they have said sometimes differ considerably.

Linguists repeatedly report in debriefing sessions that they reformulated what the patient said, adapting to the patient because they were not familiar with the situation or the therapist; did not trust him or her professionally; or thought that the therapist's utterance was too problematic, incomprehensible, complicated or cautious. Sometimes this situation occurs because of an interpreter's unspoken assumption that Western European psychotherapeutic approaches are not applicable to people of other cultures and that he or she must mediate culturally as well. Discussing such differences or different assumptions and bringing them to awareness are very helpful in working towards a successful treatment, as changing what the patient says without communicating this jeopardises a reasonable diagnosis and responsible therapy (Pourgourides 2006).

Thus, it is also necessary for the interpreter to develop sufficient confidence in the therapist and his or her professional expertise. Again and again, concern arises – for example, if patients dissociate or talk about suicidal thoughts, if their formal thinking is disturbed and misconduct is expected or if they complain of headaches or cry – as to whether the therapist is really aware of how serious the situation is and will really intervene. The question of responsibility for the patient is not usually spoken about formally but remains emotionally unclear for the interpreter: if a patient starts to cry, does the interpreter have to just sit back and let him cry if the therapist doesn't pass him a tissue? How can the interpreter endure and accept such inaction, one which can represent a real act of discourtesy in the context of daily life?

Only when it becomes clear through debriefing that there is a therapeutic meaning in offering a tissue in the therapeutic context and in whether another form of evasion or defence is allowed or encouraged or whether the therapist is attempting to prevent this. Interrupting the conversation to get a glass of water can be very beneficial in some cases, while in others, it can prevent a major breakthrough in the therapeutic conversation. When they understand that the therapist is acting deliberately and accepts full responsibility for these actions, interpreters feel more able to give up trying to steer the therapeutic process or to take on therapeutic responsibility. This is only possible if confidence-building measures, conversations about the setting and about their own ideas of the aims thereof, can take place to a sufficient degree between the interpreter and therapist.

To support the success of the therapeutic conversation, it is therefore necessary that the interpreter and therapist together develop a professional therapeutic relationship which is characterised by trust, so that in spite of their different cultural and professional work backgrounds and experiences, they can succeed in finding a common language for the problems which are to be expected in the course of the treatment and so that they can discuss realistic objectives. However, even if these conditions are met, confusing situations occasionally occur even when a trusting working relationship exists with the interpreter; in such cases, a quick exchange of glances and a more or less silent agreement on how the process should continue may be required. Especially at the very beginning of a process, with patients who speak very quietly and are very fearful, interpreters often give a questioning look to the therapist, and either they silently decide together or the therapist decides whether or not to ask the patient to speak louder.

Another prerequisite for cooperation is the neutrality of the interpreter. In accordance with this, contact with the patients outside of the therapy sessions is not allowed; interpreters therefore use a different waiting area. This also secures the interpreter's privacy protection.

The conversation can of course only be successful if the patient also trusts the interpreter. To support this, it may be important that the patient is given the opportunity to ask the interpreter certain details about his or her origin. For example, for a patient who was traumatised in Iraq, it may be important to know whether he or she is able to speak confidently in front of the interpreter or whether the interpreter belongs to a political camp related to his or her perpetrator. The therapist and interpreter should also agree on whether and how such questions are asked beforehand.

Ultimately, a therapeutic bond between the therapist and patient should be established, something which primarily takes place nonverbally, of course. The style of interpreting can either promote the formation of such a relationship or influence it negatively. As such, close communication between the interpreters and therapist is also required in this regard. When a patient asks a question, the interpreter either can answer it or can translate the question for the therapist; in the former instance, the patient then regards the interpreter as the interlocutor rather than the therapist, while in the latter, if the interpreter gives a consistent literal translation (e.g. passes the patient's question towards the interpreter 'what did he say?' on to the therapist), the patient and therapist communicate 1:1, and therefore the bond starts to take place between these two, whereas the interpreter stays as a mediator.

The interpreters with whom we work in the PIA are usually highly professional and thoughtful, so it is often possible to successfully clarify potentially confusing situations in conversations with patients before they occur, in the preliminary meetings; if not, this is always done in debriefing meetings through a high level of professionalism and cooperation.

Interpretation Costs

Only with a reasonable case history is an accurate and early diagnosis possible; therapy instructions can only be discussed in detail with the patient when a professional interpreter is on hand. Adequate fulfilment of medical responsibility is often only possible with the aid of appropriate linguistic mediation. Such an interpreting service must of course be financed. The current law in Germany makes this path difficult: according to the Benefits for Asylum Seekers Act, §§ 2,4,6 (German Social Security Code, Book V), treatment costs should be covered for 'acute or painful illness, … or indispensable treatment to safeguard the health' not only of asylum seekers but also of those who are obliged to leave, tolerated or even 'illegal' in the country. However, the health insurance is not obliged to cover interpreting costs according to German law. In a verdict about the financing of a sign language interpreter, the Federal Social Court argues that interpreting costs do not have to be financed as part of the treatment services provided by the health insurer but can if necessary be financed as an auxiliary means by the social insurer, i.e. social services (verdict of the German Federal Social Court 1995).

Within the health-care system, depending on the contractual agreement, one unit of interpreting is usually paid at a rate of approximately 25–40 euros for 45–60 min, occasionally with travel costs on top of this. Although this is a low rate compared to what is paid for interpreting in the private sector or in judicial processes, for refugees and patients who finance their life from benefits obtained under the Benefits for Asylum Seekers Act, this is almost impossible to pay.

In Germany, hospitals are legally required to provide all services that are necessary for the fulfilment of its treatment order (Social Security Code Book V); a certain budget should therefore be reserved to finance interpreting or sign language intermediaries. In some highly specialised facilities, interpreting costs are financed by donations. Individual GP practices pay a limited amount of interpreting costs themselves, and there are also some dedicated people who carry out some of their interpreting for free, although they are professionally trained. Very rarely, and in individual cases, employees of the social services grant funding for a limited number of interpreted therapy sessions. Overall, the situation remains unsatisfactory in this respect (based on own experience).

Besides this, according to the Benefits for Asylum Seekers Act §§ 4,6, for the first 48 months of their stay, in principle, people in this category may be financed only for treatment of acute illness that cannot be postponed; psychotherapy is therefore not funded in the majority of cases, assuming that psychiatric diseases which could be treated by psychotherapy never tend to be this kind of 'acute illness' per definition (Classen 2013).

Conclusion

If a therapist who has embarked upon difficult treatment of a traumatised refugee or asylum seeker recognises a difference between the patient's initial state of health and that which has been achieved, in hindsight, he or she will certainly see and feel that the effort was worthwhile. When complex psychotherapeutic treatment involving an interpreter/therapist team is successful, it is always an incredibly enriching and moving experience.

Such experiences increase our desire for more and more therapists to dare to familiarise themselves with the possibility of treatment which is supported by interpreters and, indeed, to work in this way themselves. All therapists and institutions should be aware that demands for regular funding of interpreting expenses (German Society of Psychiatry, Psychotherapy and Nervous Diseases, Position Paper 2012) should be secured either by those who pay the patient's living expenses or by the patient's health insurance.

References

Bauer AM, Alegría M (2010) Impact of patient language proficiency and interpreter service use on the quality of psychiatric care: a systematic review. Psychiatr Serv 61(8):765–773

Bezirksamt Mitte von Berlin: Migration und Gesundheit im Bezirk Berlin Mitte – Gesundheitliche und soziale Lage der Bevölkerung unter Berücksichtigung des Migrationshintergrundes: Beiträge zur Gesundheitsförderung und Gesundheitsberichterstattung, Band 17. April 2011; 53–76

Bundesamt für Migration und Flüchtlinge: Aktuelle Zahlen zum Thema Asyl Ausgabe April 2014: 1–11. URL: http://www.bamf.de/SharedDocs/Anlagen/DE/Downloads/Infothek/Statistik/statistik-anlage-teil-4-aktuelle-zahlen-zu-asyl.html;jsessionid=01F84D3B775FFEAD49DF84BFC13C0246.1_cid359?nn=1367522. Download 13.06.2014

Bundessozialgericht: Urteil vom 10.05.1995, Az.: 1 RK 20/94. URL: https://www.jurion.de/de/search?q=Bundessozialgericht+Urt.+v.+10.05.1995%2C+Az.%3A+1+RK+20%2F94&sort=1. Download vom 09.06.2014

Chu T, Keller AS, Rasmussen A (2013) Effects of postmigration factors on PTSD outcomes among immigrant survivors of political violence. J Immigr Minor Health 15(5):890–897

Classen G (2013) http://www.fluechtlingsinfo-berlin.de/fr/asylblg/AsylbLG-Leitfaden.pdf

Coffey GJ, Kaplan I, Samson RC, Montagna Tucci M (2010) The meaning and mental health consequences of long-term detention for people seeking asylum. Soc Sci Med 70:2070–2079, Elsevier

Das Statistische Bundesamt (2009) Micocensus, Bevölkerung mit Migrationshintergrund – Ergebnisse des Mikrozensus – Fachserie 1 Reihe

Das Statistische Bundesamt (2012) Micocensus. Bevölkerung mit Migrationshintergrund – Ergebnisse des Mikrozensus – Fachserie 1 Reihe 2.2

DGPPN-Positionspapier (2012) URL: http://www.dgppn.de/fileadmin/user_upload/medien/dokumente/referate/transkulturelle-psychiatrie/2012-09-12-dgppn-positionspapier-migration.pdf

Drożđek B, Bolwerk N (2010) Evaluation of group therapy with asylum seekers and refugees – the Den Bosch model. Traumatology 16(4):117–127

Federal Statistical Office, 2008. https://www.destatis.de/DE/Publikationen/Thematisch/Bevoelkerung/MigrationIntegration/Migrationshintergrund2010220087004.pdf?__blob=publicationFile

Foulkes SH (1992) Gruppenanalytische Psychotherapie, Das Individuum in der Gruppe. Klett-Cotta, München

Gesellschaft für Psychiatrie (2000) Psychotherapie und psychosoziale Gesundheit e. V. (DTGPP). Lambertus-Verlag, Freiburg im Breisgau, pp 68–79

Gierlichs HW (2003) Begutachtung psychotraumatisierter Flüchtlinge. Deutsches Ärzteblatt 100(34–35):1098

Haenel F (2002) Behandlungszentrum für Folteropfer Berlin. Der Psychotherapeut 47:185–188

Haus C (2012) Interkulturelle Psychotherapie – Psychotherapie mit Asylbewerbern in Vorarlberg aus Sicht der Existenzanalyse. Abschlussarbeit für die fachspezifische Psychotherapieausbildung in Existenzanalyse

Heeren M, Wittmann L, Ehlert U, Schnyder U, Maier T, Müller (2014) Psychopathology and resident status – comparing asylum seekers, refugees, illegal migrants, labor migrants, and residents. Compr Psychiatry 55(4):818–825

Koch-Stoecker S (2011) Psychiatrische Institutsambulanzen in Deutschland. Aufgaben und Perspektiven Psychiatrische Praxis 38:29–31

Memorandum of the BDK – German Federal Conference of Psychiatric Hospital Directors (2011) Psychiatrische Institutsambulanzen in Deutschland – Aufgaben und Perspektiven. Psychiatry Praxis 38(4):210–212

Mirdal GM, Ryding E, Essendrop Sondej M (2012) Traumatized refugees, their therapists, and their interpreters, three perspectives on psychological treatment. Psychol Psychother 85(4):436–455

Morina N, Maier T, Schmid M (2010) Lost in translation? Psychotherapie unter Einsatz von Dolmetschern. Psychother Psych Med 60:104–110

Pourgourides C (2006) Dilemmas in the treatment of asylum seekers. Psychiatry 6(2):56–58

Reddemann L (2002) Imagination als heilsame Kraft. In: Reddemann L (ed.) Leben lernen 141. Pfeiffer bei Klett-Cotta 6. Imagination als heilsame Kraft. Zur Behandlung von Traumafolgen mit ressourcenorientierten Verfahren. Klett-Cotta, 6. Auflage

Schouler-Ocak M (2000) Kultursensibles Angebot für türkeistämmige Patienten in der Regelversorgungseinrichtung Institutsambulanz des NLKH Hildesheim. In: Koch E, Schepker R, Taneli S (Hrsg). Psychosoziale Versorgung in der Migrationsgesellschaft. Deutsch-Türkische Perspektiven. Band 3 der Schriftenreihe der Deutsch-Türkischen Gesellschaft für Psychiatrie, Psychotherapie und psychosoziale Gesundheit e. V. (DTGPP). Lambertus-Verlag. Freiburg im Breisgau, 68–79

Schouler-Ocak M (2014) Interkulturelle traumazentrierte Psychotherapie unter Einbeziehung eines professionellen Sprach- und Kulturmittlers. Swiss Arch Neurol Psychiatry 165(3):85–90

Schouler-Ocak M, Bretz HJ, Hauth I, Heredia Montesinos A, Koch E, Driessen M, Heinz A (2010) Patienten mit Migrationshintergrund in Psychiatrischen Institutsambulanzen – ein Vergleich zwischen Patienten mit türkischer und osteuropäischer Herkunft und Patienten ohne Migrationshintergrund. Psychiatr Prax 37(8):384–390

Schubert CC, Punamäki RL (2011) Mental health among torture survivors: cultural background, refugee status and gender. Nord J Psychiatry 65(3):175–182

Von Lersner U, Wiens U, Elbert T, Neuner F (2008) Mental health of returnees: refugees in Germany prior to their state-sponsored repatriation. BMC Int Health Hum Rights 8:8

Wenk-Ansohn M, Gurris N (2011) Intercultural encounters in counselling and psychotherapy – communication with the help of interpreters. Torture 21(3):20

Psychotherapy with Immigrants and Refugees from Crisis Zones

15

Ljiljana Joksimovic, Monika Schröder, and Eva van Keuk

Introduction

Offering appropriate care to refugees requires temporal and structural resources, specific competence in diversity and cross-cultural issues and expertise in the fields of psychosocial and socio-medical assessment and treatment. In our experience, the absence of appropriate structures within such care often leads to a delay in identifying mentally ill or traumatised victims of torture in particular; such a delay has medical, psychological and social consequences for the individuals affected as well as for their families.

As members of the healing professions, we must do our utmost to ensure that all patients receive the treatment they need as soon as possible on the basis of their symptomatic profile. The steps towards this end must be carried out with transparency and clinical diligence. This sometimes means campaigning for structural change in order that the structures within which we work enable a patient-oriented approach (e.g. by being able to attend a specialised training course or supervision, by employing language and integration mediators or through contact and cooperation with specialised institutions).

The number of people who have had to leave their home countries for fear of war and persecution is currently on the rise once again. At the time of writing, almost 50 million people have had to flee their homes on a worldwide scale; around 15.4 million of these can be defined as refugees according to the definition of international

L. Joksimovic, MD, MPH (✉)
LVR Klinikum Düsseldorf, Heinrich-Heine-University Düsseldorf, Düsseldorf, Germany
e-mail: Ljiljana.Joksimovic@lvr.de

M. Schröder
LVR-Klinikum Düsseldorf, Düsseldorf (Registered society), Germany

E. van Keuk
Psychosocial Centre for Refugees, Düsseldorf, Germany

© Springer International Publishing Switzerland 2015
M. Schouler-Ocak (ed.), *Trauma and Migration:*
Cultural Factors in the Diagnosis and Treatment of Traumatised Immigrants,
DOI 10.1007/978-3-319-17335-1_15

law. Most of them (about 80–85 %) can escape either to neighbouring countries or within their own countries, becoming so-called 'internally displaced persons'.

Through the regulation of the European Parliament which determines which member state is responsible for processing an asylum application (the 'Dublin III Regulation', updated in July 2013), it has over recent years become increasingly difficult to enter the Federal Republic of Germany as a refugee, since the country is surrounded by officially 'safe' third countries. Germany is nonetheless seeing a steady increase in the number of asylum applications. In the 44 rich industrialised countries that were investigated by the United Nations High Commissioner for Refugees (UNHCR), over 610,000 asylum applications were registered in 2013, this being the highest level since 2001 ('Deutschland erhält die meisten Asylanträge' 2014).

In 2013, 110,000 asylum applications were made in Germany, meaning that for the first time since 1999, Germany occupied the pole position in terms of applicant countries. In second place came the United States, with 88,000 applications, followed by France (60,000), Sweden (54,000) and Turkey (45,000). The causes for this rise can be found in ongoing wars and violence, such as the civil war in Syria. Accordingly, in 2013, the most asylum seekers came from Syria (over 56,000). In 2010, before the outbreak of the conflict, Syria was only twentieth in terms of countries of origin of those applying for asylum in other countries, according to the UNHCR.

Following Syria in terms of the countries of origin of asylum seekers in 2013 were Russia with 40,000, Afghanistan with 39,000, Iraq with 38,000 and Serbia (including Kosovo) with almost 35,000 applications. In the period from January to May 2014, 62,602 people had applied for asylum in Germany. Compared with the same period in 2013, this represents an increase of 61.4 %. The main countries of origin in 2014 were Syria (10,046), Serbia (7,789) and Afghanistan (3,858) (Bundesamt für Migration und Flüchtlinge 2013).

Not all of those who apply for asylum in Germany can remain in the country. In July 2014, the overall protection rate for all countries of origin (recognition of right to asylum, refugee protection according to § 3 para. 1 of the Asylum Procedure Act, subsidiary protection according to § 4 para. 1 of the Asylum Procedure Act and ban on deportation according to § 60 para. 5 or 7 of the Residence Act) was 25.3 %.

Mentally Ill Refugees and the Health System

Rising numbers of refugees mean that in the course of their daily professional lives, doctors and psychotherapists increasingly come into contact with patients who suffer from the psychological and physical consequences of war, persecution and displacement. Addressing trauma-related mental illness and psychosocial problems among migrants from crisis areas can place high demands on doctors and psychotherapists in terms of culture- and migration-sensitive communication skills as well as knowledge of current and historical social contexts.

For example, an assessment or treatment situation might call for knowledge of other countries in terms of the specific characteristics of communication, taboos and gender roles, and behaviour when dealing with authority and rules. Diversity competence, moreover, is also required; this must be understood as an extension of the usual social and cross-cultural communicative medical/therapeutic expertise. Such competence allows the practitioner to understand the effects of so-called 'diversity dimensions' such as age, gender, sexual orientation, disability, religion, sociocultural background and skin colour on the illness, in both the society of origin and in the host society (Joksimovic 2010).

When dealing with diversity dimensions, it is important that they do not describe character traits, but rather the categories by which people experience exclusion or discrimination regardless of individual skills. Diversity competence explicitly includes the willingness to self-reflect on ones own cultural embeddedness, prejudice-conscious communication, perception of power asymmetries and discriminatory structures in the host society. The knowledge required for such competence, including active skills and specific attitudes in dealing with people from crisis zones with psychological and psychosomatic problems, is barely touched upon within medicine and psychology degrees nor through further training. Unfortunately, the few existing training opportunities are utilised only insufficiently as yet.

This leads many doctors to assume that their medical intervention and the medical profession are neutral (Beagan and Kumas-Tan 2009; Berger 2008). In so doing, they overlook the fact that Western medicine has its own culture, in that it contains values, beliefs, norms and language that directly influence their medical practice (in terms of preventive, diagnostic and therapeutic treatment as well as the formulation of reports, certificates, attestations, etc.) (Smedley et al. 2009). In the health system, awareness for this is only occasionally available so far. As such, the medical and psychotherapeutic care of mentally ill immigrants from crisis areas remains a particular challenge for health services.

General practitioners play a key role in the initial stages of detecting indication of mental illness in patients who have had to flee their home countries. They are often the first point of contact for refugees entering the health system of the host country. Many GPs feel insufficiently educated and trained regarding this task. A study conducted in Switzerland, for example, found that torture and its consequences were not mentioned explicitly as a problem by patients, nor named as such by the doctors, in any of the consultations examined, despite the fact that 110 of 1,477 diagnoses among refugees in primary care consultations were clearly associated with maltreatment (Junghanss 1998). There is an especially great risk of traumatic experiences being overlooked as a potential cause of physical complaints for which there is no adequate organic explanation.

Mental and Psychosomatic Disorders in Migrants from Crisis Zones

Scientific studies seem to indicate an increased risk for mental and physical disorders in refugee populations (Fazel et al. 2005; Johnson and Thompson 2008; Kruse et al. 2009; Laban et al. 2005). This risk is increased in comparison with both the native population (Sundquist 1993a, b) and so-called 'voluntary' migrants (Cervantes et al. 1989; Klimidis et al. 1994; Lin et al. 1985; Sundquist 1995). Above all, increased rates of post-traumatic stress disorder (PTSD), depression, pain and somatoform symptoms are found among refugee populations. A systematic review of 20 studies showed that a high rate of PTSD is approximately ten times more likely to be found among refugees than among an age-matched native population (Fazel et al. 2005). Chronic forms of PTSD are often reported. In a study by Marshall et al. (2005), for example, symptoms of PTSD were found in 63 % of refugees from Cambodia, 20 years after fleeing to the United States.

PTSD (ICD-10: F43.1) is the result either of a brief but highly stressful or disturbing event or of a longer-lasting period of such events, accompanied by feelings of fear and helplessness. According to the criteria of ICD-10, the symptoms can occur days or months after such an event, which is one that would be stressful for almost anyone. PTSD is characterised by the following symptoms: repetitive re-experiencing of the traumatic event through intrusive memories (flashbacks), dreams or nightmares; avoidance of activities and situations that might trigger memories of the trauma; and (in most cases) a state of autonomic hyperarousal, startle response ('jumpiness'), impaired concentration and/or sleep disturbance. A feeling of emotional dullness or numbness also commonly occurs.

PTSD is associated with a high risk of co-morbidity, the most common co-morbid disorders being depression and substance abuse. Somatoform disorders are also often co-morbid with PTSD (van der Kolk et al. 1996). However, only a few studies have dealt with these co-morbidities among refugees (Cheung 1993; Hinton et al. 2008; Kruse et al. 2009), although it is known that somatoform disturbances among war veterans and refugees lead to an increased utilisation of health services (Engel et al. 2000).

The literature on mental disorders among refugees increasingly reports psychotic disorders. There is empirical evidence to suggest that cumulative traumatic events may actually be a causal factor for the later development of psychosis (Fisher et al. 2010; Larkin and Read 2008; Shevlin et al. 2008). The co-morbidity between PTSD and psychosis among traumatised refugees is now being studied in more detail (Gerritsen et al. 2006; Kroll et al. 2011; Schreiber 1995). But the way psychotic symptoms are perceived, expressed and healed are also often strongly linked to sociocultural traditions.

From our clinical practice, we observe that traumatised people from crisis areas often report altered experiences and perceptions that have strong similarities with psychotic disorders. The basic similarities between traumatic disorders and psychotic disorders lie in a distortion of perception and a (usually temporary) loss of reality – in the form of vivid intrusions in traumatic disorders and hallucinations in psychotic patients. Viewed superficially, the symptoms may seem identical (hearing voices, paranoid experiences, hallucinations); the aetiology and symptom development are however different.

Cultural differences and language problems can make it difficult to differentiate between the two, meaning that there is an increased danger of overlooking possible traumatic origins of such symptoms in refugees who have recently arrived and have an insufficient knowledge of the language of the host country. Misunderstandings are more likely when doctors and therapists are unaware of the difficulty described and lack the relevant experience and skills in this field. Usually, the symptoms are then treated exclusively through psychopharmacology. Since these substances have side effects and may adversely affect the long-term prognosis of PTSD, clinical differentiation and critical diagnosis are of urgent necessity.

Another consequence of war- and torture-related trauma is the profound personality changes which can be associated with the diagnosis of 'enduring personality change after catastrophic experience' (ICD-10: F62.0). Such changes may have been preceded by the clinical picture of PTSD. The former disorder is characterised by a hostile or distrustful attitude towards the world. In addition, social withdrawal and feelings of emptiness or of constantly being threatened are all part of the pattern of symptoms. Traumatised refugees and their relatives frequently perceive disturbing changes in character traits which are particularly important to them, such as their sense of responsibility towards their family. For example, a traumatised patient might observe an indifference towards his children and grandchildren but report that they had been particularly active and interested in the development of their children before the trauma and used to be perceived as such by others. Such changes may lead to serious internal destabilisation and insecurity, especially if these changes relate to characteristics that had been central to their identity. This can lead to conflicts in the refugee's family environment (which is often stressful already) and can thus produce a severe psychological strain not only on the affected individual but also among relatives and for the next generation. In extreme cases, these changes can be experienced by the affected individual as a personal failure and thus as a victory of whoever caused them suffering. It is important to remember that the psychological and psychosomatic consequences of traumatic experiences are subject to broad individual differences and cannot always be clearly mapped with the current classification systems.

Factors that come into consideration as predictors of the above-mentioned trauma-related disorders include stress and traumatic experiences in the person's country of origin, living conditions in the host country and personal resilience. Stress factors before migration include rape, being a prisoner of war, combat experiences in war, house searches, unlawful detention, physical and psychological abuse, living in hiding, witnessing injury or death of people one is close to and/or the loss of these people and being unexpectedly confronted with corpses and body parts. In 2012, people were abused and tortured in 112 countries across the world (Amnesty International 2013). Torture, thus, should not be seen as an exception among the refugee population (Eisenman et al. 2003; Holtan et al. 2002). Undoubtedly, such experiences increase the risk of mental disorders in refugees several times over (Mollica et al. 2001; Silove et al. 1997).

Another risk factor for the development of illness and/or the illness taking an unfavourable course can be the treatment of asylum seekers by the host society; this is often marked by exclusion. Many of the impairments to (mental) health become manifest only after a certain latency, in connection with the living conditions in the host country (Laban et al. 2004). Levels of psychological distress after migration therefore differ between comparable refugee populations, depending on conditions in the host country (Warfa et. al. 2012). Silove et al. (2007) give a detailed description of the role of post-migration risk factors in psychological problems among populations exposed to mass trauma and displacement.

Diagnostic Approaches with Patients with a History of Displacement

Since the current diagnostic criteria do not adequately reflect the wide range of possible psychological and psychosomatic consequences of flight and migration, a so-called progressive diagnosis is preferable when working with patients from crisis areas who have such a history. Only through a detailed exploration of the course taken by the disorder is it possible to avoid an overhasty, incorrect 'spot' diagnosis upon which basis a potentially inappropriate treatment might otherwise be initiated.

In our work, an in-depth, psychodynamically oriented diagnosis (involving taking a disorder-specific biographical and social history as well as a culturally sensitive survey of psychopathological findings) has proven its worth. In so doing, especially in cases where the clinical picture is unclear, the aim is to gain an overview of the following aspects (Joksimovic 2009):

- What is the patient suffering from (detailed survey of the symptom profile and psychopathological findings)?
- How should the development of the disorder be understood within the context of traumatic experiences (history of trauma/displacement), the current life situation (taking a social case history), the triggering situation (current stressors) and the personality of the patient (biographical history)?
- What factors lead to the perpetuation and chronification of the illness (survey of previous health conditions and data on the current life situation)?
- Which therapeutic approach is indicated?

In our experience, refugees are rarely consulted sufficiently about their medical history and are prescribed medication even in the absence of improvement. In practice, this generally leads to an increased use of various substance groups among traumatised patients (SSRIs; tricyclic antidepressants, sleep-inducing antidepressants with a dual mode of action; neuroleptics and hypnotics) when the traumatic origin of the symptoms is not recognised (Joksimovic et al. 2013). The risk of this increases with the presence of linguistic and sociocultural barriers. Therefore, when disease-related problems of understanding occur because of linguistic difficulties, language and integration mediators must be used in the diagnostic procedure. In addition, in a cross-cultural treatment setting, the patient may interpret the context in a markedly different way from that of the practitioner.

This point can be clarified through the example of hallucinations: as an isolated symptom, especially in cross-cultural settings, hallucinations initially have very little meaning. They may occur in psychotic, depressive, traumatised and physically ill people but also in healthy individuals. Ivezic et al. (2000) found 'psychotic' symptoms such as auditory hallucinations in approximately one fifth of Croatian war veterans who were diagnosed with PTSD in psychiatric inpatient care. These hallucinations were described by the patients as being more intense than typical traumatic intrusions, but their content was still related to the trauma. 'Hearing voices' alone, then, should not limit the potential diagnosis too rashly (such as an immediate diagnosis of an illness from the schizophrenic group). For patients who come from a sociocultural milieu in which strong spiritual connections (such as to the ancestors) do not represent anything extraordinary, hearing the warning voice of the ancestors, for example, is not to be clinically regarded as auditory hallucination per se. Of course, this would be assessed differently if it occurred in combination with sleep disturbance and a sense of being driven to fulfil an order.

Making an overhasty diagnosis can be a way for practitioners to circumvent or resist the uncomfortable feelings associated with diagnostic uncertainty and engaging in patients' horrific traumatic experiences. Regular supervision under the guidance of cross-culturally competent colleagues can be of great help and support in such cases.

Specifics in Psychotherapeutic Work with Refugees

In the treatment of mentally ill and traumatised refugees, the following problem areas in the cross-cultural context are often identified:

- Language barriers
- Different conceptions of disease
- Different coping strategies and health risks
- Different senses of what represents health
- Lack of knowledge about the health-care system

On top of this, specific problems (such as doctors' and therapists' lack of knowledge on refugees' living conditions and the resulting health risks) exacerbate the problems above. Refugees' living situation is of special complexity, particularly due to restrictive conditions as pertaining to residence and basic social security. Only a small proportion of all asylum applicants receive official recognition or subsidiary protection by the German Federal Office for Migration and Refugees (BAMF) and thus a residence permit, and often only after several years; only such a permit allows the attendance of an integration course, receipt of unemployment benefits, choice of which health insurer to register with and uptake of work or a training course, etc.

Without or prior to receiving such a permit, many refugees with an immigration status such as the 'toleration' status usually have to endure very poor living conditions, often over a number of years; this commonly includes living in extremely cramped accommodation as well as having no legal right to work, attend language or integration courses or receive normal social benefits (being subject to the separate Asylum Seekers Benefits Act). In terms of psychotherapeutic care, this means that the social welfare offices are the authority responsible for reviewing the necessity of health department services. All measures that go beyond the treatment of acute and painful conditions require prior approval by the social welfare authority (i.e. not health professionals); in practice, this represents a high bureaucratic hurdle that often triggers resignation on the part of those affected and incomprehension and anger on the part of professionals. In some cases, treatments which are strongly indicated are delayed or made completely impossible.

Another specific feature of working with people who come from conflict areas is working on the consequences of the overwhelming force of traumatic experiences; as a rule, such experiences can only be stored in human memory in fragments due to the impairment of regulatory subcortical and cortical exchange processes. Traumatic experiences are stored as discrete sense impressions and usually stay insulated from contexts of experience which would otherwise be potentially conducive to relativising and processing the traumatic experience (Brenneis 1998; Markowitsch 1998; van der Kolk et al. 1998; Wessa and Flor 2002). As such, stored traumatic material can be reactivated by relatively weak cues and is re-experienced in direct, film- and image-like form or through reactivated body memories or unregulated and endlessly repeating streams of thought (intrusions, flashbacks). The ease of triggering of traumatic material alongside the relatively undeveloped verbal memory traces represents a major obstacle to the subsequent processing of traumatic experiences (Kunzke and Güls 2003).

This type of re-experiencing, no matter what the traumatic background, has no healing or processing effect; from a neurobiological point of view, information above a certain emotional intensity – here mostly fear or anger – can no longer be used in a new way. In such cases, the cortical processing mechanisms are turned off, so to speak, and more 'primitive' subcortical processes step in and take over (Acheson et al. 2012; Yehuda 2002). This must be taken into account in considerations pertaining to intervention techniques in psychotherapy. If there is evidence to suggest past experiences of torture, it is also important to avoid treatments and postures (if medically justifiable) that trigger re-experiencing the trauma. Dental examinations of people who have suffered tooth torture, gynaecological and urological examinations in cases of sexual violence and ECG studies in people who have experienced torture by electric shock must all be performed with great sensitivity to the patient. This is only possible if a relationship of trust has been created between a doctor and a patient; otherwise, treatment intended to heal could lead to re-traumatisation or serious misunderstandings. Collaboration between a patient's psychotherapist and their doctor could help in such cases.

Over the years, the following procedure has been relatively widely adopted in the treatment of trauma-related disorders, according to a division into three phases based on Janet and Paul (1925):

I. Stabilisation
II. Confrontation with the trauma, i.e. the actual trauma processing
III. Integration, i.e. implementing that which has been learned into everyday life, reviewing current relationships, working on conflicts and reconciliation with ones fate and sometimes with perpetrators.

For these reasons, special attention is paid to the first (stabilisation) phase when treating traumatised refugees. Only when patients are able on the whole to prevent and regulate intrusions and flashbacks or are at least trained in strategies to come out of states of arousal after intrusions, flashbacks and dissociative processes can trauma-confronting methods (such as EMDR) be employed to start the processing of the trauma itself (Baars et al. 2010; Hofmann et al. 1999; Kunzke and Güls 2003; Reddemann 2004; Wöller et al. 2012). If traumatised refugees remain too unstable to allow trauma processing, e.g. through a constant threat of imminent deportation (Joksimovic et al. 2011), trauma-specific group psychotherapy with other refugees alongside one-to-one therapeutic measures could be seen as a further and necessary component of the stabilisation phase of trauma therapy (Reddeman 2004).

The advantage of groups for traumatised refugees is that their members can usually connect to one another relatively quickly through common themes such as their displacement history and the living conditions in the host country. By holding the group in such a way that regressive processes are limited, preventing group members from sliding into traumatic experiences and offering safety through interventions that lend structure, the group therapist can create the conditions necessary for the group to be experienced as a safe place. The group context allows its members to explore social norms and ways of engaging with each other and how concerns and stress factors can be voiced and shared within the group. The aim of stabilising group psychotherapy is to strengthen coping skills in conflict situations in interpersonal relationships and difficult social situations, as well as to reduce social isolation. Individual psychotherapy has its limits in dealing with these problems. Modified, trauma-specific group psychotherapy, when offered after initial stabilisation in an individual setting, opens up the possibility of further stabilisation through the improvement and correction of dysfunctional interpersonal patterns.

In our clinical experience, premature confrontation with the trauma is also discouraged when PTSD is associated with psychosis-related symptoms and severe personality changes. Furthermore, traumatised and politically persecuted refugees often regard psychotherapy with suspicion; in such cases, an intensive phase of preparation and psychoeducation may be required.

A controversial discussion is currently as to whether psychotherapy that aims at processing the traumatic content itself can be effective or helpful when working with traumatised refugees. While some consider confrontation with the trauma as the preferred tool in treatment, other trauma therapists consider this position as very problematic (Reddemann and Sachsse 1998, 2000).

The process of establishing a trusting working relationship with survivors of torture and structural violence can lead to therapists experiencing feelings of incompetence. The willingness to involve oneself actively and show genuine interest and understanding in patients' problems can be of great help to the process. Clear rules and principles of trauma therapy must be explicitly introduced and adhered to; examples of such principles are the rule of 'protection first', using the stop sign when under high stress and the rule that talking about stressful material should always be voluntary. In the absence of such rules, discontinuation or irregular attendance of the therapy sessions may occur.

Taking the patient's very real uncertainties regarding their residence status/asylum application seriously (including issuing any certificates that may be required and validating negative experiences with authorities) promotes a basic sense of security and confidence among refugees. Therapists are confronted relatively quickly with the problem of whether the therapeutic conditions should also offer action-oriented support or only offer space for reflection and emotional support. According to Tucker and Price (2007), in addition to purely medical measures, appropriate services for these patients should also include case-specific advice for practical, health-related issues.

Psychotherapy with Interpreters

Language barriers in particular make it more difficult for mentally ill refugees to access adequate medical and psychotherapeutic treatment; in addition, socioculturally based misunderstandings are a common occurrence. These may often occur in everyday interactions without obvious consequences; in the psychiatric or psychotherapeutic treatment context, however, such misunderstandings can have serious consequences. They may, for example, lead to misdiagnosis, thus creating unnecessary suffering for those affected and/or requiring a great deal of time and correspondingly high costs for the health and social system. Since native language treatment services are only occasionally available in Germany currently and even in psychiatric and psychotherapeutic facilities with multilingual therapists, not all languages can be covered and the utilisation of interpreters or language and integration mediators remains as an alternative.

From a professional standpoint, the use of language and integration mediators is to a large extent justified because it facilitates patients who have an insufficient grasp of the language of the host country to utilise psychiatric/psychotherapeutic help, reduces diagnostic uncertainty on the part of practitioners and therefore often helps to prevent hospital admission (Kluge and Kassim 2006). The presence of a third person in such a treatment situation is however often unfamiliar for professionals; it can produce feelings of insecurity and the loss of control and is not infrequently rejected as a possibility. However, given the lack of alternatives, it seems appropriate to us to focus less on the question of *whether* and more on *how* this treatment setting can be made as trouble-free as possible. Firstly, the knowledge of certain principles and rules helps in making this 'trialogue' communication situation successful; secondly, attention should be paid to the typical errors in the use of language and integration mediators in order to minimise possible distortions.

Possible errors include an unsuitable interpreter being selected, too little time for briefing and debriefing, a lack of clear role clarification, inappropriate language, indirect speech, neglect of non-and para-verbal behaviour and neglect of confidence-building measures in the 'trialogue'. Professional language and integration mediators are 'bridge builders' in health, education and social services. Their task is to improve the linguistic and sociocultural understanding between professionals and patients with a migration background and thus goes beyond pure translation.

In Germany, the training to become a language and integration mediator takes place according to uniform quality standards. In addition to knowledge of the health, social and education systems, language and integration mediators also possess medical, psychosocial and legal knowledge. Furthermore, because of their own migration experience, they are familiar with the culture of origin as well as specific differences about the host country in terms of health and social care. They can therefore also mediate in socioculturally sensitive issues, such as when dealing with mental illness, gender roles, religious issues and so on. This makes an important contribution to improving the quality of treatment. However, the practitioner is still very often faced with the unsolvable problem of the absence of an interpreter or lack of funding thereof.

Clinical Certificates and Statements in Psychotherapy with Refugees

In Germany – as in most European host countries – refugees are subject to separate regulatory requirements. This includes the 'duty to cooperate': the asylum seeker must 'cooperate' by submitting certificates to substantiate any claims which are made.

Example: A 54-year-old Kurdish patient asks her psychiatrist for a certificate which was required by the immigration office – without it, they refused to renew her residence permit. The psychiatrist responsible reacts with annoyance – 'Has the patient just been coming to her appointments so that she will get a certificate one day? I'm not paid to write certificates for authorities, I'm paid to treat my patients', he says in a supervision group.

It turned out that the patient had applied for a permanent residence permit and the immigration authority was checking to see whether the reasons that had led to residence on humanitarian grounds 20 years ago (continued arrests, serious sexual violence because of her husband's political activities in Turkey (her native country), PTSD as a result of experiences with violence) were still valid. For her psychiatrist, this was a strange situation – and yet the reality of the patient's life.

Some doctors and therapists justify their position as follows: 'I don't write certificates on principle, because the therapeutic space must be protected'. This is an understandable position but is simply not applicable to the legal context in which refugees find themselves in. If the health professional does not produce a certificate, this will likely have negative consequences for the patient. Unfortunately, the protected therapy room does not apply to refugees to the same extent as for domestic patients; professional and effective treatment is nonetheless possible. In the following, the key issues relating to certificates and statements will be named and workable solutions that have emerged in specialised treatment centres for refugees presented.

Why Do Clinical Certificates Play an Important Role in Asylum and Immigration Law Procedures?

Since the war in the former Yugoslavia, which was associated with high numbers of refugees in Germany, serious war trauma was recognised by the refugees' countries of origin and had found its way into German jurisprudence. Rape, for example, was classified as an instrument of warfare, and illness due to this trauma could make return impossible. The presence of PTSD became important to asylum claims and thus of practical relevance to the legal decision-makers at the Federal Office for Migration and Refugees and courts. The focus on clinical disease in the right of abode led to a high level of suspicion on the part of legal decision-makers. Hearings before court involving disease are met with sceptical attitudes. At the same time, very few reports are commissioned, so that a high number of refugees with PTSD remain without clinical assessment. In addition, not infrequently, the certification provided by health professionals is often classified as inadequate and accordingly receives little attention.

It is legally enshrined that asylum seekers should speak credibly themselves about their reasons for fleeing their home country: 'As an essential prerequisite (...), a substantiated and essentially non-contradictory and unchanging factual report is required on the part of the applicant with respect to those circumstances that relate to his own life circumstances' (BverfG, InfAuslR 91.94). However, we know from psycho-traumatology that trauma symptoms can significantly impair the ability to deliver a verbal, noncontradictory, detailed representation of the grounds for asylum at the Federal Office for Migration and Refugees (first instance) and the Administrative Court (second instance). At the same time, we have to assume that more than one third of asylum seekers suffer from psychological traumatic disorders (Gäbel et al. 2006). Therefore it is not surprising from a clinical point of view that a very high proportion of traumatised refugees do not initially specify their trauma history in the asylum procedure and that it often becomes evident only during the course of treatment.

This complex and problematic situation means that many questions are left unanswered until the threat of deportation is presented and that refugee patients then pass on the authorities' demands, arising out of their duty to cooperate, to the professionals who are treating them. However, in our experience of treating refugees, there are quite feasible approaches as to how this dilemma can be encountered.

We distinguish between certificates and attestations, statements and expert reports. *Certificates and attestations* require brief reference to a specific question (e.g. ability to work, travel expenses, etc.). For the addressee (e.g. immigration authorities), it is important that central information such as duration and frequency of treatment, clinical picture and diagnosis and a specific clinical response to the authority's question can also be found in short certificates.

Statements are significantly more detailed and contain a thorough history of the person's displacement, a symptomatic survey, diagnostic evaluation, differential diagnosis and prognosis. These are requested by patients or by their lawyers and are to be filled out by the health professional who is treating them; such documents play an important role in decisions on humanitarian stay.

Lastly, *expert reports* are requested by the legal decision-makers: either the Federal Office for Migration and Refugees, the Administrative Court, or the immigration authorities. Here, the case file is made available to the expert, usually someone who is specially contracted for the purpose and is not the health professional who is treating the patient.

In contrast to clinical documentation for other patients, the following aspects concerning contents play a prominent role in terms of the effectiveness of a certificate/statement written for refugee patients:

- *Are there inconsistencies with previous hearings in the asylum process?* In patients with mental disorders, the course taken by the symptom development often leads to significant changes in terms of what information is presented. A patient might perhaps only become capable of speaking about experiences of sexual violence through the context of a trusting psychotherapeutic relationship and did not therefore talk about this in the interview with the Federal Office for Migration and Refugees when they entered the country. Therefore, when writing more detailed statements, it is important to ask the patient for the documents from the Protocol of the Federal Office and any court hearings beforehand – this is not very time-consuming and yet can significantly increase the efficiency of clinical documentation.
- *Can an estimation be made as to which stressors a current clinical picture is linked to?* For example, the question of whether a patient only became mentally ill after his imprisonment, or was already ill in advance of persecution, may in some individual cases have legal consequences in terms of the right to asylum. Here, a significant factor is to preserve ones own framework for clinical competency while making the most differentiated assessment possible.
- *Can the extent be assessed to which the presenting clinical picture actually exists or could it also be simulated?* Legal decision-makers are often faced with a multitude of similar-sounding pleas by asylum seekers and identical certificates from health professionals and therefore often read these clinical reports with a dose of scepticism. For example, if a patient has already been in treatment for a year, and a variety of clinically relevant information is available, the risk of simulation is far lower than after one initial meeting. Birck (2002) has dealt in depth with this complex issue (see also Gierlichs et al. 2005). Clinical practitioners are familiar with the problem of simulation in their patients and should also proceed with professionalism among refugees – and note in this case, especially in the certificates, that the question of the simulation was investigated.

Mandatory Conditions for Clinical Professionals

In 2007, the Federal Administrative Court set out minimum requirements for clinical documentation in the asylum procedure (judgement of the Federal Administrative Court from November 9, 2007): attestations should therefore include the following points:

- Basis of diagnosis
- Details on treatment, symptoms and objectification of complaints through examination

- Information on the severity of the disease, necessity/urgency of treatment and treatment thus far
- If PTSD is diagnosed and was not mentioned in the initial application: explanation of why the illness was not mentioned before

It is recommended that clinical certificates, attestations and statements addressed to the immigration authorities, Federal Office for Migration and Refugees or the Administrative Court refer to the criteria of the Administrative Court in one sentence.

In addition, on an almost annual basis, the *German Medical Association* makes decisions that relate to refugees and their treatment. In order not to go beyond the scope of this chapter, only the following decisions from the last German Medical Assembly will be mentioned here (see 276f in the minutes: http://www.bundesaerztekammer.de/downloads/)

The 117th German Medical Assembly in 2014 called on the Federal Government.

- *...To create the necessary conditions in order to meet the requirements set by the UN Committee Against Torture (CAT) in 2011 for medical and psychological examinations of refugees undergoing an asylum procedure where there is evidence to suggest torture or trauma (Top VII-65)*
- *...To grant asylum seekers as well as other foreigners in a similar position (such as people without a legal residence status) the same rights to health care as regular citizens (Top VII-66)*
- *...to urge the individual federal states of Germany to ensure that, like the role models of Bremen, Hamburg and Rostock, contracts with health insurance providers are made on a nationwide basis according to § 264 para. 1 SGB V, allowing asylum seekers uncomplicated access by means of a health insurance card to the health treatment which to which they are entitled according to the Asylum Seekers Benefits Act (AsylbLG) (Top VII-67)*

The National Chamber of Psychotherapists also regularly makes statements on the treatment of refugees (June 2013: reprimand about the Federal Government's attitude of refusing to enable psychotherapy in traumatised refugees' native languages; March 2014: call for fewer bureaucratic barriers for traumatised refugees wishing to access treatment), as well as the Professional Association of German Psychologists (most recently in the press release on 6 June 2014, International Day of the Torture Victim, see Tschischka 2014).

In 2004, in North Rhine-Westphalia, the so-called 'NRW decree: Information and Criteria Catalogue IuK NRW' was issued and made binding. This was the result of a nationwide working group with representatives of the German Federal States and Medical Associations (November 2004) and can be accessed under:

http://www.aekno.de/downloads/aekno/kriterienkatalog_nrw.pdf. According to this document, in questions of deportation, an assessment may not be limited solely to whether someone is medically capable of taking a flight, but must also take into account and portray both *obstacles to deportation in the destination country* (why a refugee with a mental health problem cannot return to their homeland) and *domestic obstacles to enforcement* (to what extent a person can cope in terms of fitness to travel from A to B in the case of deportation); this is especially important if these reasons were not put forward during previous hearings. Since it explicitly refers to medical and psychological statements and certificates, a knowledge of this decree is well within the remit of the clinician – whereas anything pertaining to legal competence should of course be left to the patient's lawyer and legal decision-makers.

There is therefore no lack of binding conditions and demands on the part of the professional associations. We highly recommend that clinical practitioners have a knowledge of these fundamentals and refer confidently to them.

Standards for Expert Assessment and Examination According to the Istanbul Protocol

This chapter is not about a detailed assessment of refugees as this topic is beyond the scope, but for the particularly interested reader, we would like at least briefly to point out which mandatory standards have been developed:

- *Standards for the assessment of people with psychosocial trauma* (revised by Wenk Ansohn et al. 2013; first publication: Haenel and Wenk Ansohn 2004). After the deportation, imprisonment and re-entry of a Kurdish asylum seeker from Aachen, general practitioners and psychotherapists in 2001 developed a statement of position from the professional clinical societies. The goal was to achieve quality assurance of the clinical reports in asylum and immigration law. Currently, this is the official training curriculum of the German Medical Association; such training is available on a regular basis in different Federal States. On the homepage www.sbpm.de, not only the current dates can be found but also a plethora of specific professional literature and structuring statements and assessment reports.
- *The UN's Istanbul Protocol* was developed by international experts under the auspices of the UNHCR in Istanbul and published by the UN in 2004. Here, the focus is on the documentation of mental and physical signs of torture rather than on the general consequences of experiencing violence, for example, in the context of displacement. The Istanbul Protocol provides clinicians in countries of origin with suggestions for professional action in the case of torture and provides clinicians in host countries treating refugees who have experienced torture with approaches for the detection of torture experiences. In the long term, a unified document should also allow the prosecution of the torturers; the necessary medical and legal structures are unfortunately still to be created for this purpose. The homepage www.istanbulprotocol.info is recommended in this context.

References

Acheson DT, Gresack JE, Risbrough VB (2012) Hippocampal dysfunction effects on context memory: possible etiology for posttraumatic stress disorder. Neuropharmacology 62(2):674–685

Amnesty International (2013) Amnesty report 2013: Zahlen und Fakten. Retrieved 22 Oct 2014, from http://www.amnesty.de/2013/5/22/amnesty-report-2013zahlen-und-fakten?destination=n ode%2F23307

Deutschland erhält die meisten Asylanträge (2014) Retrieved 22 Oct 2014, from http://www.welt. de/politik/deutschland/article126035894/Deutschland-erhaelt-die-meisten-Asylantraege.html

Baars EW, van der Hart O, Nijenhuis ER, Chu JA, Glas G, Draijer N (2010) Predicting stabilizing treatment outcomes for complex posttraumatic stress disorder and dissociative identity disorder: an expertise-based prognostic model. J Trauma Dissociation 12(1):67–87

Beagan BL, Kumas-Tan Z (2009) Approaches to diversity in family medicine "I have always tried to be colour blind". Can Fam Physician 55(8):e21–e28

Berger JT (2008) The influence of physicians' demographic characteristics and their patients' demographic characteristics on physician practice: implications for education and research. Acad Med 83(1):100–105

Birck A (2002) Traumatisierte Flüchtlinge: wie glaubhaft sind ihre Aussagen? Asanger, Heidelberg

Brenneis CB (1998) Gedächtnissysteme und der psychoanalytische Abruf von Trauma-Erinnerungen. Psyche 52(9/10):801–823

Bundesamt für Migration und Flüchtlinge (Federal Office for Immigration and Refugees) (2013) Aktuelle Zahlen zu Asyl. (Current Statistics on Asylum). Retrieved 23 Dec 2013 from http:// www.bamf.de/SharedDocs/Anlagen/DE/Downloads/Infothek/Statistik/statistik-anlage-teil-4-aktuelle-zahlen-zu-asyl.pdf?__blob=publicationFile

Cervantes RC, Salgado de Snyder VN, Padilla AM (1989) Posttraumatic stress in immigrants from Central America and Mexico. Hosp Community Psychiatry 40(6):615–619

Cheung P (1993) Somatisation as a presentation in depression and post-traumatic stress disorder among Cambodian refugees. Aust N Z J Psychiatry 27(3):422–428

Eisenman DP, Gelberg L, Liu H, Shapiro MF (2003) Mental health and health related quality of life among adult Latino primary care patients living in the United States with previous exposure to political violence. JAMA 290(5):627–634

Engel CC Jr, Liu X, Clymer R, Miller RF, Sjoberg T, Shapiro JR (2000) Rehabilitative care of war-related health concerns. J Occup Environ Med 42(4):385–390

Fazel M, Wheeler J, Danesh J (2005) Prevalence of serious mental disorder in 7000 refugees resettled in western countries: a systematic review. Lancet 365(9467):1309–1314

Fisher HL, Jones PB, Fearon P, Craig TK, Dazzan P, Morgan K (2010) The varying impact of type, timing and frequency of exposure to childhood adversity on its association with adult psychotic disorder. Psychol Med 40(12):1967–1978

Gäbel U, Ruf M, Schauer M, Odenwald M, Neuner F (2006) Prävalenz der posttraumatischen Belastungsstörung (PTSD) und Möglichkeiten der Ermittlung in der Asylverfahrenspraxis. Z Klin Psychol Psychother 35(1):12–20

Gerritsen AA, Bramsen I, Devillé W, Van Willigen LH, Hovens JE, Van Der Ploeg HM (2006) Physical and mental health of Afghan, Iranian and Somali asylum seekers and refugees living in the Netherlands. Soc Psychiatry Psychiatr Epidemiol 41(1):18–26

Gierlichs HW, van Keuk E, Greve C, Wenk-Ansohn M, Flatten G, Hartmann C, Wirtgen W (2005) Grenzen und Möglichkeiten klinischer Gutachten imAusländerrecht. ZAR–Z Ausländerrecht Ausländerpolitik 158:163

Haenel F, Wenk-Ansohn M (eds) (2004) Begutachtung psychisch reaktiver Traumafolgen in aufenthaltsrechtlichen Verfahren. Beltz, Weinheim

Hinton DE, Hinton SD, Loeum RJR, Pich V, Pollack MH (2008) The 'multiplex model' of somatic symptoms: application to tinnitus among traumatized Cambodian refugees. Transcult Psychiatry 45(2):287–317

Hofmann A, Fischer G, Koehn F (1999) Traumatic antecedents questionnaire (TAQ). Deutsches Institut für Psychotraumatologie, Köln

Holtan N, Antolak K, Johnson DR, Ide L, Jaranson J, Ta K (2002) Unrecognized torture affects the health of refugees. Minn Med 85(5):35–39

Ivezic S, Bagaric A, Oruc L, Mimica N, Ljubin T (2000) Psychotic symptoms and comorbid psychiatric disorders in Croatian combat-related posttraumatic stress disorder patients. Croat Med J 41(2):179–183

Janet P, Paul E (1925) Psychological healing: a historical and clinical study, vol 1. G. Allen & Unwin, London

Johnson H, Thompson A (2008) The development and maintenance of post traumatic stress disorder (PTSD) in civilian adult survivors of war trauma and torture: a review. Clin Psychol Rev 28(1):36–47

Joksimovic L (2009) Ethnosoziokultureller Leitfaden für die interkulturelle Psychotherapie mit Migranten aus dem ehemaligen Jugoslawien. In: Erim Y (ed) Klinische Interkulturelle Psychotherapie. Ein Lehr-und Praxisbuch. Kohlhammer, Stuttgart, pp 288–292

Joksimovic L (2010) Diversity-Kompetenz bei der ärztlichen Untersuchung: Von Symptomen zur Diagnose. In: van Keuk E, Ghaderi C, Joksimovic L, David DM (eds) Diversity: transkulturelle Kompetenz in klinischen und sozialen Arbeitsfeldern. Kohlhammer Verlag, Stuttgart, pp 135–145

Joksimovic L, Woeller W, Happ M, Tress W, Kruse J (2011) Group psychotherapy with traumatised refugees. Gruppenpsychotherapie Gruppendynamik 47(3):192–210

Joksimovic L, Kunzke D, Wöller W (2013) Pharmakotherapeutische Interventionen in der Psychotherapie von schweren Traumafolgestörungen: Grundsätzliche Überlegungen anhand einer Fallstudie. Z Psychosom Med Psychother 59(4):378–384

Junghanss T (1998) Asylsuchende und Flüchtlinge: Gesundheitsversorgung einer komplexen Minderheit. Soz Praventivmed/Soc Prev Med 43(1):11–17

Klimidis S, Stuart G, Minas IH, Ata AW (1994) Immigrant status and gender effects on psychopathology and self-concept in adolescents: a test of the migration-morbidity hypothesis. Compr Psychiatry 35(5):393–404

Kluge U, Kassim N (2006) Der Dritte im Raum – Chancen und Schwierigkeiten in der Zusammenarbeit mit Sprach- und KulturmittlerInnen in einem interkulturellenpsychotherapeutischen Setting. In: Wohlfart E, Zaumseil M (eds) Transkulturelle Psychiatrie – Interkulturelle Psychotherapie. InterdisziplinäreTheorie und Praxis. Springer, Heidelberg, pp 178–198

Kroll J, Yusuf AI, Fujiwara K (2011) Psychoses, PTSD, and depression in Somali refugees in Minnesota. Soc Psychiatry Psychiatr Epidemiol 46(6):481–493

Kruse J, Joksimovic L, Cavka M, Wöller W, Schmitz N (2009) Effects of trauma-focused psychotherapy upon war refugees. J Trauma Stress 22(6):585–592

Kunzke D, Güls F (2003) Diagnostik einfacher und komplexer posttraumatischer Störungen im Erwachsenenalter. Psychotherapeutische 48(1):50–70

Laban CJ, Gernaat HB, Komproe IH, Schreuders BA, De Jong JT (2004) Impact of a long asylum procedure on the prevalence of psychiatric disorders in Iraqi asylum seekers in The Netherlands. J Nerv Ment Dis 192(12):843–851

Laban CJ, Gernaat HB, Komproe IH, van der Tweel I, De Jong JT (2005) Postmigration living problems and common psychiatric disorders in Iraqi asylum seekers in the Netherlands. J Nerv Ment Dis 193(12):825–832

Larkin W, Read J (2008) Childhood trauma and psychosis: evidence, pathways, and implications. J Postgrad Med 54(4):287

Lin EH, Carter WB, Kleinman AM (1985) An exploration of somatization among Asian refugees and immigrants in primary care. Am J Public Health 75(9):1080–1084

Markowitsch HJ (1998) The mnestic block syndrome: environmentally induced amnesia. Neurol Psychiatry Brain Res 6(2):73–80

Marshall GN, Schell TL, Elliott MN, Berthold SM, Chun CA (2005) Mental health of Cambodian refugees 2 decades after resettlement in the United States. JAMA 294(5):571–579

Mollica RF, Sarajlić N, Chernoff M, Lavelle J, Vuković IS, Massagli MP (2001) Longitudinal study of psychiatric symptoms, disability, mortality, and emigration among Bosnian refugees. JAMA 286(5):546–554

Reddemann L (2004) Psychodynamisch imaginative traumatherapie (PITT)—das manual [psychodynamic imaginative trauma therapy—the manual]. Pfeiffer bei Klett-Cotta, Stuttgart

Reddemann L, Sachsse U (1998) Welche Psychoanalyse ist für Opfer geeignet? Einige Anmerkungen zu Martin Ehlert-Balzer: Das Trauma als Objektbeziehung. Forum Psychoanal 14:289–294

Reddemann L, Sachsse U (2000) Traumazentrierte Psychotherapie der chronifizierten, komplexen posttraumatischen Belastungsstörung vom Phänotyp der Borderline-Persönlichkeitsstörungen. In: Kernberg O, Dulz B, Sachsse U (eds) Handbuch der Borderline-Störungen. Schattauer, Stuttgart, pp 555–571

Schreiber S (1995) Migration, traumatic bereavement and transcultural aspects of psychological healing: loss and grief of a refugee woman from Begameder county in Ethiopia. Br J Med Psychol 68(2):135–142

Shevlin M, Houston JE, Dorahy MJ, Adamson G (2008) Cumulative traumas and psychosis: an analysis of the national comorbidity survey and the British Psychiatric Morbidity Survey. Schizophr Bull 34(1):193–199

Silove D, Sinnerbrink I, Field A, Manicavasagar V, Steel Z (1997) Anxiety, depression and PTSD in asylum-seekers: assocations with pre-migration trauma and post-migration stressors. Br J Psychiatry 170(4):351–357

Silove D, Steel Z, Bauman A, Chey T, McFarlane A (2007) Trauma, PTSD and the longer-term mental health burden amongst Vietnamese refugees. Soc Psychiatry Psychiatr Epidemiol 42(6):467–476

Smedley BD, Stith AY, Nelson AR (2009) Unequal treatment: confronting racial and ethnic disparities in health care (with CD). National Academies Press, Washington

Sundquist J (1993a) Ethnicity as a risk factor for mental illness. A population-based study of 338 Latin American refugees and 996 age-, sex- and education-matched Swedish controls. Acta Psychiatr Scand 87(3):208–212

Sundquist J (1993b) Ethnicity; social class and health. A population-based study on the influence of social factors on self-reported illness in 223 Latin American refugees, 333 Finnish and 126 south European labour migrants and 841 Swedish controls. Soc Sci Med 40(6):777–787

Tschischka A (2014) Viele Flüchtlinge sind auch Folteropfer!. Retrieved 11 Jul 2014, from http://www.bdp-verband.org/bdp/presse/2014/09_folteropfer.html

Tucker S, Price D (2007) Finding a home: group psychotherapy for traumatized refugees and asylum seekers. Eur J Psychother Couns 9(3):277–287

United Nations High Commissioner for Refugees (UNHCR) (2012) Displacement, the new 21st century challenge: global trends. Retrieved 23 Dec 2013, from http://www.unhcr.org/51bacb0f9.html

van der Kolk BA, McFarlane AC, van der Hart O (1996) A general approach to treatment of posttraumatic stress disorder. In: van der Kolk BA, McFarlane AC, Weisaeth L (eds) Traumatic stress: the effects of overwhelming experience on mind, body, and society. Guilford Press, New York, pp 417–440

van der Kolk BA, Burbridge JA, Suzuki J (1998) Die Psychobiologie traumatischer Erinnerungen. In: Streeck-Fischer A (ed) Adoleszenz und Trauma. Vandenhoek & Ruprecht, Göttingen, pp 57–78

Warfa N, Curtis S, Watters C, Carswell K, Ingleby D, Bhui K (2012) Migration experiences, employment status and psychological distress among Somali immigrants: a mixed-method international study. BMC Public Health 12(1):749

Wenk Ansohn A, Scheef Maier G, Gierlichs HW (2013) Zur Begutachtung psychischer Traumafolgestörungen – ein Update. In: Feldmann RE, Seidler GH (eds) Traum(a) Migration. Aktuelle Konzepte zur Therapie traumatisierter Flüchtlinge und Folteropfer. Psychosozial Verlag, Gießen, pp 283–302

Wessa ML, Flor H (2002) Posttraumatische Belastungsstörung und Traumagedächtnis – eine psy-
    chobiologische Perspektive. Z Psychosom Med Psychother 48:28–37
Wöller W, Leichsenring F, Leweke F, Kruse J (2012) Psychodynamic psychotherapy for posttrau-
    matic stress disorder related to childhood abuse – Principles for a treatment manual. Bull
    Menninger Clin 76:69–93
Yehuda R (2002) Post-traumatic stress disorder. N Engl J Med 346:108–114

A Therapy Model for Traumatised Refugees in Denmark

Marianne C. Kastrup and Klement Dymi

Resume

This chapter will present Danish 'models' of caring/treatment for traumatised refugees. It begins by covering the historical aspects of the work with traumatised refugees in Denmark, then gives a brief overview of immigration in the country; this is followed by a brief description of the general health services and the network of special services for this category of patients. The services and the treatment they offer are then described, focusing on the types of the different therapies used and the evidence of their effect and concluding with a few points on current developments and perspectives.

Introduction

There are over 450.000 immigrants, including refugees, in Denmark. About 30 % of the refugees are traumatised. For these refugees, the first contact with the Danish healthcare system often takes place in the asylum centres/facilities and is carried out by healthcare personnel employed in these facilities; alternatively, they may give the person a referral. For the rest, the first contact is with the GP/family doctors that all with a residence permit are assigned. The GPs may refer the traumatised refugees or immigrants to psychiatric specialists/services or to specialised institutions for

M.C. Kastrup, MD, PhD
Specialist in Psychiatry, Amalievej 23, DK-1875 Frederiksberg, Denmark
e-mail: Marianne.kastrup@dadlnet.dk

K. Dymi, MD, MIH (✉)
Competence Centre for Transcultural Psychiatry, Ballerup Psychiatric Centre,
Copenhagen, Denmark
e-mail: klementdymi@yahoo.com

© Springer International Publishing Switzerland 2015
M. Schouler-Ocak (ed.), *Trauma and Migration:*
Cultural Factors in the Diagnosis and Treatment of Traumatised Immigrants,
DOI 10.1007/978-3-319-17335-1_16

treating trauma. In order to understand the particular profile of the Danish health-care system and the possibilities and actual care given to traumatised patients, we will briefly describe its main features.

Historical Aspects

Human rights violations have always been part of human history. As pointed out by Eitinger and Weisæth (1998), violations including torture have long been used as a way not only to deal with the defeated enemy as a tool to demonstrate superiority, but also as a way to keep people on the 'right track'; those that abjured could be accused of being disbelievers and subjected to various violations. Over the course of history, various regimes have used such methods for the above reasons. However, these methods have also been used in order to punish criminals or extract a confession.

In many places on the Latin American continent, human rights violations have been widespread and systematic for a long time, often related to political move-ments and oppressing regimes. The victims of these violations were often affiliated with various ideological and social movements and had an above-average educa-tional and social status. Many of the survivors were compelled to emigrate and sought refuge and treatment in other countries, mainly in the West, where their cause became first known and their accounts have caused both indignation and action among those who volunteered to help as described here.

With Western society's increasing political focus on the human rights of its citi-zens, an emerging interest has developed in urging governments to refrain from practising human rights violations towards their citizens. Nonetheless, several total-itarian regimes have continued the practice (that was also practiced towards citizens in colonial settings) stating that the violations were carried out for a purpose that justified the practice.

It is worth mentioning that professional communities (e.g. physicians or psy-chologists) have shown surprisingly little concern about such practices over the years (Eitinger and Weisæth 1998). The consequences of such atrocities on the physical and mental health of the victims have also received limited attention historically.

In fact, the recognition that trauma and human rights violations have physical and mental health consequences upon those inflicted does not date back for long. Until recently, the prevailing assumption was that primarily those with a weak con-stitution or a genetic disposition would suffer long-term consequences in relation to exposure to such events and be unable to cope with it.

However, World War II meant a shift, in the sense that it became evident that the atrocities that took place in the concentration camps and the Japanese prisoner-of-war camps had deleterious consequences for those experiencing them irrespective of their background and previous health.

Research carried out in Denmark and Norway (Rasmussen 1990) demonstrated clearly that survivors of concentration camps, even years after their liberation, showed a higher mortality and more serious morbidity than the remaining population (Eitinger and Strøm 1973). Nevertheless, despite this knowledge, violations and torture have continued as a means to suppress the opposition in a given society, or under the name of the 'fight against terror', to violate persons suspected of terrorist activities.

Democracy and civilisation *progress everyday* (meaning that there is a movement towards democracy as the optimal system of government all around the world), but war, persecution and torture continue to be present, and all those with a conscience and a will to fight for justice have a duty to continue their struggle. From this perspective, it is crucial to remember these objectives and the history to which they relate. Immigration and trauma are dynamic social phenomena that are here to stay, and books such as this one will be needed increasingly, but technical and professional/medical activities cannot be separated from the human rights aspects of this issue and can only succeed by going hand in hand.

The Initiation of Therapeutic Interventions

The initiative to start therapeutic interventions directed towards victims of traumatisation is largely the result of the interest expressed by Amnesty International, surprisingly. This human rights organisation, although it does not focus on the therapeutic dimensions, has a significant interest in documenting human rights violations. Part of this documentation resulted in an appeal by Amnesty International in 1973 to the medical profession globally for help to combat torture and to participate in fact-finding investigations around the world (Kastrup et al. 1987). As a result, the first medical group in Amnesty International was founded in Denmark in 1974, with the primary aim of verifying and providing documentation, through systematic investigations of persons who reported having been submitted to human rights violations, whether or not such violations had indeed taken place. The main reason for such investigations was to be able to document – based on solid medical evidence – that violations had occurred and subsequently to use these findings in later court cases directed towards the perpetrators. In other words, the focus was not on treatment per se, but on achieving justice for the victims by bringing their perpetrators to court.

However, these many medical investigations carried out by concerned physicians in several countries revealed that, to a large degree, those who had been subjected to violations manifested a number of both physical and psychological sequelae and that these health problems required medical interventions. Having documented this, an obvious question followed: how and where should such treatment take place?

Following an international Amnesty International seminar in 1978, an international working group was established with the objective of outlining a treatment proposal for the victims. In 1979, a subsequent seminar took place in Copenhagen, organised again by the medical group of Amnesty International (Kastrup et al. 1987) with the main objective of outlining practical initiatives to help the victims. One of the conclusions was that the establishment of an institution with the aim of rehabilitating these victims was needed but that such an organisation was seen as being outside the authority of Amnesty International. As the Danish medical group was so prominent in the work, it was decided that members of this group should take the initiative to found this establishment, and subsequently the International Rehabilitation and Research Centre for Torture Victims (RCT) was established in Copenhagen in 1983.

Since then, the treatment approach that was established in 1983 has undergone continuous development to evolve into the treatment that is offered today. There was also a focus on monitoring the health and rehabilitation of torture survivors (Bøjholm et al. 1992). The present reality was made possible by the efforts and dedication of a group of people, mainly medical professionals, who for decades have worked to collect evidence about violations, help the victims in many ways and fight against impunity for the perpetrators of human rights violations who are the cause of trauma and suffering of thousands. The pioneers of this field in Denmark are Inge Genefke and others – they have inspired many and created a tradition in this highly humanistic battle and still continue to inspire many today. Further, we have seen the establishment of a number of other organisations, both in Denmark and internationally, which focus on the treatment of traumatised refugees. Some of them use the same approach to treatment and rehabilitation as the International Rehabilitation and Research Centre (now DIGNITY – Danish Institute Against Torture) (Jaranson and Quiroga 2011; www.dignityinstitute.dk); some use other approaches.

Statistical and Brief History of Immigration in DK

At the beginning of 2013, around half a million immigrants (including refugees and their descendants) were living in Denmark – out of a total population of 5.6 million people. Up until 1998, the majority of immigrants and refugees had a Christian background, followed closely by Muslims, the share of which was approaching that of the Christians. In 1999, the curves crossed each other, and until 2008, the largest proportion had a Muslim background. In 2009, the picture changed again, and since then, Christians once again make up the largest group of immigrants.

From 2005, Denmark has operated a flexible quota of 1,500 places for refugees (foreign citizens who are at immediate risk of refoulement to their country of origin or who risk assaults in their country of stay) and an extramedical category (foreign citizens with special medical needs).

Of the current immigrant population, approximately 18 % come from EU countries, 35 % from other European countries, 10 % come from Africa and a further 31 % from Asia and Middle Eastern countries. A large proportion of refugees have been subjected to human rights violations. This group is culturally mixed, and there is a high prevalence of post-traumatic stress disorder (PTSD) and co-morbid illnesses. A study from 2007 among Danish asylum seekers found 33 countries of origin, the largest groups coming from Afghanistan, Iraq, Iran, Syria and Chechnya (Masmas et al. 2008). Of the 142 examined asylum seekers, 45 % had experienced torture and 63 % of these lived up to the diagnostic criteria for PTSD. Moreover, co-morbidity of anxiety, depression and chronic pain, both somatic and musculo-skeletal, respectively, has a high prevalence among traumatised refugees with PTSD.

Outline of Health Services in Denmark (With Focus to Treatment of Trauma)

The Danish health system is characterised by being decentralised and single-funded.

The hospital sector is public, and hospitals are financed and run by the five regions (with only a very small private hospital sector alongside). General practitioners are private entrepreneurs but work under contract for the regions. Hospitals are financed by national/governmental budgets, while general practitioners are paid by a mixed remuneration system. During the past 20 years, the government has repeatedly imposed budget ceilings on the regions, limiting growth in the healthcare sector.

Family doctors (i.e. general practitioners) are usually refugees' first contact with the health services; they therefore function as gatekeepers to psychiatric institutions and/or trauma centres.

The five regions provide the vast majority of mental health services in the country and are responsible for the provision of psychiatric care by psychiatric centres with inpatient and outpatient facilities as well as community psychiatric services.

Denmark has 98 municipalities, which span from small island communities of only a few thousand inhabitants to the city of Copenhagen with more than 500,000 inhabitants. Given these differences, the conditions for fulfilling their obligations in relation to provision of social and primary health services vary considerably.

Public and Private Institutions, Organisations and Units Offering Specialised Treatment to Traumatised Refugees in Denmark

Previously, immigrants and refugees with PTSD were neglected by the Danish general psychiatric services, and even now, the present treatment capacity in the specialised, interdisciplinary treatment facilities is insufficient. The effectiveness of the treatment and rehabilitation programmes has yet to be studied and documented.

In 2001, a working group under the auspices of the Ministry of Health concluded, in relation to the rehabilitation of traumatised refugees, that treatment possibilities in Denmark were unevenly distributed by the healthcare system as a whole. Furthermore, long waiting lists were reported for the treatment facilities. Overall, there was a need to develop and improve treatment services to this population. Since then, many initiatives have taken place. According to the National Board of Health Specialisation Plan for Psychiatric Care, all five regions should run a specialised service focusing on the treatment of traumatised refugees as part of the public mental health services. Highly specialised services to this population should further be provided by one to two of the regional services. The treatment is offered mainly to refugees with residence in Denmark or Danish nationals who formerly had a refugee status and have been exposed to trauma and/or torture as a result of war or other political or organised violence.

Patients with PTSD, including traumatised refugees, generally have a higher incidence of both somatisation and physical disorders than the general population. This may mean an increased consumption of primary healthcare, increased prescriptions and ultimately excess mortality, as well as indirect costs such as reduced quality of life, long-term disability and the social and family burden constituted by the suffering.

There are specific and persistent physical, medical and social problems for those living as a traumatised refugee in exile, in addition to the symptoms that are included in the diagnosis of PTSD. To diagnose a traumatised refugee with PTSD does not include the whole range of complexity of the effects of torture and traumatic events; life in exile is in itself associated with problems concerning social adjustment and isolation, loss of socioeconomic status, separation from family members and the like.

Furthermore, there is evidence that if left untreated, PTSD may run a chronic and life-long course. As a consequence, this may lead to mental, physical and social disability, in turn resulting in considerable human and social costs.

Institutions in Denmark Focusing on Traumatised Refugees

The institutions that either are part of the Danish public health services or have a contract with them include:

1. *Capital Region*:
    1.1. Competence Centre for Transcultural Psychiatry (CTP)
        Treatment comprises contact with psychiatrist, psychologist and social worker. It includes psychopharmacological therapy, psychoeducation, structured cognitive therapy and psychosocial support.
        Treatment lasts approximately 6 months and is individual. It is highly *manualised* and all data is used in research with the purpose of demonstrating evidence of the treatment offered.
        Apart from the public organisations, two other organisations in the capital region treating traumatised refugees have a contract allowing public funding:
        DIGNITY (Danish Institute Against Torture) and Oasis
    1.2. DIGNITY (former RCT)
        DIGNITY is a self-governing institution that has gained specialised knowledge and experience on the basis of which the interventions of DIGNITY's partners in the South are developed and targeted.

The interdisciplinary treatment includes contact with medical doctor, psychologist, social worker and physiotherapist and possibility for referral to psychiatrist.

Treatment includes psychotherapy, physiotherapy and psychopharmaco-logical therapy, may be individual, group or family-oriented and typically lasts between 6 months and 1 year.

DIGNITY carries out a number of projects and programmes within research and international development, some of them financed by DANIDA (www.dignityinstitute.dk). In addition to providing hundreds of torture survivors from all world regions with rehabilitation, DIGNITY is a leading research and documentation centre on the methods of torture and its effects on human beings.

1.3.   Oasis

Treatment includes contact with a psychologist, social worker and body therapist. Therapy may include somatic experiencing, cognitive therapy, systemic therapy, psychodynamic, narrative therapy and mentalisation-based therapy. Referral to a psychiatrist is possible. Treatment is individual, in groups or family-based. Treatment usually lasts between 6 months and 1 year.

2. *Zealand Region*

Clinic for Traumatised Refugees

Treatment consists of psychoeducation, individual psychotherapy, body therapy, music therapy, acupuncture and psychosocial support. There is a possibility for referral to a medical specialist for psychopharmacological treatment. Treatment lasts 6–18 months.

3. *Middle Denmark Region*

Clinic for PTSD and Transcultural Psychiatry (KFTF)

This is a treatment institution under Aarhus University Hospital, for traumatised refugees, transcultural patients and Danish war veterans. It has a new, revised treatment concept and also offers treatment to young refugees with war-related trauma. This centre has a broader scope, compared to CTP or DIGNITY, for example, these being focused almost solely on traumatised refugees.

The clinic treats refugees and migrant patients who have a need for an interdisciplinary treatment approach, with grave psychosocial and health problems following imprisonment and torture or other war-related experiences. The treatment includes contact with a psychologist, physiotherapist and social worker and includes psychotherapy, physiotherapy, psychoeducation, health issues interview and contact with a psychiatrist for psychopharmacological treatment. It may also include workshop activities and other social activities. The treatment period is around 4–6 months. The clinic invites the relevant partners to cooperation meetings – most often the patient's own doctor and the communal case supervisor, e.g. for treatment of co-morbid somatic illness.

4. *Northern Region*

Rehabilitation centre for refugees

Treatment is interdisciplinary and includes contact with a psychologist and physiotherapist.

Further contact with a social worker and psychiatrist is offered according to need.

Treatment may be combined with a municipal offer to socially rehabilitate the patient.

The treatment duration is around 9 months.

5. *Southern Denmark Region*

ATT Department for Trauma and Torture Survivors

Based upon the results from the MTA report (see below), patients are divided into three groups, whereby those with:

1. High bio-psychosocial resources will be offered initial mentalising psychother- apy and then individual treatment.
2. Medium bio-psychosocial resources will be offered mentalising psychotherapy and symptom-based group therapy.
3. Low bio-psychosocial resources will be offered individual psychoeducation and resource-supportive treatment at home. Treatment combines psychological, somatic and social aspects.

Psychotherapy includes individual home-based treatment, mentalising-based group treatment with B-BAT physiotherapy, group therapy and possibility of referral to psychiatrist and possible psychopharmacological treatment.

An important source of information and guidance on matters related to treatment and care for traumatised refugees is a website called 'trauma.dk', which was established and maintained by a group of organisations active in the field (www. traume.dk).

Outside mental health services, a recent development has been the establishment of two migrant health clinics as part of departments of infectious medicine services at two university hospitals in Copenhagen and Odense. Both clinics provide gen- eral medical help to migrants exhibiting complicated medical problems, these frequently having a prominent psychiatric component, but there is no direct clini- cal connection to psychiatric clinics.

Medical Technology Assessment

In 2008, the Southern Denmark Region published a report (Lund et al. 2008) that was an outcome of inquiries on a literature review of evidence on treatment and rehabilitation of patients with PTSD, with particular reference to traumatised refu- gees. The review is summarised from a medical technology assessment perspective, a concept that covers the procedures and methods for examination, care, prevention, treatment and rehabilitation. The purpose of this MTA report was to clarify and summarise the current evidence on the treatment and rehabilitation of patients with PTSD, including traumatised refugees, based on a systematic literature review. Among multidisciplinary, specialised efforts, what forms of treatment improve the outcome for patients with PTSD? What kind of organisation is optimal for the inter- disciplinary specialised treatment of patients with PTSD, including traumatised refugees?

The report is not intended as a guideline for the diagnosis, treatment and rehabilitation of patients with PTSD or as a thorough discussion and analysis of the concept of PTSD in relation to traumatised refugees. The report should be seen as a statement of the evidence for treatment and rehabilitation of patients with PTSD, including traumatised refugees, based on a systematic literature review supplemented by expert knowledge.

The MTA report is a major contribution in the field, but has also drawn criticism from professionals for accepting guidelines on the treatment of traumatised refugees which are not grounded in sound evidence-based knowledge (Nyberg et al. 2011). The report is also criticised for being a basis for promoting unqualified decision-making in a political context with diminished economic resources where there is risk that decision makers would easily fall for the illusion that complex problems can be solved in an easy and far too cheap way – it is cheaper to pay a 'mentalising therapist' than an interdisciplinary treatment team. In relation to the length of the treatment period, the illusion is already a reality in several places as several regions have shortened their treatment: the report promotes one favoured treatment model, but does not take into account some good and relevant literature sources, for example, such as the conclusions from the meta-analysis in the Cochrane Collaboration review on psychological treatment for PTSD (Bisson and Andrew 2007).

An Overview of the Different Therapies for Traumatised Refugees Used in Denmark

As is described above, the different organisations have chosen different therapeutic approaches based on tradition, clinical experience or focus on scientific evidence.

Evidence for effective treatment of traumatised refugees is indeed limited, and the need for studies in this field is as great and urgent as the human and societal consequences of costly and ineffective treatments.

The Cochrane review concludes that individual trauma-focused cognitive behavioural therapy (TFCBT), eye movement desensitisation and reprocessing (EMDR), stress management and group TFCBT are all effective in the treatment of PTSD (Buhmann 2014). It highlights that trauma-focused treatments are more effective than non-trauma-focused treatments.

A couple of follow-up studies on traumatised refugees from Denmark without a control group have been published finding limited evidence for improvement in the condition of the patients.

The Competence Centre for Transcultural Psychiatry (CTP)
(www.psykiatri regionh.dk)

The following centre is described in somewhat more detail than other current actors in the field, because from the very beginning of its activity, it has used treatment and research as an integrated well-established practice in the way it functions, with the aim of offering the best known interdisciplinary treatment to its patients. At the CTP, the target group is traumatised refugees with PTSD, depression and anxiety, living in the capital region of Denmark. Patients are referred to CTP by general practitioners or psychiatrists. CTP treats approximately 200 patients per year. The treatment is interdisciplinary and consists of consultations with a psychiatrist whereby pharmacological treatment is prescribed according to best practice in the field and supplemented with cognitive behavioural therapy by a psychologist. Manuals are used both for the treatment given by the medical doctor and by the psychologist. With the aim of increasing knowledge about the effect of different types of treatment for traumatised refugees, several randomised clinical trials have been completed or are being undertaken at present in parallel with the treatment since 2009.

Treatments in CTP include a combination of sertraline, mianserin, psychoeducation and trauma-focused cognitive behavioural therapy (TFCBT). The treatment administered to each patient is monitored in detail, and changes in outcome and predictors of change are analysed.

The manualised treatment consists of weekly sessions with a psychiatrist and/or psychologist over a period of 6 months. The treatment effect is evaluated through a combination of self-ratings and blinded and non-blinded observer ratings. Outcome measures include symptoms of PTSD, depression, anxiety, pain and somatisation, quality of life and level of functioning (HTQ, HSCL-25, SCL-90, WHO-5, SDS, VAS, Hamilton, GAF). Treatment is offered using professional interpreters, and screening instruments are translated into the six most common languages in the patient group.

CTP has developed TRIM ('Treatment and Research Integrated Model') – a system that takes the data that clinicians normally entered into medical records and organise the information into checklists instead. From here, the data can be entered directly into a research database. TRIM makes it possible to carry out research on a shoestring budget, and another advantage is that the patients who agree to take part in the research are not stressed by extra activities in connection with their participation. This model also ensures that refugee patients consistently receive best practice treatment based on the latest research findings. This has so far led to revisions of the psychologists' treatment manual for the cross-cultural target group and also to the development of a questionnaire which will improve the understanding of how physiological, psychological and social factors affect the outcome of the treatment for the individual patient. This data will be used to create a culturally adapted and effective treatment for traumatised refugees.

The CTP's primary objectives are to increase our understanding of the effect of medical and psychological treatment for traumatised refugees, to shorten waiting lists and to make treatment more cost-effective. CTP's work has also attracted interest internationally, and on that basis, it is currently setting up collaboration with researchers in Australia, Germany and New Zealand (Sonne 2013).

Since the start of the clinic, systematic data collection is integrated into the daily clinical work, and the patients' condition is evaluated through self-rating scales before and after treatment. Treatment has been manualised from the beginning (manuals based on treatment with sertraline and TFCBT, the best practice treatment of PTSD at that time).

Several studies with code names PTF1–PTF4 (2008 to the present) are also going on in CTP on transcultural trauma patients in Denmark.

The following paragraphs are taken from the newly defended thesis by Buhmann (2014).

PTF1

Buhmann (2014) was a large randomised clinical trial that evaluates the effect of the treatment of a representative sample of chronically traumatised refugee patients living in Denmark, with sertraline in combination with mianserin and psychoeducation TFCBT and a combination of pharmacotherapy and psychotherapy. PTF 1 is the first study with sufficient power and one of the first studies with the strength of a waiting list comparison, as well as being one of the first studies separating pharmacotherapy and psychotherapy in traumatised refugees. It thereby accounts for any effects due to spontaneous recovery, and treatment modalities are examined separately and in combination.

Two hundred seventeen patients completed treatment. A small but significant effect of treatment with antidepressants sertraline and mianserin and psychoeducation was found in depression and anxiety symptoms, headache and self-rated level of functioning. A large significant effect was found in level of functioning after treatment with medicine compared to waiting list controls. No effect of psychotherapy was detected, and there was no interaction between psychotherapy and medicine. No effect was found of TFCBT as it is implemented in this trial, and there was no interaction between treatment with antidepressants and psychotherapy and therefore no added effect of psychotherapy. Treatment with antidepressants, sertraline and mianserin is promising, and adverse reactions associated with the treatment are limited.

Moderate changes in symptoms of PTSD, anxiety and depression, level of functioning and quality of life on self-rating scales were found. This stands in contrast to the otherwise scarce evidence of the treatment of traumatised refugees and other PTSD patients, which indicates that an added effect can exist when combining psychotherapy and medicine in the treatment of PTSD. PTF 1 found no effect of treatment on PTSD, in contrast to other studies of traumatised refugees.

Despite methodological limitations, the finding of a significant improvement on all rating scales is important, considering that previous follow-up studies of comparable patient populations have not found significant change in the patients' condition after treatment. The study showed statistically significant changes in the condition of the patients from assessment before treatment to follow-up. Other Scandinavian studies have found little or no change in patient condition after treatment.

PTF2

Studies of treatment efficacy in PTSD suggest an effect of cognitive behavioural therapy (CBT) including primary trauma-focused cognitive behavioural therapy (TF-CBT). Some studies among traumatised refugees also suggest that cognitive therapies can be effective in this patient group. However, there are no studies of whether any form of cognitive therapy is better suited than others for traumatised refugees. This study aims to investigate the efficacy of CBT with a focus on stress management and, respectively, cognitive restructuring. Patients are randomly assigned to psychotherapy focusing on either stress management or cognitive restructuring, and everyone also receives standard medical treatment as described in PTF's medical manual (2011) (www.psykiatri.regionh.dk).

PTF3

Overall, there are recommendations for larger studies of a homogeneous group of patients with PTSD, a combination of evidence-based pharmacological treatment and psychotherapy and assessment of social functioning. These are the recommendations this study will attempt to address. The effect of two different types of pharmacotherapy (sertraline and venlafaxine) is being studied in combination with manual-based cognitive behavioural therapy (MB-CBT). Changes in social functioning in the course of treatment will be compared with changes in PTSD and depression symptoms. At the same time, the MTA report's recommendation on the division of patients into groups according to expected gains in relation to resources is addressed, and the question of whether such a division is related to real treatment benefits for patients will be examined (www.psykiatri.regionh.dk).

PTF4

Treatment of traumatised refugees: the effect of basic body awareness therapy versus mixed physical activity as add-on treatment

The aim of the study is to examine whether physical activity as an add-on treatment to the usual psychiatric treatment gives an increased effect compared to psychiatric treatment only, in terms of mental symptoms (PTSD, depression and anxiety), quality of life, functional capacity, coping with pain and body awareness (www.psykiatri.regionh.dk).

Future Perspectives for Treatment of Traumatised Refugees in Denmark

As is evident from the overview, the various treatments available in the regions and the various institutions in Denmark have many similarities, but also some differences:

Similarities	Differences
Assessment is typically done by using structured interviews, ratings scales, e.g. Harvard trauma questionnaire, SCL-90, GAF, WHO-5	Access to psychiatrist
Multidisciplinary work – all provide this	Availability of physiotherapy
Individual psychotherapy is provided by all	Treatment of somatic complaints
Psychosocial counselling is provided by all	Availability of group therapy
Psychoeducation provided by all	Other kinds of therapy, e.g. music, body workshop training

In a country the size of Denmark, one may wonder why there are such differences in the treatment provided for the same population, namely, traumatised refugees, and why there are no national guidelines available.

Several reasons may be given. One reason is that the five regions have a high degree of autonomy when it comes to provision of healthcare in their region, so differences may be due to their prioritising of this treatment.

Another reason could be that the differences are a reflection of different sizes of the traumatised population and thereby different needs in the different regions.

A third reason could be that the treatment offered reflects differences in the availability of professionals, e.g. a shortage of qualified psychiatrists in some areas of the country.

A fourth reason may be historical, namely, that a new treatment facility was originally established as a contrast to another treatment model that was, for example, too medically oriented.

A fifth reason may be that, despite having a multidisciplinary approach, different centres nevertheless have a particular interest or expertise in a certain treatment (e.g. music therapy) that may not be available elsewhere.

All in all, this shows that there is still a long way to go until we have a uniform approach to treatment which is based on evidence and acceptable for all.

Concerns

When wanting to optimise treatment, a number of concerns arise, as listed below:

1. Re: the target population

   We have to be aware that the population of traumatised refugees is far from a homogeneous population, although this is often how the group is perceived by administrators. On the contrary, it includes persons with very different backgrounds in terms of education, religion, economic status, etc. as well as very different resources that need to be taken into consideration when planning services.

2. Re: staff

   There is a need to ensure that staff possess the necessary cultural competence to manage patients of different cultural and ethnic backgrounds and that there is an awareness of the important impact that trauma may have on the general psychiatric morbidity and manifestation of symptoms, also among patients suffering from other psychiatric disorders. Working more frequently with interpreters requires that staff are trained to do so.

3. Re: services

   Treatment of traumatised refugees started outside the public health services at highly specialised institutions. Over time, however, we have seen a movement of the therapeutic activities towards mainstream public services, thereby providing the possibility of inspiring the mental health services in general to have a larger focus on the impact of trauma as well as cultural matters. It is also important to be aware that working with interpreters requires extra time and resources.

4. Re: research

There is an urgent need for robust research focusing on determining which interventions show maximum evidence. Furthermore, there is a need for identifying factors that have predictive value in determining who may benefit from a given intervention and thereby providing the possibility of focussing interventions on those patients.

In relation to the population	In relation to staff	In relation to services	In relation to research
Traumatised refugees are a multifaceted group with diverse needs – not a uniform population or a homogeneous group as there is tendency to see them	Enhancement of the cultural competence of staff	Complexity of clinical cases presented – compared with local population	Need for robust results related to evidence of treatment
Lack of data about the size of the population, its socio-demographic profile, its utilisation of services	Language barriers with training in the use of interpreters	Patients may have difficulty choosing the appropriate service for a given problem	Evaluate short-term treatment in order to fulfil unmet needs
	Training in specific topics related to the diagnostics and treatment	Extra resources of manpower and time in clinical management	Need to identify factors that predict who may benefit from intervention
		Need for information, etc. in different languages	CTP's model of treatment and research, focus on predictors, etc. should be promoted and expanded
		There is no information on whether it is better to be part of public system services or outside them – such as Oasis, etc.	

International Collaboration and Networking

The humanistic attitude and a high level of solidarity are characteristics of the Danish healthcare system in general and especially of the array of institutions and organisations mentioned above that are involved in the care and treatment of traumatised refugees in Denmark.

A broad understanding of the issues and an open and active attitude are among those factors that characterise the activities in this field in Denmark and that make it an obvious and necessary obligation to communicate and network with colleagues and institutions in other countries, related to treatment and research exchanges and mutual support. In this era of globalisation, this feature is increasingly important and is a factor that promotes and helps the cause of a world without torture and with proper care of the victims of violence worldwide.

References

Bisson J, Andrew M (2007) Psychological treatment of post-traumatic stress disorder (PTSD). Cochrane Database Syst Rev 3, CD003388

Bøjholm S, Foldspang A, Juhler M, Kastrup M, Skylv G, Somnier F (1992) Monitoring the health and rehabilitation of torture survivors. RCT, Copenhagen

Buhmann CB (2014) Traumatized refugees: morbidity, treatment and predictors of outcome. PhD thesis (code PTF1) defended/approved by the University of Copenhagen on 9.4.2014

Eitinger L, Strøm A (1973) Mortality and morbidity after excessive stress. Humanities Press, New York

Eitinger L, Weisæth L (1998) Torture: history, treatment and medical complicity. In: Jaranson J, Popkin M (eds) Caring for victims of torture. APA Press, Washington

Jaranson J, Quiroga J (2011) Evaluating the services of torture rehabilitation programmes: history and recommendations. Torture 21(2):98–140

Kastrup M, Lunde I, Ortman J, Genefke I (1987) Victimization inside and outside the family: families of torture – consequences and possibilities for rehabilitation. PsychCritique 2(2):337–349

Lund M, Sørensen JH, Christensen JB, Ølholm A, Center for kvalitet, Region Syddanmark (2008) Medical Technologi Vurdering (MTV) om Behandling og Rehabilitering af PTSD – herunder traumatiserede flygtninge. Vejle, Version 1.0. www.regionsyddanmark.dk

Masmas TN et al (2008) Asylum seekers in Denmark – a study of health status and grade of traumatization of newly arrived asylum seekers. Torture 18(2):77–86, Author info [1]Medical Group, Amnesty International, Copenhagen, Denmark

Nyberg V, Nordin L, Harlacher U, Sjölund BH (2011) Hvordan er kvaliteten i de danske MTV-rapporter? Ugeskr Laeger 173(23):1676

Rasmussen OV (1990) Monograph, medical aspects of torture. DMB 37(suppl 1):1–88

Sonne CK (2013) A new competence centre for transcultural psychiatry will integrate research with the treatment of traumatised refugees. The Competence Centre for Transcultural Psychiatry; at www.sciencenordic.com

www.dignityinstitute.dk

www.psykiatri-regionh.dk/menu/Centre/Psykiatriske+centre/Psykiatrisk+Center+Ballerup/Undersogelse+og+behandling/Kompetencecenter+for+Transkulturel+Psykiatri/

www.traume.dk is a web portal developed in collaboration by the Rehabilitation and Research Centre for Torture Victims (RCT Copenhagen), Danish Refugee Council, Centre for Transcultural Psychiatry (VfTP) and Centre for Trauma and Torture Survivors (CETT) Vejle

Printed in the United States
By Bookmasters